14- 120 - 357

WORLD HEALTH AND HISTORY

WORLD HEALTH
AND HISTORY

BY

W. HOBSON, M.D.

Chief, Education and Training, W.H.O. Regional Office for Europe, Copenhagen
Formerly Professor of Social and Industrial Medicine, University of Sheffield

BRISTOL: JOHN WRIGHT & SONS LTD.

1963

614.09
H 653w

Distribution by Sole Agents:
United States of America: The Williams & Wilkins Company, Baltimore
Canada: The Macmillan Company of Canada Ltd., Toronto

PRINTED IN GREAT BRITAIN BY
JOHN WRIGHT & SONS LTD., AT
THE STONEBRIDGE PRESS, BRISTOL

To Heather

ACKNOWLEDGEMENTS

The author acknowledges his indebtedness for the use of illustrations to the following bodies: The World Health Organization (*Figs.* 3–13; 15–18; 21–31; 35, 36; 42–46; 48, 49). The Wellcome Historical Medical Museum (*Figs.* 1, 2; 14; 32). The United Sheffield Hospitals (*Figs.* 19, 20). The National Smoke Abatement Society and Aerofilms Ltd. (*Figs.* 38, 40). Davy and United Engineering Co. Ltd. (*Fig.* 34). The Sheffield Telegraph (*Fig.* 39).

PREFACE

THE inspiration for this book first came from my reading the story of typhus fever in that classic book by Hans Zinsser, *Rats, Lice and History*. I was a Major in the R.A.M.C. in those early days of the Second World War, training and preparing for the Second Front. My job as an officer commanding a field hygiene section was to look after the health of a division in the field, being mainly concerned with the prevention of illness and the maintenance of health rather than with the treatment of illness or war casualties. In those days we were preparing for possible outbreaks of typhus fever when our troops invaded Europe and we expected widespread infestation of the civilian population with lice. I had already experienced this as a Medical Officer of Health dealing with refugees from bombed cities. Our method of attack was slow and laborious—treatment of the hair with various medicaments and steam disinfestation of clothing. In our training for overseas we had mobile disinfestators and an elaborate scheme for dealing with infested persons. We practised our drill assiduously until we had it perfected, but we never took our bulky apparatus to Normandy; the whole concept of the control of lice was changed overnight by the discovery that DDT was an effective residual insecticide.

At the end of December, 1943, DDT was used for the first time to control an epidemic of typhus when in a few months over 3,000,000 people were dusted with DDT in Naples. Our troops were completely free from lice, but most of our German prisoners were louse-ridden and typhus was common on the Eastern Front. It is remarkable that the Germans did not know of the effectiveness of DDT, even though it had been discovered in 1874.

The army which invaded Europe and defeated the Germans was the most healthy army the world has ever known. DDT also controlled flies in North Africa, mosquitoes in India, and ticks in Malaya, and certainly prevented millions of casualties. At the time of the battle of El Alamein, 40 to 50 per cent of enemy troops were affected by dysentery, 'glued to the commode', largely because of the lack of fly control. The result of the war could have been very different if the enemy had known about DDT and we had not.

Later on I was concerned with the terrible outbreaks of typhus and dysentery at the Belsen concentration camp, with the control of malaria in West Africa, and with cholera in India. All this only served to strengthen my own firm belief in the importance of preventive medicine. Alas, few people are interested in the subject and doctors tend to neglect this branch of their profession. No one is interested in the millions of cases of diphtheria that *don't* occur because of immunization, or of cholera that is prevented because of a pure water supply.

DDT has, within the last ten years, prevented many millions of deaths from malaria, and is the basis of the World Health Organization malaria eradication programme. This is one of many examples given in this book of the effectiveness of preventive medicine.

This book is an attempt to make the subject of preventive medicine interesting; it is addressed to all who should be concerned with the subject, politicians, administrators, doctors, students, and the intelligent lay public.

In the future, prevention will depend more and more upon international co-operation by means of such agencies as the World Health Organization and especially on individual action by influencing the habits of people.

This book describes how disease has changed and determined the course of world history; there are some lessons to be learnt from this as we enter the space age.

The world cannot have too much health education and that is what this book is really all about. I hope it will prove to be more interesting than most books on health education!

Copenhagen,   W. HOBSON
12 *October,* 1963

CONTENTS

ix

LIST OF ILLUSTRATIONS

xi

STATEMENT

Apart from a few additions this book was written when the author was Professor of Social and Industrial Medicine in the University of Sheffield.

The views expressed in it are purely personal ones and do not in any way purport to express the official views or policy of the World Health Organization.

WORLD HEALTH AND HISTORY

CHAPTER I

INTRODUCTION

The health of the people is the foundation upon which all their happiness and all their power as a state, depends.—DISRAELI

THIS book is concerned with the war against disease which has been raging since pre-historic times, ceaselessly and unremittingly. It describes how the course of world history has been shaped by the rise and fall of epidemics, and shows how the future course of world events may be influenced not only by the skill and knowledge which we display in regard to the control of disease but also by the level of population growth. Some major battles have been won so far in the fight against communicable disease but there are still many to come; in addition, new weapons of attack must be forged against such conditions as the degenerative heart diseases, cancer, and mental ill health.

The application of knowledge to the welfare of the whole community has always lagged a long way behind the discovery of some salient scientific fact, unless there has been some impelling need or force of circumstances which required a solution. Despite the fact that preventive measures against small-pox have been known for over two hundred years, the disease continues to take its regular toll of victims in many countries in the East, but it is only when a large-scale epidemic occurs that public opinion begins to demand, and is willing to accept, measures for its control.

The history of community health development shows that no country has ever reached a high standard of health mainly because it possessed the necessary medical knowledge concerning the cause of disease; it requires in addition a people whose social development is such that they will persist in the necessary practical measures for the control of disease even in the absence of epidemics. In the words of Emerson: 'The health standard of a nation is a fair gauge of its intelligence, and its degree of social development.' In many parts of the world today lack of an efficient form of local self-government is the greatest bar to health progress. Millions of pounds are being spent on new hospitals and medical colleges, but in the towns and villages, apart from a few show places, there is a woeful lack of sufficient funds to carry out the simplest of sanitary measures. Taxes are, naturally enough, unpopular and the local politicians elected to office are loath to carry out any measure which might cause them to lose favour in the eyes of the electorate, whilst the Public Health law, if it exists, is usually ignored.

Not only is it important to remove many old taboos and prejudices based often on deep-rooted aspects of folk-lore, but, in addition, it is necessary to develop a public opinion clamorous for high standards of health. For this, literacy and education are essential.

In countries all over the world, governments are introducing measures for improving health, but the success of these measures will depend ultimately upon the co-operation of each individual. People the world over need to know more and more about the part they can play in the fight against ill health. Some need to know a great deal, in particular politicians, administrators, doctors, teachers, and parents. Unfortunately most people are distressingly ignorant of what has happened in the past. This is hardly surprising when one realizes how little has been written on the subject; in the words of Wilson Smillie (1952), 'Historians have paid little or no attention to the impact of disease upon our civilization. Public Health is not even mentioned as a social phenomenon.'

Medicine is a social science, and its progress depends upon a knowledge and understanding of social processes. During the nineteenth century, men like Benjamin Disraeli and Sir John Simon had sufficient vision to see the importance of this concept. By their courage and far-sightedness, they produced a system of Public Health which became the envy of the civilized world and which has long remained a model for future development. But the world as a whole is faced today with completely new problems which must be tackled by methods of control as vigorously as the old problems were tackled. In the battles of the future the individual person will have to play an ever-increasing part. The doctors of the future must be trained to think in this way and to realize that they have a duty to the community as well as to the individual. This is a point of view which needs to infiltrate the whole of teaching, not only of doctors but of all citizens. Unfortunately, doctors themselves are trained mainly to treat the sick person, and the increasing specialization in medicine fosters the importance of this idea. Alas! who shall teach the teachers? It is a sad thought that so many of the leaders of medicine and of politics are imbued with the idea of palliatives, and the tendency is to glorify the super-specialist as the ultimate in prestige in the field of medicine. Today no citizen can afford to think only in terms of his parish; he must think in terms of a new public health which embraces the whole world. What better description of this concept than that quoted in *The First Ten Years of the World Health Organization* (W.H.O., 1958)?—

Public Health is the science and the art of preventing disease, prolonging life and promoting physical health and efficiency through organised community efforts for the sanitation of the environment, the control of community infections, the education of the individual in principles of personal hygiene, the organisation of medical and nursing service for the early diagnosis and treatment of disease, and the development of the social machinery which will ensure to every individual in the community a standard of living for the maintenance of health.

Against this ideal, let me quote the words of James Mackintosh (1953), formerly Professor of Public Health in the University of London:—

Everyone says that prevention is better than cure and hardly anyone acts as if he believes it, whether he is attached to Parliament, Central or Local Government, or the commonalty of citizens. Palliatives nearly always take precedence over prevention and health services today are too heavily loaded with salvage. Treatment—the attempt to heal the sick—is more tangible, more exciting and more immediately rewarding, than prevention.

In these pages I have tried to show that a study of disease prevention and control can be exciting and more rewarding in the long run than treatment. I believe that when people are well informed about health matters, they will generally take the long view; that is why the world cannot have too much health education; and that is really what this book is all about.

CHAPTER II

HEALTH AND HISTORY

The heritage of the past is the seed which brings forth the harvest of the future.—INSCRIPTION ON THE ARCHIVES BUILDING, WASHINGTON

IN prehistoric days the health of the family depended upon the physical prowess of the individual. The prime necessity for life, as indeed it is today, was food. In order to survive, the men of the household had to hunt to provide food and clothing. Death was usually from accidents and the survival of the fittest was a natural law which brooked no interference from man. The Polar Eskimoes today still depend upon the animals they kill for food and many of them die in the prime of life from hunting accidents. The weakly, the deformed, and the aged cannot survive under the harsh conditions of life in the Arctic. Life in those far-off prehistoric days must have been very similar.

As knowledge grew and the climate became milder, men began to turn to agriculture and to follow a more settled way of life. The more adventuresome, and those better fitted to survive physically and mentally, passed these qualities on to their offspring, and gradually the village way of life began with the problem of law and order and health. Moses was one of the first leaders of men who realized the importance of health and his rules for a healthy way of life are laid down in the book of Deuteronomy. The increase in populations meant that people had other problems to solve: how to cope with human enemies who were seeking better pastures and hunting grounds and an easy way of getting something for nothing, by plunder. So life in walled villages began. Since those days the world has seen the rise and fall of many civilizations in China and in India, but perhaps the greatest have been centred around the Mediterranean, often called the cradle of civilization. Crete, Egypt, Persia, Carthage, Babylon, Palestine, Greece, and Rome, all have had their turn. The relics can be seen today, the ancient palaces, amphitheatres, and remains of fine public buildings. Historians have argued for generations about the cause of the fall of many of these famous civilizations, Gibbon, for example, in his *Rise and Fall of the Roman Empire*. The history books are full of descriptions of wars and famous battles, of internal strife and corruption, but little has been said about epidemic disease as a potent factor in determining the course of history. There can be little doubt, however, that pestilence played a great part in the fall of many of these civilizations. Malaria, plague, and typhus were the 'men of death' in those days. One of the greatest enigmas still to be explained is why almost overnight

4

the great cities of the Roman Empire disappeared and crumbled into ruin, desolate and empty of people. Bubonic plague, the 'Black Death', as our ancestors called it, was largely responsible for wiping out great centres of population, leaving the empty ruins to be covered by the sands of the desert or by the newer towns which subsequent generations built. The Romans had great ideas about personal health and cleanliness; they built houses, baths, and aqueducts for water. At Segovia, in Spain, the Roman aqueduct is still in use for bringing pure water to the town. The standards of personal health, however, deteriorated when debauchery and sexual licence increased; sophistication became the order of the day and the old ideas of Sparta gave way to the sloth and luxury of Nero's court.

GREEK MEDICINE

The Greeks were devoted to the pursuit of health and owed much of their knowledge to Hippocrates who studied the control of disease in the Greek islands and in particular on the island of Cos, his birthplace. He set down his observations in his famous books, *Airs, Waters, and Places*, which stressed the importance of the environment as far as the health of the community was concerned. He studied such things as climate, race, water supply, housing, clothing, habits of eating and drinking, and the effect they had in producing ill health and disease. In the four books entitled *Regimen* he developed the theory that health depends upon a proper balance between food and exercise. He gave the following counsel:—

Exercises should be many and of all kinds; running on the double track increased gradually; wrestling after being oiled, begun with light exercises and gradually made long; sharp walks after exercises, short walks in the sun after dinner; many walks in the early morning, quiet to begin with, increasing till they are violent and then gently finishing.

Hippocrates stressed two ways of preserving health and preventing disease: (1) By ensuring a healthy environment; (2) by personal habits. He also studied the rise and fall of epidemic disease. He showed, for example, that pulmonary diseases were common in the spring and that warm, moist weather was unhealthy because of malaria. The great contribution of the 'father of medicine', as he has been called, was to stress the importance of preventive medicine as distinct from curative medicine and to point out the ancient truth 'that prevention is better than cure', a dictum, unfortunately, which is often forgotten by many of our modern physicians.

Of course, Hippocrates wrote also upon the value of treating the sick patient, depending upon nature to achieve the cure and relying on certain methods of study. These were the 'Tripod of Empirics' which taught one to rely upon (1) one's own observations; (2) the observations of others; (3) analogy. He also formulated the Hippocratic oath which ever since has stood as a code of ethics of the medical profession, although few doctors actually take the oath. The following translation is from Loeb's Classical Library.

5

Hippocrates his Oath which he gave unto his disciples and scrollers which professing Phisicke and Chirurgerie is very worthie to be observed and kept faithfully.

I swear by Apollo the Healer, and Aesculapius, and Hygieia, and Panacea.

And I call all Gods and Goddesses to witness, that I will, according to my power and judgment, make good this oath, and this covenant which here I sign.

To think of him who taught me this art as I think of my parents. To hold my life as his life, and to give him, in the time of his need, a share of my belongings. To consider his sons as my brothers, and to teach this art, to such of them as wish to learn it, without payment or agreement.

To impart the doctrine, and the interpretation, and the whole learning to my sons, and to my master's sons, and to students enrolled and sworn under medical law, and to nobody else.

And I will use all ways of medical treatment that shall be for the advantage of the sufferers, according to my power and judgment, and will protect them from injury and injustice. Nor will I give to any man, though I be asked to give it, any deadly drug, nor will I consent that it should be given. Likewise I will not procure abortion. But purely and holily I will keep guard over my life and my art.

Nor will I cut them that have the stone, but will send them to men whose work it is to perform that operation.

And, into whatever houses I enter, I will enter into them for the benefit of the patients. I will refrain from any wilful hurt or wrong, and from falsehood, and especially from all lewdness, whether it be my chance to deal with men or women, freeman or slave. And, whatever, in practice, I see or hear, or even outside practice, which it is not right should be told abroad, I will be silent, counting as unsaid what was said.

Therefore, as I faithfully observe and keep this my oath, may I have enjoyment in my Art and living, being in good repute among all men for ever and ever; but, if I transgress and break the same, let all things fall out unto me contrary.

Hippocrates died in 377 B.C. and in A.D. 13 Galen was born in Pergamon. He also stressed the importance of personal hygiene in the maintenance of health and the prevention of disease. His book *De Sanitate Tuenda* has only recently been translated into the English language. Both Hippocrates and Galen knew a great deal about personal health from their own observations, but unfortunately they had no real scientific knowledge on which to base their ideas of community health.

In those days medicine was for the aristocratic few, and they had little idea of applying the benefits of this knowledge to the welfare of the whole community. Although the Romans were great law-makers they produced little in the way of social legislation or public health law. The Greeks, on the other hand, were some of the greatest philosophers of all time, but Plato and Socrates, with all their theorizing and their brilliant discussions of logic and philosophy, could not prevent the plague from devastating their land.

The aqueducts and baths and high standards of personal hygiene were of no avail against the Black Death and so their civilization disappeared, leaving behind a rich tradition in writing of philosophy and logic. Europe was plunged into the Dark Ages, and the lessons of those 'dead' civilizations were forgotten for centuries. Epidemic after epidemic swept across Europe, wiping out populations and affecting the course of wars. The history of Europe in those days is the history of typhus and plague, of rats and lice and men.

6

WESTERN EUROPE

Gradually new civilizations and cultures grew up in Western Europe, in which men lived in walled cities for protection against their fellow men. This overcrowding in cramped living quarters, this life in closed communities, brought with it community diseases, not only typhus and plague, but cholera, typhoid, tuberculosis, syphilis, influenza, and diphtheria. Medicine vainly tried to cope with these problems by the art of black magic and the use of secret remedies concocted from weird and expensive ingredients. The art of curative medicine was dependent upon the idea of the high priest who knew everything, who was infallible, and who was all-powerful.

Even in the earliest days of living in communities men had learnt from their own observations that contagion, and hence overcrowding, played a large part in the spread of disease, but it was not until the nineteenth century that any real progress was made in prevention. The battle against ill health and disease took place on two main fronts. On the one hand, the scientists and technicians were making further advances in knowledge in their particular spheres, and on the other, the politicians and administrators were endeavouring to overcome the forces of prejudice, inertia, and apathy to bring about the necessary reform and apply the knowledge which scientific study had made available. Advances in knowledge relating to the control of the environment depended upon the advances in several basic sciences and in particular those of physiology, bacteriology, and statistics, and it was not until real progress had been made in these sciences that it was possible to achieve worth-while progress in the prevention and control of disease. In the first place, however, it did not need any profound scientific knowledge to realize that ill health and disease were associated with bad housing, unhealthy work places, inadequate water supplies, defective sanitation, and the overcrowding and poverty associated with life in the slums.

In England the first Sanitary Act of Parliament was passed in 1388, its purpose being to prohibit the pollution of rivers, ditches, and open spaces in an effort to prevent disease, but apart from the Elizabethan Poor Law Act of 1601, there was little effort made by Parliament to improve communal health until well into the nineteenth century. During the eighteenth century, there were made two scientific discoveries of very great importance in preventive medicine. The first was the discovery by James Lind in 1747 that fresh oranges and lemons could prevent scurvy. The second was the demonstration by Edward Jenner in 1796 that inoculation with the harmless virus of cow-pox could confer a high degree of immunity against small-pox. These two discoveries paved the way for the great triumphs of preventive medicine in controlling malnutrition and epidemic disease.

Before any real advance could be made in the control of disease, it was necessary to have some means of measuring vital phenomena. John Graunt had collected mortality statistics from the London Bills of Mortality compiled by the Company of Parish Clerks and in this way information was collected about the Great Plague of London in 1665, but this information was incomplete. Efforts made by John Fothergill in 1753 to take a census met with failure. In 1801, however, the first English census was taken, and in 1836 the registration of births, marriages, and deaths became compulsory.

In the realm of vital statistics, undoubtedly the greatest figure was that of William Farr, who was appointed Compiler of Statistics to the General Register Office from 1840 to 1880. His methods for the measurement of mortality statistics have proved a most important weapon in improving communal health, and his classification of the causes of death has been in use until comparatively recently. He realized that mortality statistics alone did not supply sufficient information concerning the diseases of the community and recommended a complete return of all the causes of sickness.

It is not always realized what great effect economic changes have on the health of the community. During the early part of the eighteenth century the way of life of agricultural England had changed little from the Middle Ages. The people were largely self-supporting and lived on their home-grown products; their diet was mainly wheaten wholemeal bread, oatmeal, potatoes, milk, butter, cheese, and vegetables. Drummond (1939) analysed this diet in the light of modern scientific knowledge on nutrition and found that by modern standards it was adequate in all respects and a better diet than the average today. Providing the harvest held there was no malnutrition, and the only food problem that the people had to face was a bad harvest. All this was altered, however, by the discovery of steam power which heralded the Industrial Revolution. In the reign of George III (1760–1820), the population of Great Britain rose from 7,500,000 to 14,000,000. The country had to import grain to feed the ever-increasing industrial population which was flocking from the country to the new towns. A duty was imposed upon cheap wheat from America and the price of bread increased. People were no longer able to live on the produce of their own gardens, and a great change came about in the food habits of the people. The consumption of milk decreased and few fresh vegetables were eaten; the staple foods of the people became adulterated and sophisticated. Thus the health-giving wholemeal flour was replaced by the better-looking but less nutritious white flour. The feeding of the industrial areas brought with it its problems of supply and distribution, and inevitably, due to the increased handling of the food and delay in distribution, there were great facilities for contamination and spoiling.

The yearly consumption of refined sugar, which has neither vitamins nor minerals, rose from a few pounds per head at the beginning of the nineteenth century to nearly 1 cwt. per head by the end of the century. Hence the diet of the people came to consist mainly of the cheap energy-producing foods poor in both vitamins and minerals.

The changes in food habits were not the only evils. In order to get cheap labour, women and children were employed for long hours in the mines and factories, labouring and toiling like beasts of burden. The distress of the time has been described by Thomas Hood in his poem, 'The Song of the Shirt':—

Oh! God! that bread should be so dear,
And flesh and blood so cheap!

8

and by Arthur Young's tranquil observation, 'Every one but an idiot knows that the lower classes must be kept poor or they will never be industrious.'

One of the greatest difficulties in these new towns was the disposal of solid human excreta; in the country it had been of value as a fertilizer for the land, but in the new towns, as the piles of human dung grew, they became dangerous to health as well as disgusting. They were, in addition, an economic burden, since it became necessary to pay to have them cleared away. There were regular dumping grounds in London on sites now occupied by University College, Gower Street, Hyde Park Gardens, and Belgrave Square. With the development of water sanitation, refuse was flushed away into cesspools, whose contents soaked through into the earth, polluting the wells.

The water closet had already been known for two centuries; it was rediscovered in England by Sir John Harington who installed a flush closet in Richmond Palace for Queen Elizabeth I. The increasing use of water for baths was disastrous for this system, because the cesspools filled up too quickly and overflowed. The solution to this evil was to drain the sewage into the nearest river; the Thames became an open sewer and the Serpentine took the whole of the drainage from Bayswater, Kilburn, and Paddington.

During the Industrial Revolution the slum landlords and jerry-builders had thrown up large numbers of hovels around the factories in order to provide cheap dwelling-houses for the workers. There was no control over this *laissez-faire* attitude which favoured the motives of self-interest in place of the general happiness of the community. The philosophy of the nineteenth century was the Darwinian one, of the survival of the fittest and the devil take the hindmost. The window taxes, only repealed in 1803, encouraged the boarding-up of windows, with a resultant lack of light and adequate ventilation. Over all this was a dense pall of smoke from the nearby factories. Cod-liver oil and ultra-violet lamps were then unknown; small wonder that rickets was known throughout Europe as 'the English disease'. The scene is described by the Earl of Shaftesbury in the following words: 'What a perambulation I have taken today in company with Dr. Southwood Smith; what scenes of filth, discomfort and disease. No pen or paint brush could describe the thing as it is—one whiff of Cowyard, Blue Anchor or Baker's Court outweighs ten pages of letterpress.' Under these conditions epidemic disease was rife, and the pressing need of the time was for widespread sanitary reform.

Although the work of John Howard on prison reform had stirred public conscience, it was the great cholera epidemic of 1832 which first led to positive action. In the words of Trevelyan: 'The sensational character of the novel visitation scared society into the tardy beginning of sanitary self-defence.'

The cholera epidemics of 1832 stimulated Edwin Chadwick to investigate the health of the inhabitants of the large towns with a view to improving the conditions under which they lived. The report on this inquiry was published

9

under his name in 1842 and entitled *A General Report on the Sanitary Conditions of the Labouring Population of Great Britain.* It is certainly one of the greatest texts of social pathology that have ever been published. Chadwick investigated the homes of the labouring classes and first showed that mortality was greatest in the slum areas. This report revealed conditions of filth and disease which Parliament received 'with astonishment, dismay, horror and even incredulity'. This report led to the Public Health Act of 1848, and the acceptance of the principle that the State is responsible for the health of the people, a principle which had first been enunciated by Johann Peter Frank (1745–1821) many years before. The Act set up a General Board of Health for five years in the first instance and provided for the creation of Local Boards of Health. The General Board of Health was unpopular from the start. It had to try to cope with a severe outbreak of cholera as soon as it was formed; it survived until 1858 when its medical duties were taken over by the Privy Council. The Act was permissive rather than compulsory and had very little real powers to enforce reforms that were needed. There was a lack of a regular Civil Service and no adequate machinery for Local Government; moreover, the knowledge of the causation of disease and methods of prevention were very inadequate. A lot of hostility that Chadwick encountered was due to his own intransigent personality. Despite his enthusiasm and zeal, he lacked the tact which was necessary to enable legislation to become effective. He ignored the views of others and rode rough-shod over vested interests, and there was widespread complaint of too much authority from London.

The torch had already been lit by the earnestness and fervour of Chadwick, but the man who was responsible, more than any other, for sanitary reform in England was Sir John Simon (1816–1904) (*Fig.* 1). He was able to gain reforms by his skill, eloquence, and tactful approach. Not only was he a skilful surgeon, but he was appointed a Fellow of the Royal Society at the early age of 29 years, for his work on the pathology of the thyroid gland. He later became President of the Royal College of Surgeons. He was a great friend of the literary giants of the day, and Thackeray, Tennyson, Rossetti, and Burne-Jones were all frequent visitors to his house. His greatest work, however, was in the field of preventive medicine. After his appointment as Medical Officer of Health to the City of London he was appointed as Medical Officer to the General Board of Health and to the Privy Council. He built up a system of public health which became the admiration of the rest of the world.

During the last one hundred years we can trace two phases in the growth and development of public health. During the latter half of the nineteenth century the main efforts were concentrated on the improvement of the physical environment. During the first half of the present century, the developments have been more concerned with the provision of personal medical and social services. One of the chief difficulties in the way of public health legislation was the lack of any competent administrative system, and it was necessary to achieve this before there could be any real progress in public health matters.

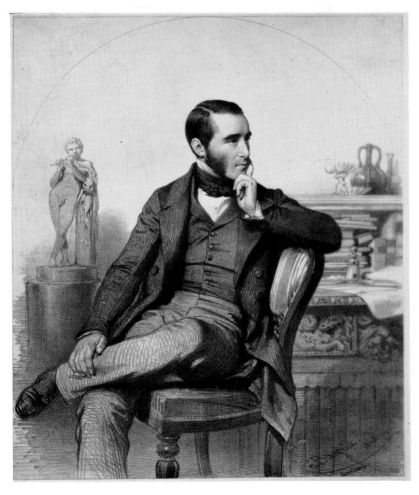

Fig. 1.—Sir John Simon (1816–1904), pioneer in public health. From the lithograph
by C. Baugniet, 1848.

The most pressing needs were for the removal of the slum conditions and for the provision of adequate water and sewerage schemes.

The appointment of Medical Officers of Health by all local authorities was made compulsory in 1872. The great Public Health Act of 1875 dealt with many aspects of sanitation and was the greatest measure yet brought before Parliament for the control of the physical environment. Its main provisions related to the drainage and wholesome condition of houses, sewerage, the scavenging of streets, the removal of refuse, the control of slaughter-houses and offensive trades, and the isolation of infectious disease. Its importance can be judged by the fact that it remained in force until 1936, when it was replaced by a new Public Health Act; for over sixty years it remained the most important single enactment dealing with the control of the public health; it has rightly been called the 'Magna Charta of Public Health'.

There was a much higher incidence of disease amongst the poor, and even in 1900 the infant mortality was still very high (150 per 1000 live births). Chadwick had shown that poverty and ignorance were important causes of ill health and disease, and in 1901 Seebohm Rowntree tried to estimate the poverty factor. In his report, *Poverty, a Study of Town Life*, he showed that 28 per cent of the people in York were living in poverty. Charles Booth in his *Life and Labour of the People of London* also showed that 31 per cent of the people in London were living below the poverty line. Poverty and all that went with it still remained a potent cause of ill health and premature death.

The low standards of physical fitness were revealed by the disclosures of the Army Recruiting Office for the South African War, when 40 to 60 per cent of recruits were unable to pass the preliminary medical examination. This led to the introduction of school meals and the start of the School Medical Service in 1907.

The work of Florence Nightingale in the Army had already established the importance of nursing as such, but she maintained that a nurse could do more by teaching household hygiene than in the hospital. It was the development of this idea which led to the provision of health visitors to advise mothers on the care of children. This was a direct attempt to combat the high infant mortality-rate. The first attempt in this direction to be undertaken by Local Authorities took place in 1890 when the home visitors of the Ladies Sanitary Reform Association came under the control of the Medical Officer of Health for Manchester. The first welfare centres were called Schools for Mothers, indicating that the chief function of the health visitor is an educational one. In 1915 the notification of births became compulsory and this gave the necessary information to enable the health visitor to contact mothers soon after childbirth.

The work of the hospital almoner developed in relation to the old charitable institutions such as the Royal Free Hospital and St. George's and St. Thomas's Hospitals in London. Her function was to assess poverty and the means to pay for hospital treatment, in addition to dispensing alms. Gradually, however, she has played an ever-increasing part as a medical auxiliary, helping the doctor in diagnosis and in treatment by investigating and prescribing the appropriate remedy for social ills.

Legislation was passed to deal with such subjects as the provision of midwives, maternity and child welfare, school medical services, special services for infectious diseases, including tuberculosis and venereal disease, and the care of mental defectives and blind persons. There was still, however, a great deal to be done in relation to the physical environment and important enactments were passed to improve the working conditions in factories, to raise housing standards, and to control the cleanliness and purity of food and drugs.

At the beginning of the century there was a great need for a Simon or Disraeli to co-ordinate the two great branches of medicine, preventive and curative. 'The hour came but not the man', and the gulf between the general practitioner, the hospital specialist, and the medical officer of health became wider.* General practitioners often resented the intrusion of public authorities on medical matters, whilst many of the ablest members of the profession of medicine were attracted to the remunerative prizes of consulting practice.

Before 1911 the poor could only obtain medical services through the Poor Law. Medical attention was provided by District Medical Officers and vaccination was carried out by Public Vaccinators; these duties were carried out by general practitioners on a part-time salaried basis. The workhouses and Poor Law Infirmaries were drab, cheerless buildings, built with the idea that life in them should be made less attractive than work, and in those days work was unattractive enough. With the dawn of the twentieth century, a new philosophy became apparent in relation to the poorer classes of the community; this more enlightened philosophy recognized the duty of the State to provide certain basic essentials as a right rather than as a form of charity.

The first step in this direction was taken as a result of the deliberations of the Poor Law Commission which was set up in 1905. There was sharp division between its members, and the famous Minority Report published in 1909 advised the abolition of much of the old Poor Law and visualized its eventual break-up. This Minority Report was largely the work of Sidney and Beatrice Webb, but its proposals were not put into effect until 1929. The existing provision of medical services was inadequate and the idea of a public medical service had been very much in the minds of liberal thinkers. Bismarck had already organized a scheme of National Insurance in Germany, and when Lloyd George visited that country in 1908 he was so impressed with its success that in 1911 he introduced the first National Insurance Act in Britain. This provided insurance against ill health for many of the working population. At first there was considerable opposition, particularly from the general practitioners, but by 1913 there were 12,000,000 insured persons and 10,000 general practitioners were operating the scheme. There were certain drawbacks to this Act, however. Firstly, it made no provision for specialist

---

* The work of the health visitor, which was largely preventive, was divorced from the work of the hospital almoner, which was largely therapeutic.

services; secondly, the wives and children of insured persons were not included in the scheme; and thirdly, there was little association between the preventive work of the public health departments and the work of the general practitioner.

In 1918, an important step was taken when the Ministry of Health was formed with a Minister responsible to the Crown. The aims of this Ministry have been described in the *Annual Report of the Chief Medical Officer of the Ministry of Health for 1934* as follows: 'To bring every advance in medical science, every measure calculated to maintain health and to prevent disease, to the service of the people and to make health the birthright of every inhabitant of this country'. So at last, the step which had been advised one hundred years before by Jeremy Bentham, and later by Sir John Simon (1890), was taken. Today the Ministry of Health has so increased its power that it exercises control over most of the medical services, including the work of general practitioners, hospitals, and public health services.

Between the two world wars great advances were made in the knowledge of nutrition. The work of Gowland Hopkins and Edward Mellanby demonstrated the importance of vitamins and the need for a well-balanced diet. Standards were laid down for optimum health. These standards were low enough; for example, the British Medical Association calculated in 1933 that if the right food was bought in the cheapest markets and prepared in the best way, 5s. 10d. per head per week would provide a diet sufficient for health, but it was quite a different matter to apply this knowledge and ensure that everyone had an adequate health-giving diet. John Boyd-Orr (1937) and G.C.M. M'Gonigle (1936) had shown that a high proportion of the inhabitants of this country were unable to afford an adequate diet. This state of affairs was particularly bad in North-east England and South Wales following the depression of 1929. Again, poverty was shown to be an important cause of ill health.

The provision of free milk and the extension of the meals in schools service were attempts to combat these evils. The stimulus of the Second World War led to further improvements in the nutrition of the people. These included the provision of priority foods, of vitamin supplements for expectant mothers and for children, and the raising of the extraction rate of flour and its fortification with calcium. The rationing system also ensured a more even distribution of the food available.

The discovery of sulphonamides and antibiotics revolutionized the prevention and treatment of communicable diseases, but unfortunately most of the virus diseases are unaffected by antibiotics and are still as resistant to treatment as before. We must therefore look to other methods for their control.

In 1929, the Local Government Act helped further to break up the Poor Law by bringing many of the old Poor Law hospitals under the Local Health Authority. The criterion for admission to these hospitals was not that of poverty, but medical need, irrespective of income. The culmination of this new attitude was the publication of the Beveridge Report and the passing of a series of Acts, which, considered together, are an attack upon what Lord Beveridge calls 'the five giants on the road to reconstruction, want, disease, squalor, idleness, and ignorance'. These Acts are: the Education Act (1944), which in addition to the educational provisions set up a free comprehensive medical service for schoolchildren; the Disabled Persons Employment Act (1944); the Family Allowances Act (1946); the National Insurance Act (1946); the National Health Service Act (1946); the National Assistance Act (1948); and the Children's Act (1948). By 1948, therefore, one hundred years after the passing of the first Public Health Act, there was a comprehensive system of social security for every person in Britain, and the maternal and infant mortality-rates were lower than at any time in history. Unfortunately, the practice of public health is still largely divorced from the work of the general practitioner and the hospital specialist. It is hoped that in the future the health centre, as envisaged in the Act, may provide a place where the work of preventive and curative medicine can be co-ordinated.

Suggestions for a reorganization of the health services have been made in the report of the Porritt Committee (1962) in *A Review of the Medical Services in Great Britain*. The focal point will be the Area Health Board which will have an overall responsibility for the planning and administration of all the medical services in an area, thus bringing out the co-ordination between preventive and curative services which is so very necessary.

The centenary year of the passing of the first Public Health Act marked the entry of a third and new phase, the development of social medicine, characterized by a new outlook in relation to medical and social care.

The basic sciences on which the practice of social medicine depend now include, in addition to physiology, bacteriology, and statistics, the study of sociology and psychology. As the physical factors in the environment have been brought more and more under control, so have the psychological and emotional factors assumed an increasing importance in the causation of ill health and disease. Malnutrition and epidemic disease have been brought under more effective control, but there still remains the ever-increasing problem of the psychosomatic and psychoneurotic illnesses, the degenerative diseases of older people, and cancer.

C. E. A. Winslow (1951) described the difficulties for the world as a whole to provide for the continually mounting cost of medical services. In the U.S.A., for example, comprehensive medical care is so expensive that few can afford to pay for it without some form of medical insurance scheme. Certainly one way of tackling the problem is to reduce the burden of sickness by concentrating most of our effort on preventive services.

Let us turn now to a more detailed study of some of the great killing diseases of the world. Of these, by far the most terrible are plague, typhus, and malaria; all of them spread by insects, which together are responsible for more than half the deaths which occur each year in the world.

14

CHAPTER III

THE BLACK DEATH

THE HISTORY OF PLAGUE

ALTHOUGH man has been plagued by epidemics since the dawn of history, the earliest records of pestilence and disease are often so lacking in detail that we cannot always be sure of their nature. There are many such epidemics recorded in Biblical history. The Plague as we know it today can take several forms, but the most easily recognizable is that known as bubonic because of the large swellings or buboes which appear in the groin and under the armpits from the infection of the lymphatic glands. It is spread by the rat-flea and at the same time as the human epidemic there is also large-scale mortality amongst rats. This type of plague can be easily recognized from recorded descriptions. The first recorded epidemic of plague occurred after the great battle between the Philistines and the Israelites.

The Philistines conquered the Israelites and captured the Ark of the Covenant. Their triumph was short-lived, however; terrible epidemics broke out and a large proportion of the population was killed. The following quotations from the Bible clearly show the nature of the affliction: 'In Gath the Lord smote the men of the city, both small and great, and they had emerods in their secret parts', and again, 'and mice sprang up in the midst of their country and there was great and indiscriminate mortality in the city'. The disease no doubt came in via the numerous seaports which were in communication with other parts of the ancient world and then spread inland via rodents, finally attacking man. The skeletons of rats and mice have been found on Neolithic sites at Mount Carmel in Palestine and rats and rat-fleas capable of spreading plague are to be found in Palestine today. There is a painting by Poussin (1594-1665) in the Louvre depicting the plague of the Philistines.

The sorcerers of the Philistines recommended that golden images of 'mice' and 'emerods' be made as offerings and that the Ark should be returned. The cause of the plague was thought to be the sins of the people who had offended the Lord and He in His anger had caused the visitation of the plague. The remedy was to be sought in prayer and sacrifice, and the means of preventing it from occurring again were to exhort the people to repent and not to sin in the future. This sort of attitude to disease persisted from Biblical times right up to the end of the nineteenth century when the real physical causes were discovered.

Although there were probably many other outbreaks the next great plague recorded in history was in the time of Justinian. An account of the outbreak was given by Procopius and it clearly gives a clue to diagnosis: 'The first symptom was a sudden temperature followed by a bubo in the groin, under the armpits or behind the ears. Some died at once, in others black blisters appeared on the skin and many were quickly killed by the vomiting of blood.' There can be little doubt that this was bubonic plague. It probably originated in central Asia; by A.D. 542 the great pestilence was well under way and had spread as far as Scotland; it eventually spread throughout the whole of the ancient world. In Constantinople at the height of the epidemic more than 10,000 people died each day and it was impossible for the dead to be buried.

According to one observer half the inhabitants of the Byzantine Empire were killed by A.D. 565, and Gibbon put the total mortality at 100,000,000. No part of Europe escaped and the profound effect it had is to be seen in the many paintings of that time depicting plague. Again the Lord was held responsible; many of the paintings of the period show arrows of disease falling from above and piercing the victims. Even today this sort of belief persists in the East, sometimes making it difficult to set in motion preventive measures based on modern science.

Cities and villages were abandoned as the people fled from the scourge, agriculture stopped, and famine followed in the wake of pestilence. Many parts of the Middle East never recovered from the loss of life which resulted, and the whole of the Roman Empire was thrown into confusion. One of the most amazing events of history is the complete disappearance of ancient civilizations and many historians have tried to explain the cause. Certainly epidemic disease in the form of plague must have played a large part.

Between the plague of Justinian's era and the Black Death in the Middle Ages Europe sank into the Dark Ages, life becoming mainly agricultural, and the large cities of the ancient world disappeared. Epidemics rage when there are large numbers of people living in dense, overcrowded conditions with free communication between one centre and another; pestilence travels along the trade routes and flourishes in the centres of trade.

We know now that the wild rodents of the Asiatic steppes form a permanent reservoir of infection for the disease, and probably the great outbreak of the Black Death in the Middle Ages originated, like the others, in the centre of Asia. Recently a Russian archaeologist discovered a large number of graves dating back to 1338 near Lake Issyk-Kul. Inscriptions on the graves clearly indicate that the persons had died of plague.

By 1346 plague had reached the shores of the Black Sea. At first the disease spread slowly, but as it gained in momentum and horror people began to flee westwards in terror and from thenceforth the spread of the disease was rapid. As in many other epidemics, we can state with exactitude when and where the disease entered this country; in the case of the Black Death the date was July, 1348, and the place, Melcombe Regis in Dorsetshire.

Hecker (1844) considered that one-quarter of the inhabitants of Europe died, and in some parts of England studies of manorial documents indicate that

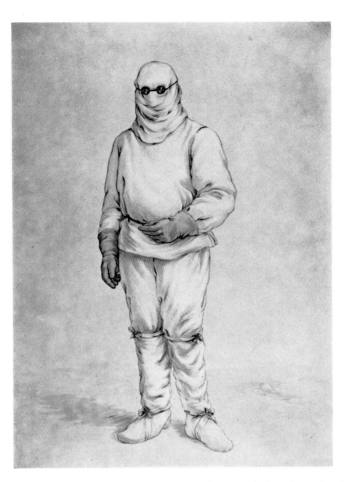

Fig. 2.—Plague doctor. Costume used by the Japanese during the outbreak of pneumonic plague in Manchuria, 1909.

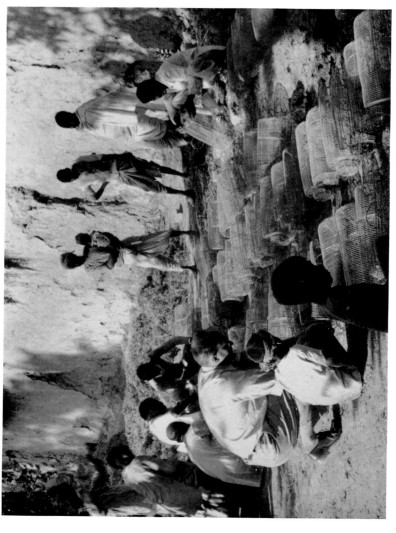

Fig. 3.—Plague in India. Villagers, long used to associate rats with plague, lend a hand in the baiting of the traps to a W.H.O. scientist consultant.

less than one-tenth of the inhabitants survived. The harvest of that year remained ungathered and flocks of sheep and hens wandered about uncared for. The immense loss of life must have revolutionized the whole manner of existence in England.

One of the most gruesome accounts is given by John Clyn of Kilkenny, in the following words:—

That pestilence deprived of human inhabitant villages and cities, and castles and towns, so that there was scarcely found a man to dwell therein; the pestilence was so contagious that whosoever touched the sick or dead was immediately infected and died; and the penitent and the confessor were carried together to the grave . . . many died of boils and abscesses, and pustules on their skins and under their armpits; others frantic with pain in their head, and others spitting blood, . . . I . . . waiting for death till it come . . . so I have reduced these things to writing; and lest the writing should perish with the writer, and the work together with the workman, I leave parchment for continuing the work, if haply any survive, and any of the race of Adam escape this pestilence and continue the work which I have commenced.

Plague spread over Europe in successive waves and eventually settled in the great centres of commerce, London, Marseilles, and Venice. Society by now had learnt that flight to the country was one way of avoiding infection and gradually the idea of sanitary control grew. Isolation of the sick, disinfection of clothes, and quarantine of ships were recognized as means of preventing the spread, only to be forgotten in future years after the epidemic had disappeared. At first the ideas of a natural origin of the disease conflicted with those of the teaching of orthodox religion. Mohammedans regarded the attempts to fly from the epidemic as evidence of lack of faith in the Koran. In London the first revolt against this authoritarian doctrine of the Church proclaimed itself in Orders issued by the Privy Council in 1592, which prescribed measures for limiting the spread of the disease, and a London clergyman was sent to prison in 1603 for proclaiming that plague was a punishment for sin. Throughout the great plagues of London, however, the clergy continued to preach sermons calling on the people to repent their sins. After the Great Fire of London in 1666 the plague disappeared from England in epidemic form for good. It lingered, however, in the Middle East.

The main epidemics of the sixteenth and seventeenth centuries in London occurred in the following years:—

Year	Deaths	Year	Deaths
1563	20,136	1625	41,313
1593	10,662	1636	10,400
1603	33,347	1665	68,596

The sufferings were greatest, as usual, amongst the poor who lived in the dense and overcrowded slums of the great city. The nobility and wealthy merchants had places in the country where they could go until the epidemic had waned. Business came to a standstill as the roads from the city were blocked with panic-stricken refugees with nowhere to go. The constant tolling of the church bells and the sight of carts full of corpses must have added to the misery and confusion.

Classic descriptions of the Black Death in London have been written by Samuel Pepys in his *Diary* and by Daniel Defoe in his *Journal of the Plague Year*. Pepys's often-quoted letter tells of 'little noise heard day or night but tolling of bells'. In July a student in London writes that in St. Giles 'they have a Bellman . . . with a cart; there dye so many that the bell would hardly ever leave ringing and so they ring not at all'. Delirious men and women screamed at the windows and burst into the streets to die. The dead-carts rumbled by, at first by night, then by both night and day. The churchyards were filled; to this day they stand high above the streets; when they no longer sufficed huge pits were dug for the dead. 'It is a greate mercy now counted', wrote one John Allin, 'to dye of another disease.'

'London'—to borrow Defoe's vivid phrases—'might well be said to be all in tears. . . . The shrieks of women and children at the windows and doors of their houses, where their dearest relations were perhaps dying, or just dead, were so frequent to be heard as we passed the streets, that it was enough to pierce the stoutest heart in the world to hear them. . . . Whole families, and indeed whole streets of families, were swept away together.'

The Plague spread to many country villages and towns. A typical case in point is that of the village of Eyam in the Peak District of Derbyshire. The epidemic is supposed to have been brought in by means of a bale of cloth sent from London to the local tailor. Many families fled, but even so 259 people died out of a total of just over 300 who remained. The Rector of Eyam, the Rev. William Mompesson, realized that those who fled from the village were a source of infection to the surrounding hamlets and he urged his parishioners to stay within a specified boundary. This remarkable example of a self-imposed quarantine was imposed rigidly for over a year, and food was brought, through the help of the Earl of Devonshire, to a pre-arranged place on the boundary. Many of the victims were buried in unknown graves, but there are still some old gravestones in the churchyard which bear witness to the tragic story. Every year a commemoration service is held in Eyam on the last Sunday in August.

The great losses in man power brought about by the Black Death meant that there was a shortage of labour to till the land; the price of labour rose and the price of farms fell. This spelt the end of the feudal system and many serfs bought their freedom. A new class of yeoman farmer arose, able to rent farms of their own or even to buy land, or others remained as free labourers able to demand high wages. Parliament had to pass laws to try to keep down the price of wages. Plague changed the whole status of England from a society based on personal service to a money economy dictated by the State.

The last of the European outbreaks occurred in Marseilles in 1720. The severity of the epidemic can be judged from the fact that in the first year there were nearly 40,000 deaths out of a population of 90,000. The infection was brought to Marseilles by ship and spread by its cargo of cotton, silk, and muslin which probably harboured rat-fleas. It raised anew the controversy between two current schools of thought as to the cause of the disease.

One theory was that the infection was in the nature of a contagion and that the disease spread by direct contact from case to case. The miasmatic school believed that epidemics were due to a poison generated in nature.

In July, 1834, a great epidemic of bubonic plague broke out in Alexandria, causing at least 32,000 deaths. Again the old controversy broke out with renewed vehemence. Many of the persons employed in handling cotton acquired the disease and eight out of ten English ships had cases of plague on board. Clot Bey, an Egyptian surgeon, used criminals in experiments to try to determine the cause. In one experiment a condemned criminal died eight days after sleeping in a patient's bed and wearing his under-clothes, and Clot Bey even inoculated himself with the blood of a patient with negative results; and so the discussion went on with neither side proving its point.

The scene was now set for the development of the third great wave of epidemics in the history of plague, probably the greatest of them all. It all began as before in the remote steppes of central Asia. Explorers and missionaries were beginning to penetrate the remote province of Yunnan, in China, and outbreaks of plague had been described there in 1871 by Emile Roches. He described an outbreak of disease amongst rats and gave the typical description of bubonic plague in human beings. Eventually the epidemic reached Canton, and cases were described there by Dr. Mary Miles in January, 1894. Over 50,000 people died of the disease, chiefly those living in the poorer sections of the city where overcrowding was common. Those living on river boats escaped. Soon the infection spread to Hong Kong and it was not long before it had spread to America, Australia, and India, with a death-roll of over 13,000,000. In a later epidemic between 1 July, 1904, and 30 June, 1905, there were 1,328,249 recorded deaths from plague in India alone.

Bombay was soon infected and the population fled, thus disseminating the infection far and wide in the interior of India. The alarm created in the civilized world was enormous and numerous commissions were sent to investigate the cause of the disease. Never before had such an array of talent been assembled at one place to investigate the cause and prevention of a disease. Commissions were sent from Austria, Britain, Ceylon, Egypt, Germany, Italy, and Russia.

Some of these investigators believed that the disease was spread by the ingestion of infected food which had been contaminated by cockroaches, flies, or rats, but later feeding experiments were negative. The Plague Research Commission carried out some classic experiments which proved beyond doubt the method of spread. This, however, was not until 1905.

In the meantime the public health authorities were carrying out preventive measures on an unprecedented scale without really knowing the true cause of the disease. The Bombay Council employed a staff of 31,000 people to cleanse and disinfect the streets; 3,000,000 gallons of disinfectant were poured into the sewers each day and fire engines sprayed the inside of houses with deluges of carbolic acid. All this caused more harm than good as it drove the infected rats farther afield and so hastened the spread of the disease.*

It was clear that plague was not like any ordinary contagious disease, and direct spread of infection from case to case was hardly ever seen except in those patients who developed infection of the lung. This was known as pneumonic plague; but cases of bubonic plague could be nursed quite safely and it soon became well known that a plague hospital was the safest place in the world. The idea of the rat being responsible was not at first generally accepted and it was ten years after the 1894 epidemic before it was recognized that human plague followed rat plague; and moreover it was a particular type of rat, the black rat, that was responsible. This is an indoor rat, living often in living-rooms, in heaps of litter, in walls, roofs, or floors. Conditions in medieval England and in India were very conducive to its multiplication. The streets were full of garbage and filth of all descriptions, whilst the floors of the houses were covered in straw impregnated with food and filth. Moreover grain was often stored in the living-room.

In a series of well-controlled animal experiments the Plague Research Commission showed conclusively that plague can only be transmitted by rat-fleas and that climatic and other conditions play an important part in their reluctancy to bite man. Before this investigation little had been known of the habits of rats and fleas. Only by an intensive investigation of their habits and the way they lived was it possible to find out the precise facts about the mode of spread. One of the best guides to the danger of plague was the density of fleas. Flea-counts give a clue to variations in rat density and are much easier to carry out than rat-counts. The most dangerous flea goes by the name of *Xenopsylla cheopis*, and is essentially an indoor flea breeding only in dry situations. However, in some parts of the world such as Peru, where the climate is dry, it will breed out of doors away from houses, and so in some localities plague diffuses into the countryside amongst those working, for example, in cane sugar and cotton. The precise mode of action by which the flea infected its victims was investigated. After feeding on blood infected with plague bacilli the flea's stomach becomes blocked and the insect cannot feed normally. As a result it suffers from shortage of food and can be seen to make frequent and futile efforts to feed, inserting its pricker repeatedly into the skin of the victim, whereas the normal flea settles down to feed on one spot and enjoys a good meal of blood without delay. The efforts of the flea starved by the blockage of its stomach cause it to regurgitate masses of plague bacilli back into the wounds which it has made in its victim's skin, and so nature ensures the maximum opportunity for the flea to pass on the infection. The Commission concluded that the infection was kept going in other rodents during the off-season for plague, and by catching large numbers of rats and examining them for the plague

---

* Since the last great outbreaks there had been great advances in the science of bacteriology and on 14 June, 1894, a Japanese bacteriologist, Kitasato, working with Yersin, discovered that the disease was caused by a specific organism which he called the 'bacillus pestis'.

bacillus they were able to show the seasonal relationship between rat and human plague. The rat-flea was responsible for the spread of the disease from rats to men, for as soon as the rat died, the fleas became short of food and left the dead body of their natural host to search for food elsewhere. It was then that man was most likely to be attacked. Fleas which had entered clothing or rags would be particularly hungry if they had been cooped up without food for several days.

It was Simond who first showed that the bite of the rat-flea was responsible for the way the disease spread and so explained many anomalies in this. By examining patients who had contracted the disease he found the tiny puncture where the insect had first bitten its victim. Usually these were single punctures and the typical bubo always appeared in the glands draining the area in which the bite had occurred. He was able to recover the typical bacillus of plague from fleas which had fed on infected rats. It has been shown also that rat-fleas bite very little at temperatures over 80° F., and this explained the falling off in the severity of epidemics in the hot season. It explained also that the finding of a dead rat carcass in a house was a particularly bad sign because it indicated that the fleas were seeking a new host on which to feed. Since rat-fleas live on rat or human blood they were a means of directly transferring infected blood from a diseased animal to a healthy human being. It explained, too, why it was so dangerous to handle newly dead animals, although men could handle rats which had been dead for some time with impunity. Since fleas can live for a long time in old clothing and buildings it explained how infection could be kept alive in the body of the live insect. It was clear also why infected houses were more dangerous than patients with the disease.

Such, then, is the common mode of spread of bubonic plague in India, but investigations elsewhere were beginning to show that there were quite different problems in other parts of the world. Moreover, it was necessary to explain why these terrific outbreaks of the disease suddenly appeared and then for centuries virtually nothing was heard of them.

Our story now turns to a different sphere, the high steppe-lands of central Asia.

In 1895 two Russians described a disease which occurred amongst families engaged in trapping the Manchurian marmot in Transbaikal. Apparently the disease was contracted from sick animals, and some of the cases showed enlarged buboes in the axilla and groin whilst in others the symptoms were to be found mostly in the lungs.

The Manchurian marmot, or tarabagan, is a large rodent much hunted for its fur and for food. The Mongols have for centuries hunted the fit and healthy animals but avoided the sick animals which are easily caught. Their experience had told them that such animals spread disease. In 1909 the price of Manchurian marmot increased enormously and large numbers of Chinese flocked into the area to capture the animals, and naturally, being inexperienced, they caught mostly the slow-moving diseased animals. The disease was thought to be bubonic plague, and the outbreak soon reached epidemic proportions amongst large numbers of Chinese hunters. To complicate matters these men with their families were living in overcrowded conditions in filthy village inns and improvised hovels. A marked feature of this outbreak seems to have been the frequency of lung complications, a type of plague known as pneumonic, which spread like wildfire in the closely packed dwellings. In this type of disease the infection was spread from case to case by coughing. The infection spread along the route followed by the Chinese Eastern Railway, through Manchuria and North China to Peking and back into Siberia. (*Fig.* 2.) This great epidemic of pneumonic plague of 1910 killed 60,000 people and ten years later in 1920 it was followed by another. Undoubtedly the magnificent efforts of Dr. Wu Lien-Teh and his colleagues limited the death-roll, which even then amounted to 9300 deaths in all. (*See* Wu Lien-Teh, 1959.)

The results of the inquiry into the 1910 epidemic stimulated a large-scale investigation into plague and its relation with the wild rodents of south-east Russia, and it was found that there were many species of wild rodents which were naturally infected. This infection was given the name of sylvatic plague, from the Latin *silvaticus* meaning 'wild' or 'of the woods'. Hirst prefers the term 'campestral' (referring to a level field) as being more suitable. Fortunately many of the areas where these animals live are sparsely populated and it is only where man comes into close association with these creatures that infection spreads to human beings. The study of the natural history of the rodents of the world is therefore of enormous importance. This approach to the study of epidemic disease is known as ecological, the study of the relationship between host and environment.

CALIFORNIA

We must now leave Asia for the time being and see what had been happening in other parts of the world. In 1896 plague had spread to other important seaports, including Colombo in Ceylon, and had caused great consternation when it had appeared in Sidney and Brisbane. Extensive investigations confirmed the importance of the black rat and his flea as the culprits in the story. Our story, however, enters a new phase, when in March, 1908, plague was diagnosed for the first time in the United States of America at San Francisco. So once more infection had spread by ships along the trade routes, despite the most intensive precautions in ships crossing the Pacific from the plague areas. Infection was discovered amongst the rats and an extensive rat destruction campaign was started. A force of 400 men was employed, over £3000 was spent on rat-traps, and cheese was bought in quantities of 3000 lb. at a time; one feels that a Pied Piper of Hamelin would have been a godsend and certainly worth his fee. It soon became apparent that there was plague also amongst ground squirrels. In 1908 a boy died from plague after being bitten by a sick squirrel which he had caught as a pet, and in September, 1909, a man who went squirrel-hunting started a small epidemic of pneumonic plague in Oakland, California. This plague of wild rodents spread slowly but surely eastwards and like a forest fire nothing could stop its advance. By 1912 all the coastal countries were infected, by 1929 it had crossed the Sierra Nevada, and by 1933 it was in Montana and New Mexico. By 1942 it had entered Canada and is still spreading slowly in the Middle West. Many species of rodents have been shown to be involved, including ground and tree squirrels, prairie dogs, marmots, woodrats, mice, and rabbits.

In a few cases man has contracted the disease, but there have not been the same extensive epidemics as have been recorded from Asia. Bubonic plague caused 113 deaths in San Francisco between 1900 and 1904, mostly in Chinese and Japanese, and another small outbreak in 1907 resulted in 77 deaths. The disease also occurred in New Orleans in 1914 and spread to Texas and Florida, but there were probably less than 100 cases. Small outbreaks of pneumonic plague have occurred in California, the last in 1924. The lesson is clear; when man does not live under conditions which bring him into close contact with the wild animals which harbour the disease he will not become infected. It is only under special circumstances that this occurs in a highly industrialized country like the U.S.A. The conditions are such that these cases are limited in number and do not start an epidemic. Probably the standard of living accommodation is the most important factor. But hunters, trappers, keepers, people handling grain, and so on may be at special risk.

THE SOUTH AFRICAN VELDT

The same story has occurred in South Africa where infection entered the country from plague-infected rats on shipboard which then spread the disease to the wild rodents of the countryside, particularly multimammate mice and gerbilles. Probably the Boer War was responsible in the first place when feeding-stuffs for men and horses were imported in vast quantities bringing the rats at the same time. Human plague was first detected in January, 1899, following the importation of plague-infected commodities. For some time there were no more cases and it was hoped that the infection had disappeared, but in August, 1914, an outbreak of pneumonic plague occurred up-country in isolated farms. This was followed by small outbreaks occurring all over the country, all apparently unconnected. The outbreaks corresponded with the sandy areas in which the wild rodents had their homes. One farmer died after being bitten by rodent fleas during his afternoon siesta, near where many mice and gerbilles lay dead. They were all infected with plague. In 1923 plague spread to the Orange Free State and there were 184 deaths; altogether 2149 cases were recorded between 1919 and 1943. There was another great outbreak of plague in gerbilles in 1934, the previous summer having produced a very large crop of the favourite food of this animal. It was followed by a human epidemic which resulted in 184 deaths.

It would appear that the link between the gerbille and human beings is the multimammate mouse. It wanders at night, particularly in the summer-time, picking up fleas from the gerbille burrows and bringing them into houses. There has been a great increase in the wild rodents recently owing to destruction of their natural enemies, the wild cat, jackal, and lynx. Interference with the balance of nature can cause widespread repercussion and involve the death of man himself.

THE PAMPAS OF THE ARGENTINE

The same story has unfolded here; the wild rodent responsible is chiefly the cavy, which is rather like a guinea-pig living a colonial existence. The infection is spread from them to human dwellings by the long-tailed rat, which, like the field-mouse of Britain, may enter human habitation, particularly in the winter, but also lives in trees.

There have been 225 deaths from pneumonic plague contracted in this way recorded in the Argentine. Many of them have occurred in children who have caught sick wild animals as pets. Similarly, outbreaks have occurred in Brazil in rats, and human plague contracted from guinea-pigs which are kept as pets has occurred in natives in the high Andes.

OTHER CENTRES OF PLAGUE

Outbreaks have occurred in many other parts of the world. The islands of Java, Madagascar, Mauritius, the Philippines, Hawaii, and Formosa have had severe epidemics. It has occurred in Japan, Siam, and Malaya, in East Africa, in Uganda and Kenya, in West Africa at Accra, Senegal, and Jos, and in North Africa in Morocco and Egypt. The most recent outbreaks have been again in Calcutta. It would appear that there are very few places with warm climates which have not had plague in this last great pandemic.

Research workers are now investigating the habits of wild rodents all over the world and have already found no less than seventy naturally infected species. There seems to be a greater tendency for the development of pneumonic plague following these wild rodent infections.

Why has plague failed to establish itself in Britain during the last fifty years, despite the fact that there have been severe epidemics all over the world and considering the fact that there were severe outbreaks in the seventeenth century? In fact, plague, in epidemic form, has been absent from this country for nearly 300 years. It cannot be due to the fact that there has been no rat plague, because this has occurred at several ports, including Glasgow, Liverpool, Cardiff, Bristol, and London. Several cases of human plague occurred in 1906 in workmen in Bristol who were handling flea-infested rags in a warehouse at the docks; 201 tons of rags were destroyed and 20 tons of disinfectants used to kill off any fleas left.

There have been isolated cases of human plague in gamekeepers and rat-catchers and in some cottagers in East Anglia. In the winter of 1906 the head keeper at Woolverston Park in Norfolk noticed that rats were dying in unusual numbers. In December, 1906, 5 people died of a disease diagnosed as pneumonia; all were living in the same cottage in the village of Shotley, 3 miles from Woolverston Park. Three years later 5 more people died from pneumonia; all living in the same household, 2 miles from Shotley. All had swollen glands. The next year not far away in Freston, 4 people died under similar circumstances; death was rapid and certified as pneumonia. Fortunately, the doctor in charge of the last cases was not satisfied, and bacteriological investigation showed that the deaths were due to plague. Year after year plague-infested rodents were found in East Anglia, but no more human deaths occurred until 1918 when 2 people died from it in the village of Erwarton, 1½ miles from Shotley. The plague epidemic in rodents has died out; it is now thought that the disease was probably introduced from grain ships discharging in the river Orwell. In 1962 an experimental scientist died from plague at Porton, England.

Plague did not produce the widespread epidemics which it had done in the Middle Ages and in the present century in India. We must ask ourselves why?

It is clearly due to improvements in domestic hygiene; carpets have replaced the pile of straw on the floor, and walls and ceilings are now better constructed. The proper storage of grain has meant that rats and their fleas no longer live in close association with human beings. Moreover, we are now highly intolerant of personal parasites. But another important factor has been the ousting of the domestic black rat by the large outdoor brown rat during the seventeenth century.

France has also had a few cases of human plague recently in Paris and Marseilles. It is disturbing to note that in recent years there has been in Europe a great increase in the black rat population and the worst of the plague-carrying fleas.

Since World War II plague has been epidemic in the following countries, each of which has had more than 100 deaths during that period:—

Africa: Belgian Congo, Tanganyika, Madagascar
Asia: Burma, Pakistan, India, Java, Thailand
South America: Brazil, Peru.

Burma and Java have had over 6000 deaths and India over 150,000. In 1962, however, there were only a few hundred cases reported in the whole world, mostly in India and South America. Plague has now become a rural rather than an urban disease. (*See* Pollitzer (1954) for a full account of plague.)

CONTROL OF PLAGUE

Venice was the chief port of entry into Europe for merchandise from the East and as such she experienced many epidemics of plague. Lazarettos were set up for the isolation and control of plague patients. This procedure was called quarantine (Italian *quarantena* = forty days) because the patients were held for forty days, since it was thought that it took this length of time to dissipate the infection. Eventually they were set up in all the Mediterranean ports. John Howard, the prison reformer, gives a first-hand account of such places and of the terrible conditions which were rife there.

The chief measure now in force for the prevention of plague is the control of rats (*see Fig.* 3). This is done by rat-proofing ships and port installations and by de-ratting ships with prussic acid and poisoned baits. It has been shown that rats can be almost eliminated from ships by proper rat-proofing.

25

There still remains the danger of carrying infected fleas in cargoes brought from plague-infested areas. This is a danger which is not sufficiently realized by our port authorities. These cargoes discharged into warehouses at our ports can easily spread infection to the black rats which infest them. Grain from Burma and Ceylon is particularly dangerous and some method of disinfestation has been recommended but not put into force. The World Health Organization keeps records of plague occurring anywhere in the world, and this serves as a useful check on the possibilities of spread. The elimination of rats in ports and towns is an extremely difficult matter; they can, however, be kept down to a minimum as far as dwelling houses are concerned. It is possible to eradicate rats within a localized area, but only by the appropriate survey techniques, the use of skilled personnel, and the expenditure of considerable sums of money. The best weapon would appear to be the proper rat-proofing of buildings. This is expensive in primitive countries, but even so a great deal has been achieved in places like Java, Madagascar, and India. In fact, it has been a blessing in disguise because it has led to improvements in housing conditions which otherwise would not have occurred.

Personal protection against the bite of fleas is important in plague areas. This can be done by wearing protective clothing and dusting with DDT. Active immunization by anti-plague vaccines is also important to raise the level of immunity. These measures are particularly important in those especially exposed to risk, as in doctors, nurses, and sanitary inspectors. It is also possible now to take drugs by mouth, for example, sulphonamides, which are of great value in preventing the disease in those who have been in contact with it. Finally, treatment is now much more effective; the newer antibiotics such as streptomycin have reduced the fatality-rate of cases of moderate severity from 75 per cent to 10 per cent or less.

Today mass evacuation of areas is no longer practised. Now frequent surveys reveal the danger-spots immediately and the spread of infection is soon brought under control. This is chiefly effected by mass inoculation of the people and by the employment of insecticides. In Madagascar, for example, between 1935 and 1940 nearly 800,000 vaccinations were given against a plague. But the reservoirs of infection still remain, not only in seaport towns but in the country. Plague is now becoming a rural problem and the anti-plague work involved in outbreaks in these areas is best handled by mobile teams, who can survey the local causes, institute treatment, and plan measures for its prevention. In this way it is often possible to overcome local prejudices and ensure good co-operation.

We should never be lulled into a sense of security by the apparent success of some of these measures. We can never be sure how and when the disease will break out in some new form. Should atomic warfare destroy civilization as we know it today, we should have all the conditions necessary for another great epidemic of plague. There are reservoirs of infected rodents all over the world ready to live in close association with a highly susceptible population, which would have to exist under the most primitive conditions.

Overcrowding and shortage of human food would be common, but there would be no shortage of food for rats!

Nor should we imagine that we could necessarily rely on DDT, since many vectors have now developed resistance to this and to other insecticides. The great wars and famines of the past have encouraged the spread of epidemics and similar catastrophes in the future may do the same, but whatever happens, our knowledge of the cause and our study of the lessons of history should be potent factors in controlling such outbreaks.

Plague illustrates, perhaps better than any other disease, the need to adopt a holistic attitude to nature. Outbreaks of epidemic diseases have determined the fate of nations, and how seemingly trivial are the events on which these happenings may sometimes be based—an unusually good harvest, a rise in the price of animal skins due to changing fashions, or even the personal habits of certain kinds of fleas.

ZOONOSES

Before leaving this important killer of men and animals, let us consider for a moment some other important diseases which are spread from animals to man; they have been called, as a group, the zoonoses. Their control depends upon close co-operation between the public health worker and the veterinary specialist. One of the best known of such diseases is hydrophobia or rabies which has been known for thousands of years. It is due to a virus which is transmitted by the bite of a rabid animal, usually a dog or cat, but also by the bite of foxes, wolves, and vampire bats. Outbreaks of rabies have been followed by widespread campaigns against the animal responsible. Thus in 1837 there were 2 cases of rabies in Sheffield; as a result 2040 dogs were destroyed in a few months. It is always fatal in man unless serum can be given straightaway, and has caused some concern in recent years because of its increased prevalence in the Middle East.

In the present century, however, a number of new virus diseases of the brain have been described from various parts of the world. One of the first was encephalitis from St. Louis in 1933. This disease is spread from chickens by the bite of mosquitoes. Outbreaks of similar types of disease have occurred in many parts of the U.S.A., and from Venezuela, Japan, Siberia, India, Australia, and Africa. We still have a lot to learn about their mode of spread, but in most cases there appears to be a reservoir of infection in certain species of birds or animals, particularly the horse. The infection is usually passed on to man by the bite of blood-feeding arthropods, such as mosquitoes, ticks, and mites. These diseases show marked seasonal variations dependent upon the life histories of the various vectors and hosts which are concerned in the spread.

They are an interesting group because they have only been recognized in recent years; whether these are new diseases or not it is difficult to say; probably they went by other names in the past; moreover their control will probably be similar to that of plague. Like the latter they are diseases of rural areas, breaking out when man alters the equilibrium between himself and nature. Further study, to be profitable, must depend upon the ecological approach, taking into consideration every factor in the environment.

Other diseases which are spread to man from animals are tularaemia and toxoplasmosis, which are contracted from rabbits; glanders from close association with horses; psittacosis from contact with parrots and other birds; Q fever and undulant fever from sheep, cows, and goats. Anthrax and bovine tuberculosis which are contracted from cows are described in later chapters. The rat is a particularly dangerous animal; not only does it harbour plague but it is responsible for leptospirosis, rat-bite fever, and certain forms of food-poisoning. The pig carries numerous parasitic diseases which can be spread to man. Even the dog is not without danger; it can carry many diseases harmful to humans, the most dangerous being hydatid disease, whilst the cat is responsible, amongst other diseases, for the newly described cat-scratch fever. Fortunately many of these diseases are rare. There are more than one hundred diseases which are *common* to man and animals.

CHAPTER IV

OF LICE AND MEN

WE have shown how a small arthropod, the flea, has been responsible for great changes in the economic life of nations, particularly on the domestic front. We shall now discuss a disease which has its greatest effects when men are crowded together and particularly during war and famine. Our chief culprit in this case is the human louse, and the disease it causes is typhus fever. Although there can be no doubt that many of the earliest recorded epidemics were due to typhus fever, it is often difficult to distinguish it from other serious epidemic diseases such as small-pox, dysentery, typhoid fever, and malignant scarlet fever. In the first place typhus probably originated in Asia as a natural disease of rats and was spread by rat-fleas. A study of the present-day distribution of typhus lends support to this. There are still centres of rat-borne or murine typhus in Mexico, the U.S.A., and the Mediterranean basin. Gradually it has spread throughout the world and in the process the method of spread has become modified to include lice, ticks, and larval mites in the list of vectors.

The first recorded epidemic occurred in 1489 in Spain when the Spaniards were fighting the Moors for Granada. It was called 'malignant spotted fever' and it was thought to have been introduced from Cyprus and to be due to unburied corpses. In 1490 it was found that 17,000 had died from the disease whereas only 3000 had been killed by the Moors.

During the next fifty years the disease spread throughout Spain and from there was carried to Mexico by the explorers and conquerors of the New World. Small-pox and measles were also sent across the ocean; in return we got syphilis and tobacco. We have now conquered syphilis, but the ill-effects of tobacco are only just beginning to reveal themselves. Typhus was generally regarded by the chronicles of that day as a new disease which had come from the East. In Italy in the sixteenth century typhus fever completely changed the course of history. In 1528 the French were about to take Naples where the Prince of Orange was making his last stand on behalf of Charles V of Spain against Francis I of France. The army had been reduced to 11,000 men by disease and Charles V was heavily engaged all over Europe. There seemed little hope for Naples, but in the crowded camps of the French typhus struck and within three weeks 21,000 men were killed out of an army of 58,000. The small remnant was destroyed by the defenders of Naples and the Pope crowned Charles V as ruler of the Holy Roman Empire. The battle had been won by typhus.

From then onwards typhus fever was never absent from Europe, but one significant fact was that whilst mortality in the armies of the north and west was high, mortality in armies from the east, i.e., from Turkey and Hungary, was low, showing that the disease had already been present in the Eastern countries giving rise to a high level of immunity. This is an important piece of evidence in favour of the origin of the disease from Asia. The Thirty Years' War from 1618 to 1648 saw renewed outbreaks of the disease reinforced by dysentery, typhoid, diphtheria, scarlet fever, and small-pox. The constant movement of armies of hired soldiers backwards and forwards across Europe ensured that no corner of Europe was left without its focus of infection.

In England some of the earliest outbreaks of typhus occurred in the prisons where it was known as 'jail fever'. At Oxford in 1577 a Catholic bookbinder, being tried for profaning God's word, caused an outbreak of the disease amongst those present at his trial. There were 500 deaths in the town from this outbreak; 100 of the dead were members of the University. As we know now that infection is transmitted by the louse, all those who contracted the disease must have been louse-infested. The disease decimated both the Royalist and Parliamentary armies in 1643 at the siege of Reading. In the famous Bloody Assize of Judge Jeffreys in 1685 infection spread from the prisoners to the judges. It was probably during the Civil War that typhus spread to Ireland, which long remained a stronghold of the disease, culminating in the great Irish epidemic of 1816–19. During these four years it is estimated that there were 700,000 cases out of a population of 6,000,000. It was associated with the failure of the potato crop, hence another name, 'famine fever'. 'Ship fever' was also another name it received from the lousiness of the men impressed into the Navy by the press gangs. Dr. James Lind banished typhus fever from the British Navy when he issued strict instructions for the disinfestation of the sailor's clothing; this disease and scurvy were two of the greatest killers of seamen.

Napoleon had reason to remember typhus. As his armies advanced through Poland into Lithuania so the sickness rates increased. After the battle of Ostrowo in July, 1812, he had over 80,000 sick. When the retreat from Moscow began on 15 October there were only 80,000 left out of an original army of 500,000. Typhus was responsible for a large majority of his losses.

In 1909 Charles Nicolle made the great discovery that typhus fever was spread from man to man by the louse, not only by its bite, but by crushing it and rubbing the remains which contained the infective agent into excoriations of the skin brought about by scratching. In other words, a form of auto-inoculation.

Now, as long as we continue to live under our present-day conditions the louse is kept under control, but the moment some emergency alters this equilibrium, then there is a marked and immediate swing of the pendulum in favour of the parasite. It is amazing how quickly a community can become louse-ridden. This was seen during World War II, during the evacuation of refugees from bombed cities. They had to be accommodated under emergency measures in schools and public buildings, crowded together in close contact. One of the great problems was invariably infestation with the louse. The same sort of thing is seen during periods of famine, for example, after the failure of the potato crop in Ireland in 1847. In the nineteenth century in England epidemics occurred from the great crowds of unemployed who wandered from city to city.

A hundred years ago schools and prisons lacked adequate bathing facilities and even today there are many houses without baths. In the 1951 Census the question was first asked of householders whether they had a bath or not, and it was found in Sheffield, for example, that 44 per cent of households were without them.

Even though we may think that cleanliness is next to Godliness it can still be enjoyed without a bathroom and in many houses a bucket in front of the fire or the kitchen sink are still the only means available. People can remain clean without a bathroom, but what is important is the standard of personal hygiene in such things as care of the hair and the wearing of clean underclothing.

With the beginning of the twentieth century it looked as though typhus had disappeared for good from the civilized world, although many cases still occurred in such places as Iceland, Russia, and the Balkans. However, our complacency was soon to disappear as the greatest conflict in history changed the way of life of millions of people, soldiers and civilians alike. In 1914 as a result of the first battles in Serbia there was widespread destruction of towns and villages, and the civilian population flocked southwards fleeing from the battlefield. There was, of course, no shelter for them; the sick and wounded had to be cared for and there were thousands of prisoners too. There was a shortage of hospitals, drugs, nurses, and doctors. The typhus epidemic began in 1914 and in less than six months over 200,000 people had died, including half the Austrian prisoners. Out of 400 Serbian doctors, 126 died. Doctors and nurses are particularly liable to contract the disease because as soon as a person becomes sick with typhus, the temperature rises and the lice already infected with the organism responsible for the disease (*Rickettsia prowazeckii*) become more active and begin to leave the dying person, like rats leaving a sinking ship. When they have a chance to find a new source of food, a healthy adult, they pass the infection to their new host.

From this time on typhus took its customary toll on the Eastern front, but strangely enough it never spread to the Western front, although as all soldiers of the First World War know, there was universal lousiness. No doubt this was due to two causes. First, because of the conditions of war there was a strict barrier separating Eastern Europe from Western Europe so that it was extremely difficult for infection to be imported from the East into the West, and, secondly, it was the first war in which an army had been really well fed, and throughout the war the nutritional state of the troops was kept at a high level. There was, however, a considerable amount of trench fever, a disease which is also spread by the louse.

31

The utmost precautions were taken to control the spread of infection from the East, and delousing in prisoners from the Eastern front was carried out on a truly gigantic scale. There was nothing, however, to prevent the spread of the epidemic eastwards, and after the war revolution and famine were the aftermath, resulting in the greatest epidemic of all time in Russia. Between 1917 and 1921 it has been estimated that there were more than 25,000,000 cases of typhus in Russia with 3,000,000 deaths from the disease.

When World War II broke out it was natural enough that thoughts should be directed to the possibility of typhus, and soon, sure enough, the familiar story once more unfolded itself. In 1940 there were 4000 cases in six months in Warsaw, and it spread to Germany with nearly 2000 cases in the same year. The disease never reached the epidemic proportions of the past once the early campaign was over. The blitzkrieg technique did not give sufficient scope for the development of an epidemic and the high standards of hygiene in the German army soon brought it under control. The summer campaign in France in 1942 was soon over, but in North Africa typhus reached epidemic proportions. In 1942 there were outbreaks in Algeria (35,000 cases), Morocco (25,000 cases), Tunis (16,000 cases), and in Egypt (22,000 cases).

In the plans for the invasion of Normandy naturally one of the first considerations was the prevention of typhus amongst any troops fighting on the Continent, because it was known that typhus fever was present in the German army, particularly during 1942 and 1943. The preparations for the Second Front included large-scale preventive measures against lousiness. One of the greatest discoveries was the value of the insecticide DDT which was extremely effective in killing the louse. This had originally been discovered in 1874 in Switzerland by a student called Zeidler, but it was not until 1942 that its value as an insecticide was realized. It was incorporated into a special powder, known as AL63, which was used to spray the clothing of soldiers at regular intervals; in addition, all underclothes were impregnated with the substance. The results were highly successful, the army which invaded Europe and defeated the Germans was the most healthy army the world has ever known, and the louse was a great rarity. Not only was the army free from vermin, but it was probably better fed than any other fighting force in history.

The danger of this disease in wartime led to intensive research being carried out on the production of a vaccine which could be used to prevent the disease. By 1942 a suitable vaccine had been prepared and all troops were inoculated with it.

The first successful vaccines were prepared in Poland by the Polish doctor, Weigl. His great difficulty was to find some suitable medium upon which he could grow the tiny organism which caused the disease. The only medium he knew was in the intestine of the living louse; his experiments therefore were carried out by inoculating the living organism of typhus into the intestines of lice. He had to train his workers in the delicate task of inserting very fine glass pipettes into the anal orifice of the tiny insect, a rather unusual occupation. As can be imagined this was a very tedious and difficult business and did not produce very large amounts of vaccine. It required about 150 lice to provide sufficient vaccine for one person. This meant that extensive louse farms had to be kept going and they could only be fed on human volunteers immune from the disease. Weigl had about 200 of them who had recovered from typhus fever and so were immune. A great advance was made, however, when it was found in America that the organism could be grown on live chick embryos and the vaccine used at the present time is prepared from organisms which have been cultivated by inoculation of fertile eggs.

Naturally our knowledge of the cause of the spread of typhus did not come about without considerable research on the habits of the human louse, and one of the difficulties in this field of research is keeping them alive. Unfortunately, the louse can only feed on human blood and in a laboratory carrying out this kind of work human volunteers have to be found on which to feed the animals. These are usually placed in thin, round, metal boxes covered with fine gauze. The box is strapped to the leg of the volunteer with gauze next to the skin so that the louse can feed through the gauze but still remain a prisoner. Needless to say, volunteers are very difficult to come by and the scientist himself usually has to act as the provider of the meal for his unusual pets.

No doubt there are some who have feelings of disgust and revulsion when hearing of this work. They should remember that it was only by research of this kind that it has been possible eventually to master some of the dread diseases which have attacked man in the past.

THE NAPLES EPIDEMIC

Italy had been the scene of many epidemics of typhus in the Middle Ages, but in the years before the Second World War had managed to escape the epidemics which had occurred in the rest of Europe. There were no recorded cases between 1928 and 1943. As a result the population was highly susceptible to the disease. In 1943 there were close on a million people in a city which had been devastated by Allied bombing and by the retreating Germans. They were living largely in overcrowded shelters with lack of food and clothing and with primitive sanitary arrangements and a low standard of hygiene. Typhus had spread into Sicily from North Africa and had occurred at Bari in Italian soldiers. The first cases were in one of the Naples prisons, among prisoners from Tunisia and Yugoslavia. When the Allies entered Naples, on 1 Oct., 1943, the epidemic was under way and winter was approaching. Jail fever had once again reared its ugly head. Mass delousing was carried out on a scale which had never been attempted before. This was done with hand and power dusters using insecticidal powders. From 15 Dec., 1943, to 31 May, 1944, 3,265,786 persons were dusted in Naples and the vicinity. At the end of December, 1943, DDT was used for the first time. The epidemic reached its peak in January, 1944, and virtually came to an end in March, 1944. Altogether there were 1040 cases and deaths in Naples. That ancient city owes a great deal to Zeidler, who first discovered DDT, to the Geigy Company of Switzerland, who demonstrated its value as an insecticide, and to the Allied armies, who applied the knowledge so effectively and so quickly. At last man had found an effective answer to one of the most frightful of the 'men of death'.

Typhus was not yet conquered, however; it was still spreading unchecked in the German camps, where men and women were living under conditions far worse than those in Naples. Moreover, the efficacy of DDT was not yet known to the Nazis.

Probably DDT has been responsible for saving more lives than all the other discoveries of medical science put together, but for an effective proof of what may seem a rather wild statement we must wait until we can discuss malaria. It is remarkable that the Germans did not know of the value of this insecticide until the war was over, otherwise we might not be telling the next story.

TYPHUS IN BELSEN

No description of the horrors of typhus would be complete without an account of the concentration camps of the Nazis, particularly Belsen. Up to the invasion of Normandy in the Second World War there had been no cases of louse-borne typhus in England, although it had occurred in the Mediterranean theatres and was prevalent in Germany and on the Russian front. It was decided that a line should be drawn across Europe to isolate the West from Germany. This *cordon sanitaire* was based on the river Rhine. Up to 1945 there had been no cases reported in the Rhineland, but in February and March of 1945 a small epidemic broke out in Aachen, München-Gladbach, and Cologne. Before the entry of the Allied armies about 400 cases of typhus had been reported in the Rhineland. The area was full of displaced persons, all trying to reach their homeland. There were at least half a million of them, under-nourished, poorly clad, and used to low standards of hygiene after their years of existence under the most primitive conditions. In the words of John E. Gordon (1948): 'It was Wild West, the hordes of Genghis Khan, the Klondike gold rush and Napoleon's retreat from Moscow all rolled up into one.' Here was a situation without parallel in the history of war and wide open for the spread of typhus. The United States forces entered Cologne on 5 March, 1945; by the end of April the disease had virtually disappeared owing to the energetic measures taken for its control. German prisoners of war were kept free of lice by repeated dusting with DDT, but it was more difficult to get hold of displaced persons who were constantly on the move. Out of 693 recorded cases, 400 were in this latter group. Civilians were not allowed across the Rhine unless they had a certificate to say that they had been recently deloused. As can be imagined there was soon a thriving black market in forged certificates. After a few weeks the movements of displaced persons became more controlled. Many of them in their first flush of enthusiasm to get home had not realized the difficulties of travelling on foot with a grave shortage of food.

34

Camps for displaced persons were set up in many areas to collect these unfortunates and the majority of them were only too glad to enter these havens of refuge, where they could find food, shelter, clothing, and medical care.

As the advance continued the really serious hotbeds of typhus were uncovered in the concentration camps. First Buchenwald was uncovered by the 3rd American Army on 12 April, 1945, and then Belsen by the 2nd British Army on 15 April. This was followed by the discovery of Dachau, Flossenberg, and Monthausen.

With the liberation of these camps the first thought of their inmates was to get home as soon as possible and the few who were fit enough scattered throughout the countryside. As the cities were liberated millions of con-script workers from countries all over Europe were also released. Later there was the problem of hundreds of thousands of German prisoners rushing west as fast as they could go to avoid being captured by the Russians, and in addition the many German civilians who had fled before the Allied advance were now trying to return westward to their own ruined towns. Finally, many of the older men of the Wehrmacht were released to return home to till the land and start the wheels of reconstruction turning again. Germany was an astounding place in those early spring days of 1945; masses of humanity, some travelling east, some south, some north, but mostly westwards, carrying typhus with them, and yet typhus in the inner Reich came under effective control in a relatively short time, just as it had done in the limited area of the Rhineland.

The bulk of the cases occurred in the concentration camps. Both the American and British armies had their experiences of this. Dachau was the worst in the American sector. It was liberated by the U.S. 7th Army on 1 May, 1945. There were about 40,000 inmates, alive and dead. Extreme filth and louse infestation prevailed everywhere and the most appalling overcrowding, the dead lying with the living. The number of cases recorded was 2336 up to 1 June, with 311 deaths.

We must turn, however, to Belsen in the British sector, the most notorious of all the prison camps, infamous because of the sheer horror of the conditions imposed by the Nazis.

The camp was built in 1940 in the pinewoods near the pretty village of Belsen in Hanover. It was surrounded, like other camps of its kind, by barbed wire and guarded by the notorious S.S. troops. The inmates were housed mostly in single-story wooden huts consisting of one large room, 100 feet long and 20 feet wide. In some there was a toilet and a small washroom, but many had no such provisions, the inmates having to walk varying distances to central toilets and ablution blocks, in some cases over 200 yards. The only furniture consisted of triple tiers of wooden bunks, packed closely together. There were 82 of these human kennels. In addition there were the living quarters of the Commandant, J. Kramer, and his wife and the S.S. guards, an administrative block, several cookhouses, and, of course, a well-built crematorium.

35

The inmates were mostly Jews from Poland, Czechoslovakia, Holland, Russia, Hungary, Yugoslavia, and Roumania. They received one meal a day, consisting of black bread and mangel-wurzel soup; the calorific value was under 800 per day. The inmates were allowed out for only three hours a day and there was no artificial light. There were two meals a day for non-Jews and other privileges for block leaders who were put in charge of the huts. The possession of a book or newspaper was forbidden and punishable by lashing. Many of the victims naturally enough died under this treatment. Some of the favoured female inmates received the most remarkable privileges and lived on the fat of the land, the best food, chocolates, alcohol, and cigarettes.

Association between male and female was strictly forbidden and the molestation of female inmates by male S.S. guards was a serious offence. The females, however, had quite enough to cope with the brutalities of their female guards. I talked to many survivors of Belsen and they were all in agreement that the female S.S. were far more brutal than their male counterparts. Irma Grese was a typical example. I saw her in hospital, herself sick with typhus; she was subsequently executed. Many of these females were lesbians and had their favourite prisoner who in return received many privileges. In fact, one such guard had followed a beautiful Czech film star from the notorious Auschwitz camp* across Europe to Belsen, in order to be near her. Auschwitz was the camp where mass extermination of the Jews took place and this girl only escaped with her mother because of the intervention of this guard. Auschwitz is now kept as a national museum by the Polish Government and remains exactly as it was during the war, but the site of Belsen is being rapidly overgrown by heather and birch trees.

During 1944 the Belsen camp became overcrowded with evacuees from camps in the East which were threatened by the Russian advance.

Typhus was brought to the camp in January, 1945, by a train-load of Hungarian Jews. The trip had taken three weeks, because of Allied bombing of the railways, and during that time they had huddled together for warmth, inadequately clothed and with little food. Many were dead on arrival, but there were sufficient numbers alive to start an epidemic. The huts were already overcrowded and so the new arrivals had to be distributed round all the huts.

Some attempts at delousing were in operation, but the Germans were still using the old-fashioned system of dry heat, which was quite inadequate.

Two or more persons occupied each tier of a bunk, so that in the most crowded places there were 24 persons in a space $12 \times 6 \times 8$ feet. Others had to stand or sit crouched on the floor. The places in the bunks once lost were never regained, and when an occupant died there was a fight for the place and for his or her clothes, and the strongest won, so that gradually the weakest sank to the floor. Blankets were wholly insufficient and many prisoners were naked. There was, of course, no heating even in the depths of

---

* Much of the detail for this chapter was obtained from this girl by the author.

winter. In some huts there were no bunks at all and the mass of humanity was just piled one on top of the other. There was no attempt to remove the dead; they lay there together with the living. The few toilets were blocked and in any case the majority were too weak to leave their resting places, and those who were strong enough did not dare leave. As the huts became full to overflowing, the weakest were pushed out to die in the open. Excreta were everywhere, knee-deep on the floors and trickling down from the upper bunks. Diarrhoea was universal owing to dysentery and starvation. Under these conditions there was universal lousiness and as the typhus epidemic gained momentum, the number of dead bodies rapidly increased.

The food situation became rapidly worse owing to the large increase in numbers and the difficulty of transporting food to the camp, following the Allied bombing of communications. In the end, in some of the worst huts the inmates were eating anything they could find, including excreta and the parts of the dead which were still edible, usually the liver or heart.

Perhaps the reader has had enough of this macabre story. It might be imagined that nothing could make it worse, but about a week before the camp was liberated its power supply was cut off and there was no electricity to pump the water, so that there was no more drinking water. The need for water is well known in typhus; this and the starvation increased the death-rate.

The British first entered the camp in the evening of 15 April, 1945. There were about 10,000 dead and 45,000 living, many of whom were quite beyond hope. The smell of death and faecal matter could be detected in the village of Belsen 3 miles away. Of the 45,000 living, 13,000 died later in the camp, 3500 had typhus, 10,000 had tuberculosis, 20,000 had enteritis due to dysentery or famine, and 10,000 had famine oedema. Probably everybody in the camp had suffered from typhus at some time or other. Many had probably suffered from the disease in their native country and had a high degree of immunity. These survived more readily than others who came into contact with the disease for the first time in Belsen. It has been estimated that there were about 20,000 cases of typhus between January and April, 1945.

The first task was to provide food and drink and, what was particularly important, to control its issue. Many people died from gulping down unsuitable food in large quantities. It was necessary to erect latrines and delousing centres quickly. The selection of patients for treatment was not an easy task; examination was difficult because of overcrowding and darkness, and the living were so covered with dirt, sores, and vermin that it was impossible to make a proper clinical diagnosis. The situation was further complicated by language difficulties. Those who stood a chance of living had to be given priority, and each had to go through the delousing centre before transport to hospital. In the 'human laundry' each patient was scrubbed with soap and water and dusted with anti-louse powder, and then transported by ambulance to hospital. From the moment of release those who were fit went everywhere in search of food, clothing, and better quarters, others set out in search of loot in the neighbouring villages, whilst many, becoming impatient of inevitable delays, set out on foot for their distant homeland. The S.S. guards had fled into the neighbouring woods and a band of released Hungarian soldiers had a happy time with a little private war of their own, rounding up their enemies. Kramer, the 'beast of Belsen', had a particularly unhappy time, but was saved, to be hanged later for his crimes.

Under these conditions there was a great danger of spreading the infection and a quarantine was put on the camp.* Only those on duty were allowed to enter or leave the camp and each time they had to be dusted. Later there was the question of delousing, housing, feeding, and clothing those who were reasonably fit. Fortunately there was a large tank training school (a Panzer *Truppenschule*) nearby with well-equipped barracks, canteens, hospital, and offices, and even a theatre and other welfare facilities. Mass delousing of the living was carried out by teams of Royal Army Medical Corps personnel, using 10-gun power-dusters. The work was very slow because of the difficulties of working in overcrowded huts, and the smell was so overpowering that several soldiers collapsed and some officers refused to enter at all.

The work began on 22 April, 1945, one week after the British had entered the camp. It was slow work because most of the inmates were too weak to walk to a central point and so the dusters had to be taken into the huts. Those able to walk were dusted in the passage-ways or outside each hut; other persons, corpses, and beds were deloused in situ. The accent was on thoroughness and so, slowly but surely, the work went on until by 30 April, 30,000 living persons and their beds had been dusted. This was not expected to eliminate lice entirely, but it did reduce the incidence to a low level and stop the epidemic. It was, of course, necessary later to carry out further programmes of dusting with DDT. Altogether by the end of May over 78,000 delousing operations had been carried out. Those fit to walk were evacuated to the Panzer school barracks by lorry after passing through the delousing station; the evacuation of the sick to hospital continued. In the meantime, many others had died.

We must not forget the workers in these camps, doctors, medical students,† nurses, sanitary personnel, soldiers, and bathhouse workers, who were all at special risk. Many of the workers were recruited from Poles, Hungarians, and Germans who had already been in contact with the disease. As soon as possible an inoculation programme was started. It was most difficult to get workers from the camp to be inoculated. They nearly all claimed to have had the disease. They had the most amazing knowledge of it and were most useful in helping to make correct diagnoses. As can be expected, cases of typhus fever occurred in those responsible for looking after the inmates; these included 32 out of the 48 German nurses, 10 of the 57 Hungarian

---

* This quarantine period was imposed for a period of 21 days after delousing.

† In May, British medical students came to Belsen to help with the work of clearing up the camp and caring for its inmates.

control unit, 7 British soldiers, and 6 medical students. The latter cared for those who were sick from typhus and were at great risk. Fortunately all the British personnel had been vaccinated so their disease was mild and there were no deaths amongst them.

I have said little of the great administrative problems involved in the setting up of hospitals and services for the care of 13,834 sick patients nor of the great problem of feeding and treating such vast numbers, but the reader can judge these difficulties for himself.

The last case of typhus occurred on 14 May, and the decline in the incidence of typhus was sharp and dramatic, 14 days after all the inmates had been deloused. There can be little doubt from the evidence that delousing with anti-louse powder Mark III was the most important factor in bringing the epidemic under control. A few cases of typhus occurred in escapees from the camp, but fortunately these were few in number and no major outbreaks were reported. About 3000 are estimated to have left the camp, but most of them did so after delousing. From March to June, 1945, there were 498 cases of typhus fever reported from Allied countries, over 400 of them from France and Belgium.

The Germans were still using the old-fashioned technique of hot-air disinfestation, which can only deal with relatively small numbers at a time. But for DDT powder, there can be little doubt that we should have had a terrible epidemic in Western Europe.

This account of typhus in Belsen has been given in some detail because it brings home to us with added force the human misery and suffering which exist during war and pestilence amongst civilian populations. The reader may well ask why the Germans allowed such conditions to develop. Probably they never planned that it should be like this, things got out of hand, and the numbers of inmates became far too great for the accommodation and food supply, and there were more urgent matters to attend to elsewhere. There is evidence that they tried to combat lousiness; in the early days a regimen was laid down in which each inmate had to have delousing treatment once every three months, but the old-fashioned method could not cope with the sudden influx of people. If dusting with DDT powder had been routine, there would have been no typhus in Belsen.

Typhus in Other Parts of the World

Louse-borne epidemic typhus occurred in Japan and Korea during 1945 and 1946; over 30,000 cases were reported. It has been estimated that 2,000,000 cases would have occurred if a suitable control programme had not been arranged. Louse infestation had increased because of shortage of clothing, fuel, and soap, and there was considerable overcrowding.

A large-scale repatriation movement at the end of the Korean war resulted in the migration of millions of persons and the spreading of infection between Korea and Japan. Two million persons were dusted with DDT at the ports. As a result of the widespread use of DDT and vaccination with typhus vaccine the epidemic was brought under control. Only 28 cases were reported in the United States Army personnel; all the cases were mild and there were no deaths, no doubt due to the fact that all the patients had been vaccinated prior to their illness. Once more, as in Naples, the dread scourge of louse-borne typhus had been brought under effective control. One word of warning, however; it has been reported from Korea that lice responsible for typhus have since developed resistance to DDT and nowadays other insecticides are used, for example, BHC. (*Fig. 4.*)

Let us turn now from a consideration of the classic typhus of history to newly recognized types spread by other insect vectors. In this respect typhus is like plague. With the turn of the century there began to appear from various parts of the world descriptions of fevers which resembled typhus but differed in their method of spread.

In 1910 Dr. Brill described a disease in New York which was similar to classic typhus but much less fatal. It was particularly common in Jewish immigrants to America from the Balkans, the home of European typhus. Similar cases were described from other cities in U.S.A. They were, in fact, recurrences of typhus fever in patients who had previously suffered from attacks of the disease in Europe. We now know that the disease has been imported into the U.S.A. by these immigrants and infection has spread to the rat population by means of the rat-flea. The disease has become therefore an occupational one, found only in those persons who come into close contact with rats, and the problem of its control is the same as in plague. This type of typhus has now been found in many parts of the world including Europe, South America, Asia, South Africa, and Australia. It explains how typhus can be absent for centuries from a country and then suddenly break out in epidemic form when conditions are right.

Another interesting type of typhus fever is Rocky Mountain spotted fever, spread by an animal tick which is found on cattle, sheep, and dogs, which form a natural reservoir for the disease. It is contracted by persons living in the mountains in the spring months, and particularly by prospectors, miners, sheep herders, and cattlemen.

The eastern form occurs more in domestic animals—the horse, the cow, and the dog—and is seen more commonly in children.

Similar forms of tick-borne typhus fever occur in the Mediterranean (boutonneuse fever), in South Africa where they are spread by the dog tick, in India, Siberia, and Australia. This group includes Brazilian spotted fever, Kenya fever, North Queensland tick typhus, South African tick fever, Indian tick typhus, and Siberian tick typhus. As the various parts of the picture are being painted in, it is clear that wild rodents play an important part in maintaining reservoirs of infection, whilst domestic animals are important in the actual spread of disease to human beings.

The last group of these arthropod-borne fevers comprises those spread by the bite of small larval mites. The first to be described was Japanese river fever; it follows the bite of a mite found on the vole, and is common in many parts of Japan. Scrub typhus has been found in Malaya, Formosa, Indo-China,

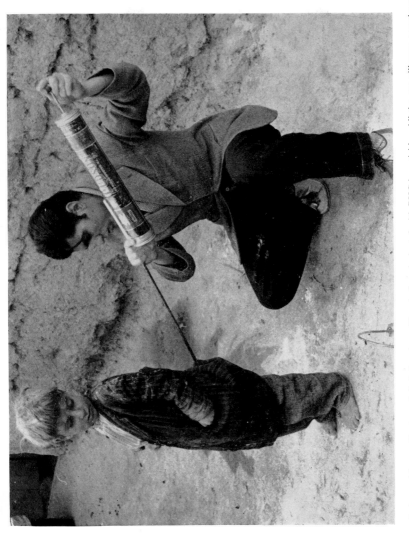

Fig. 4.—Arthropod-borne diseases. A little boy in a village in Iran is dusted with BHC insecticide. All the 400 villagers, together with their clothing and bedding, receive this treatment regularly to destroy typhus-carrying lice.

Burma, India, Java, Sumatra, New Guinea, and Northern Queensland. The rat acts as an intermediate host, and the larval mite bites man when he walks through the tall grass in which the mite lives.

During World War II there were many casualties from scrub typhus in the south-west Pacific and in China, India, and Burma. In fact, it was far more important than the classic louse-borne typhus. We were dealing with what was to us a new disease. Thus 6685 cases of scrub typhus were reported in U.S. Army personnel and only 64 cases of epidemic typhus in the same period.

The various mites live on wild rodents during the early stages of their life, but at one stage of their existence they are to be found on the soil and grasses. The disease then is seasonal and found only in those who walk through the scrub, such as explorers, prospectors, soldiers, and agricultural workers. The disease was controlled in the Allied armies by the wearing of protective clothing impregnated with insect-repellents (dimethyl phthallate). It required a high standard of discipline in the hot humid climate of Burma to get men to wear such clothing all the time, but it certainly paid dividends as the Allied armies quickly brought the disease under control. Not so in the Japanese, where there was an enormous incidence of the disease. It has been said that at one time 40 per cent of the Japanese army in Burma was immobilized by scrub typhus. This was due in part to the use of scrub typhus as a strategic weapon; the Allied armies kept out of the scrub as far as possible and so directed the course of the fighting that the Japanese were forced to operate in mite-infested areas; perhaps the first example of the use of biological warfare.

This story is similar to that of plague; in the normal course of events the disease occurs in those whose job brings them in close contact with these parasites. Today both typhus and plague are diseases of rural populations. It would appear that both originated in the rodent populations of central Asia.

For the first time in history it has been possible to control epidemic disease during a major war, and only because our armies had the best medical services ever, and because our generals had the good sense to recognize, in the words of Hans Zinsser (1935), that 'war is 75 per cent an engineering and sanitary problem and little less than 25 per cent a military one'.

When, however, there is no medical control of population then typhus will break out, as recent events in the Congo have shown, where there have been many cases of the disease following independence. The outbreak was finally brought under control by the emergency aid given by the United Nations and the World Health Organization. In 1961 and 1962 there were further outbreaks in Ethiopia.

CHAPTER V

WINGED DEATH

MALARIA

THIS story of the fight against killing diseases brings us now to the greatest of them all—malaria—a disease which has probably been responsible for killing more people in the world than any other single disease, to say nothing of the considerable amount of ill health and debility which it produces. The signs and symptoms of malaria are usually so characteristic that when they are described in ancient writings they can be easily detected as such. (*Fig.* 5.) We know, therefore, that malaria was widespread from the very earliest ages in the Mediterranean basin, India, and South China. The disease became common in Greece about 400 B.C. and it was certainly common in the Roman Empire where a goddess of the intermittent fevers, Dea Febris, was worshipped in an effort to control the disease. Some authorities believe that malaria was an important cause of the decline of both Greece and Rome. Sigerist, the medical historian, discussing the effect of malaria on Roman civilization remarked, 'the entire history of a landscape was determined by a single disease'. The disease was widespread throughout Europe, Asia, and Africa during the Middle Ages, but there is some doubt about the route which carried malaria to the New World. Some historians believe that the disease was carried by Columbus; others that it may have spread to the Americas eastwards from Asia. Today it is found mostly in tropical and subtropical countries, but it has been reported from as far north as Arkhangel'sk (Archangel) in the U.S.S.R. (64°N.) and as far south as Cordoba in Argentina. It has occurred at 9086 ft. above sea-level in Bolivia and 8500 ft. in Kenya. It was common until quite recently in Holland and Britain; the marshes round Hackney Wick had an unsavoury reputation for the ague, as it was called in the eighteenth century. Despite the fact that we have known the cause of malaria for over fifty years it still remains one of the most important health hazards in the world. It has been estimated that before present-day control methods were used over 300,000,000 suffered from the disease, that is 1 in 10 of the population of the world, and over 3,000,000 died annually. In this respect, therefore, it puts even plague and typhus in the shade. These latter act in an all-or-none manner, either the person is killed quickly or just as quickly recovers with rarely any permanent ill-effect. Not so malaria; usually the sufferer from this disease has it for life; it comes and goes, causing prolonged weakness, debility, and ill health. (*Fig.* 6.) In the areas where malaria is common, the whole life of the village is affected. A high percentage of the children born die from the disease, and those who reach adult life are permanently incapacitated by it. The men are lethargic and unable to till the land properly; consequently agriculture suffers and there is insufficient food. This aggravates the ill health, and the same thing occurs in the women, who are unable to stand the rigours of child-bearing, producing weak, sickly, anaemic infants, and so the vicious circle goes on. The harm done by this disease, then, is not to be measured in terms of death alone, but also in the vast amount of human misery which it produces. In 1911, Ronald Ross wrote the following: 'Malaria is the great enemy of the explorer, the missionary, the planter, the merchant, the soldier, the farmer, the administrator, the villager and the poor and has I believe modified the world's history by tending to render the whole of the tropics comparatively unsuitable for the full development of civilization.'

Hippocrates described how the intermittent fevers were associated with the swamplands and occurred most often during the warm months of summer. Many workers have tried to incriminate the mosquito, but it has always been difficult to explain why in some areas where they were plentiful there was no malaria. In 1880 a great step forward was the discovery by Alphonse Laveran of the specific organisms responsible. P. Manson described the various stages of the parasite in human blood and imbued a young army doctor with enthusiasm for research into the cause of the spread of malaria. This young doctor was Ronald Ross, who worked against official opposition and continued his search despite many failures. At Secunderabad, on 19 June, 1897, he discovered the parasite in the stomach of a mosquito which had been fed on a human sufferer from malaria, a patient named Husein Khan. In a further series of experiments he showed that mosquitoes were the carrying agents of the malaria parasite in birds. It was the Italian, G. B. Grassi, who first demonstrated the role in human malaria of the female anopheline mosquito. Now it became clear why others had failed. The malaria parasite will only develop in certain species of mosquitoes and it requires ten days for this development to take place after the mosquito has taken a meal of infected blood; during this time the parasites migrate from the stomach to the salivary glands and are then ready to be infected into a new victim when the mosquito takes a meal. Grassi now proceeded to show how this discovery could be used to prevent malaria. He worked at Capaccio, one of the most malarial regions in Italy, rendering ten houses mosquito-proof, and out of 112 workers sleeping in these houses only five developed malaria; in other workers the incidence was almost 100 per cent.

The most outstanding results were first obtained in the control of malaria by General W. C. Gorgas in Havana and Cuba between 1901 and 1904. The breeding places of the mosquito were destroyed, or if that was not possible they were sprayed with oil so that the larvae were suffocated. Adult mosquitoes were attacked in houses, and patients suffering from the disease were nursed under mosquito-nets to prevent the spread of infection. As a result of these efforts the incidence of malaria was reduced enormously. Unfortunately the same success was not met with elsewhere and in World

War I both the Allied and enemy armies were heavily attacked by malaria in the Mediterranean. Those who survived returned home to cause fresh outbreaks of the disease in Northern Europe. In Holland, malaria was just as common despite a great reduction in the number of mosquitoes, whilst in the southern United States there had been a great decrease in malaria, although there was no appreciable diminution in the number of mosquitoes. It was clear that the answer was not as simple as was first thought, and even as late as 1936 the problem of the control of malaria was still not completely solved.

In the years since the end of the Second World War there has been a remarkable reduction in some parts of the world, for example, in the United States of America, Western Europe, Brazil, Chile, British Guiana, Venezuela, Cuba, and Sardinia. It is still a serious menace, however, in many parts of South America, Asia Minor, South-east Europe, Africa, southern Asia, and the Western Pacific islands, despite widespread control activities. Many parts of the world are free from the particular kind of mosquito (the anopheles) which spreads the disease and so they are free from malaria. Such favoured places are the islands of the North and South Pacific and the Bahamas. In cold climates the disease only occurs occasionally; the conditions are not suitable for its spread, although the anopheles mosquito may be present.

The control of malaria demands a detailed knowledge of the mode of life of the mosquito responsible for the carriage of the disease. The habits of the species vary from locality to locality. Moreover, one species of mosquito concerned in the spread of malaria may have certain habits in one locality and yet have quite different habits in another. In one area it may prefer a shaded locality for breeding and the control will depend upon the cutting down of cover near breeding places, yet in another locality this action may have the reverse effect and encourage breeding. In order to understand the control of malaria in any locality it is first necessary to carry out detailed surveys of the area.

Although there are about 200 species of anopheline mosquitoes in the world only about 24 are of importance in the spread of malaria. The most dangerous are those which rest in dark corners during the day and come out to feed at night and so spread the disease from one member of the family to another. In some countries malaria may occur in the early winter when the mosquitoes seek the warmth of houses, although living away from human habitation during the summer. The female mosquito lives on human blood like the flea and the louse, but must have water in which to breed. Since mosquitoes do not usually fly more than one mile, the spread of malaria is limited to a radius of one mile from their breeding quarters.

Each species has its own preference in the matter of breeding sites, which are often very restricted. Most species prefer shallow, sunlit fresh water, but many prefer brackish or sea-water lagoons. Others prefer the dense shade of jungle swamps and some the margins of fast-running mountain streams (as in Greece). Quite small collections of water can be sufficient, as in old tin cans, wells, cisterns, or even in that held by growing plants.

The history of malaria shows that man himself has made the very conditions which are essential for the rapid multiplication of mosquitoes. (*Fig.* 7.) As in the case of plague and typhus man creates his own disease conditions. Thus in the colonization of the West, man's first efforts were directed at the clearing of forests, resulting in the exposure of lakes and ponds to the sunlight. Schemes for the production of water power and for the supply of drinking water result in the damming of streams and the production of lakes. Anyone who travels by train can see for himself the stagnant pits which remain when there have been excavations for embankments and the approaches to bridges. Even the getting of coal has produced large areas of stagnant lake and pond which are ideal for mosquito breeding. The most essential factor of all, of course, is man, and human habitations were built in large numbers wherever there were railways, coal-mines, and water undertakings. The presence of children has a pronounced effect upon the persistence of the disease, as they become carriers far more easily than adults; moreover, they remain carriers, that is, infective, for long periods, whilst to all outward appearances they may be perfectly fit. In the U.S.A. malaria followed the settlers westward and up the river valleys, and the same story has been seen in India, Malaya, South America, Africa, and Australia.

Malaria has appeared where the flooding of land for rice fields has been introduced as in Portugal, Spain, Italy, and the East, from India to China, and also following the development of fish culture in Siam.

However, when agriculture becomes intensive, extensive drainage of land takes place with the eventual elimination of breeding places. This resulted in its virtual disappearance before World War I in central Europe. After the end of this war malaria again appeared owing to the neglect of agriculture and the return of soldiers from infected areas, to disappear again as the people concentrated once more on agricultural drainage schemes.

In Trinidad malaria has become a problem since the growing of cocoa trees has been intensified. The local conditions so created have encouraged the breeding of the local malaria carrier.

Of course, war itself, particularly modern war, creates all sorts of opportunities for mosquito breeding near to living quarters. Trenches, bomb craters, airstrips, roads, and all the other semi-permanent construction of temporary camps form ideal places. Such operations created widespread malaria problems in the war against Japan in the Far East.

Ignorance of the breeding habits of mosquitoes is an important cause of outbreaks of malaria. In the Spanish-American war it was the usual custom to build the barracks for troops up in the hills away from the marshes and swamps of the coast region. But in Cuba this caused disaster because the only mosquito which could carry malaria bred in the mountain streams.

The modern habits of man have been responsible for other methods of transmission, not comparable to those of nature, however, in their severity or extent. Thus in the early days of blood transfusion, malaria was transmitted on several occasions from an infected donor.

45

Perhaps the most remarkable examples of man-produced malaria are those which have been described in drug addicts from the use of unclean syringes. Cases have occurred in New York and Cairo. However, cases due to drug addiction and blood transfusion are rare curiosities.

Climatic conditions have a marked effect upon malaria, a phenomenon first described by Hippocrates. Many mosquitoes will survive quite low temperatures, but the malaria parasite itself will not develop below 60° F., so that in temperate zones the spread of malaria is limited to the summer months. It is necessary to have some intermediate host or carrier who will keep the disease going during the winter. As far as we know, man is the only known host of this type to the malarial parasite. In the tropics continuous transmission of the disease occurs all the year round, because the temperature rarely falls below 60° F.

CONTROL

The best way of dealing with malaria is by complete eradication if possible or at least by bringing it under such control as to render it unimportant. Remarkable success has been achieved in the U.S.A. and tropical America in the elimination of malaria. This has been largely brought about by the simple but effective method of the widespread spraying of houses and buildings with DDT (*Fig.* 8). The success of this method is due to the fact that DDT is what is known as a residual insecticide; it leaves a fine film of powder on the walls and ceilings which remains effective for many months. The female mosquito is not infectious until 10–15 days after she has ingested blood from a sufferer of malaria. After a meal she will rest on some surface to digest her food and it is usually about two days before she will feed again. During that time any insect which alights on a surface impregnated with DDT picks up some of the powder, which is eventually lethal to it. Although it does not kill straightaway the net result is a marked decrease of mosquitoes and other insects in the habitation of the people. Moreover, the method is simple to use and relatively cheap to apply. Respraying only needs to be done at regular intervals and the powder itself, now that it is mass-produced, is cheap. At first the method was hailed with great enthusiasm, but more controlled studies showed that it did not always cause the eradication of the disease. There was a considerable decrease immediately after spraying but after several weeks the numbers again increased. From a practical point of view, however, it was shown that the method caused a marked diminution in the incidence of malaria.

In British Guiana and Venezuela the local vector has been entirely eliminated, and it is considered that residual spraying once every eighteen months will be sufficient to keep the area free from mosquitoes. In the Philippines, however, there is a totally different story. Residual spraying of houses has not affected the numbers of mosquitoes or the incidence of malaria, because the particular species of mosquito does not enter houses to any large extent and so remains unaffected by the spraying. In Jordan, spraying of houses has been ineffective because the mosquitoes live in caves and fissures in the rocks and much of the population is nomadic.

It is clear that residual spraying is not the answer to the eradication of malaria in those areas where the mosquitoes do not feed in houses to any appreciable extent, and there is some disturbing news that both flies and mosquitoes are developing resistance to DDT and other insecticides such as gammexane and dieldrin. In 1946 only one insect of public health importance was known to be resistant, but by the end of 1956 there were thirty-seven species known to be resistant to insecticides. On the north coast of Java, in Greece, and on the Persian Gulf DDT is no longer able to control the malaria vector, whilst resistance has been encountered in India near Delhi and in northern Nigeria; in Mississippi resistance to dieldrin has developed. In Florida, California, and parts of Central America the larvae of many kinds of mosquito are showing high degrees of resistance; in Trinidad, for example, the larvae of the 'tiger' mosquito, *Aëdes aegyptii*, are now a thousand times more resistant than normal laboratory-bred strains.

There are reports, too, of recent outbreaks of malaria in Greek villages where the disease had been eliminated by DDT spraying; the local population have lost their immunity and the mosquitoes are becoming resistant. Apparently under continuous spraying, it takes six or seven years for malaria-carrying mosquitoes to develop resistance. There is a great need therefore for effective eradication within five years; if, on the other hand, the programme is carried out in a half-hearted fashion, spraying must go on indefinitely. For this reason, during the last ten years the tendency has been to concentrate on eradication of malaria instead of control. In addition to residual spraying it is necessary to attack the breeding areas of the 'wild' mosquitoes. Moreover, a country can easily be reinfected from adjacent 'uncontrolled' areas; concentrated action on a global front is therefore necessary.

An East Asia Conference on Malaria was held in 1953 in Bangkok to review the results of the post-war period. A remarkable improvement in health was apparent. There was a greater demand for land where formerly there had been apathy, and there was better school attendance. Similar reports were received from most of the Asiatic countries. The removal of this drain on public energy of the people of Asia must have an enormous effect upon the economics of these countries, particularly in the agricultural field. The increased expectation of life is already greatly affecting the population; the birth-rate still remains high, but death-rates are falling rapidly, causing large increases in the population and producing a more vigorous and virile people. Out of 23 South-east Asia countries with a total population of 659,000,000, one-quarter live in malarious areas; 30 per cent were protected against malaria in 1953. In Ceylon where 3,000,000 people—one-third of the population—live in highly malarious areas, the disease has been almost eradicated. India, with 200,000,000 persons exposed to infection, plans to clear infection from the country within the next ten years. In Africa the problem is more complex, and experimental control centres are testing the various methods. By the end of 1955, however, 14,000,000 out of the 116,000,000 at risk had been protected by spraying. In Brazil there has been remarkable success in finally eliminating the malaria carrier introduced into that country from Africa.

Extensive attempts have been made to eradicate malaria from the island of Sardinia (so far the cost has been over £4,000,000), and in Corsica, as a result of similar efforts, there have been no primary cases reported since 1953 and no deaths.

The world distribution is certain to show considerable changes in the next few years as a result of the widespread malaria control programmes which are being organized in many countries with the help of the World Health Organization.

It seems certain that in some areas special defensive measures are necessary. This is especially so in wartime when soldiers may be exposed to exceptional risks, or where the population is largely nomadic.

Other measures for defence include the use of screens and nets in houses, particularly at night, the avoidance of danger spots at night, such as native villages, and the use of protective clothing and insect repellents. The regular taking of antimalarial drugs in small amounts can also protect against infection even from bites by an infected mosquito. (*Fig.* 9.) Such drugs (for example, pyrimethamine) can be supplied in table salt.

The pre-war insect repellents, such as oil of citronella, have fallen into disuse because they were largely ineffective. During World War II great stimulus was given to the study of insect repellents because of the danger from insect-borne disease. Research into the discovery of new and more effective insecticides was intensified and as a result some very efficient ones were discovered, namely, methyl phthallate, dibutyl phthallate, indalone, and Rutgers 612. A mixture known as 6-2-2 is a most effective combination and consists of six parts of dimethyl phthallate, two parts of indalone, and two parts of Rutgers 612. This will protect for two or more hours, even when the person is sweating. It can be smeared on the skin and used in impregnated clothing.

Several new drugs have been discovered for the treatment of the disease recently, but still the most important principle is to prevent mosquitoes from feeding on infected cases, as man is the only vertebrate host in which the parasite can develop. Before 1946 malaria used to kill about 1,000,000 people every year and there were 100,000,000 cases. By spending £10,000,000 a year for five years malaria could be eradicated altogether from the sub-continent of India.

What an enormous bill would be saved, not only in terms of cash, but what is much more important, in terms of human health and happiness! Although the cost of eliminating malaria may involve the spending of large sums of money, the cost per head is low; for example, it costs 7d. per head per year for two sprayings. In the words of Paul Russell (1952) (W.H.O. consultant on malaria): 'Whereas formerly many countries could not afford to control malaria now they cannot afford not to eradicate it.' (*Fig.* 10.) By 1958 about one-third of people exposed to the disease had been protected. It is confidently expected that malaria will be eliminated from Europe within the next few years. Unfortunately when the disease becomes rare governments are unwilling to spend large sums of money on its final eradication. The final

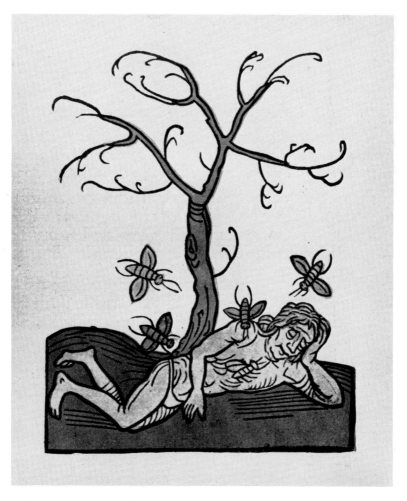

Fig. 5.—Malaria. *Hortus Sanitatis,* 1491. Mosquitoes shown in a fifteenth-century book on natural history.

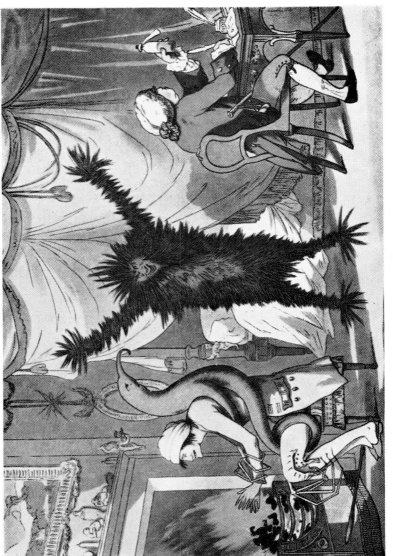

Fig. 6.—The chill and fever of malaria as imagined by Rowlandson (1756–1827).

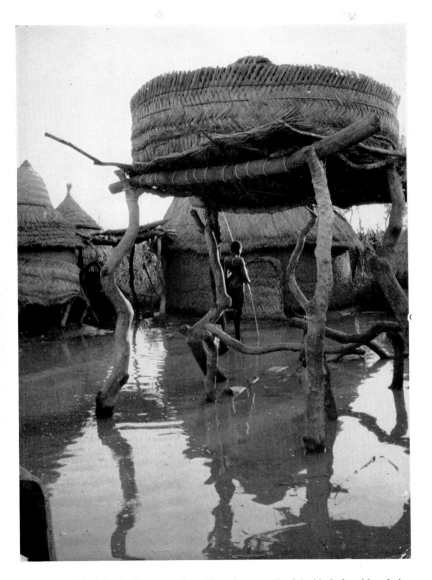

Fig. 7.—Malaria in the Cameroon Republic. An example of the kind of problem facing the malariologist. The houses of the Banana tribesmen shown here are built on stilts above a swamp, ideal breeding place for mosquitoes.

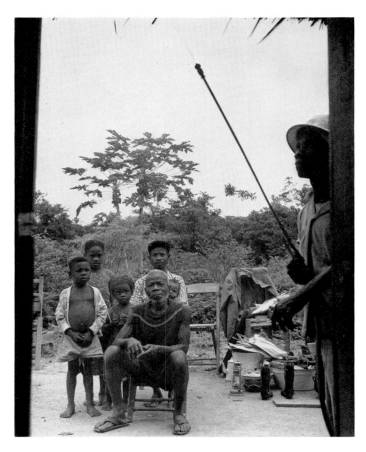

Fig. 8.—Malaria in Liberia. In the village of Gehtar, Liberia, the village chief and his family look on while the W.H.O. team sprays their house with DDT.

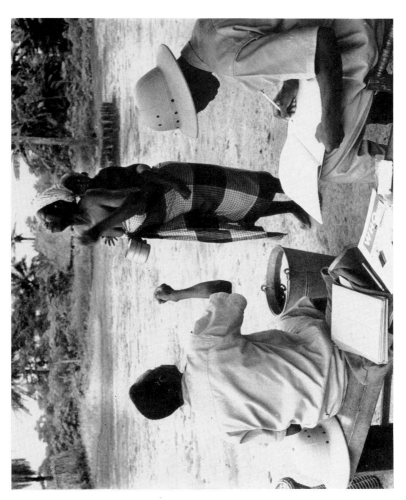

Fig. 9.—Malaria in Liberia. In the village of Gehtar, Liberia, anti-malaria tablets are distributed which children and grown-ups swallow with enthusiasm.

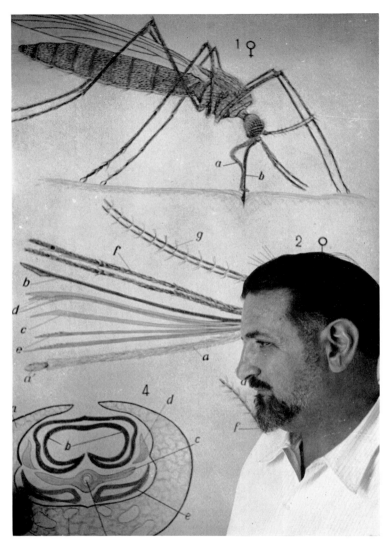

Fig. 10.—'Here's the dawn, Dr. Malaria.' Dr. Luigi Mara has spent the last four years in a relentless mosquito hunt all across malaria-ridden Kurdistan in Iraq. He has managed to win the confidence of the Kurds, traditionally one of the most hostile peoples in the world, and is known among them as 'Dr. Malaria'. For the last fifteen years, 'Dr. Malaria' has led a nomadic life himself, going 'on his rounds' in Eritrea, India, Switzerland, Liberia, Sierra Leone, Gambia, the Sudan and Iraq—first on behalf of the Health Department of Italy and more recently as a malariologist of the World Health Organization. It was four years ago that Iraq, worried because her economic development was threatened by malaria, applied to W.H.O. for help. And it was to 'Dr. Malaria' that there was entrusted the most seriously threatened part of the country, Kurdistan.

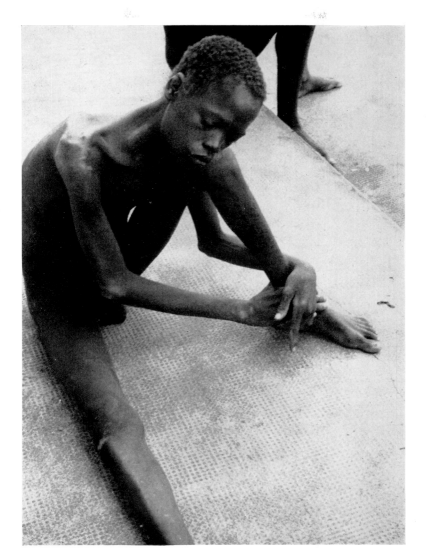

Fig. 11.—Victims of sleeping sickness in an institution in the Cameroon Republic. From the southern edge of the Sahara desert to Zululand in the Union of South Africa, the peoples of tropical Africa are afflicted by a number of diseases carried by tsetse flies. Tsetse-fly control in Bechuanaland is one of the W.H.O.-assisted projects in the African regions.

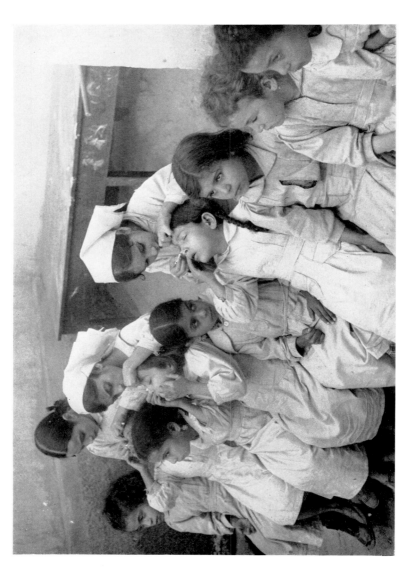

Fig. 12.—Trachoma in Egypt. Members of the health committee apply antibiotic ointment to their fellow pupils at a girls' school at Sindion.

stages require the setting up of special 'surveillance teams' with the object of discovering the remaining few cases and bringing them under effective treatment. The application of insecticides can then be discontinued, and eradication is declared, when, despite intensive search, no indigenous cases have occurred for three consecutive years. If eradication can be declared in all countries of the world then the disease should never occur again, even though mosquitoes increase, because the parasites have been eliminated from all human population, and since the mosquito only carries the parasite for a short time it cannot act as a reservoir. All this of course requires large sums of money and co-operation on an international scale.

YELLOW JACK

The story of the mosquito would not be complete unless it included an account of yellow fever and the dramatic events which led to the discovery of the cause of this fatal disease.

The first outbreak that can be identified as yellow fever occurred in Yucatan in 1648, but whether it originated in Africa or America is not known. Up to the end of the nineteenth century it was common in the Caribbean islands and the coastal regions of North, Central, and South America. Yellow Jack, as it was known in the days of sail, was one of the most dreaded of the diseases of the Atlantic trade routes; probably the legend of the Flying Dutchman, as described by Sir Walter Scott, was inspired by stories of this disease, which could wipe out whole ships' companies.

The disease was particularly common in the ships trading with West African ports, especially in the Bight of Benin, which had an unsavoury reputation, particularly for those who slept on land. For this reason ships used to anchor some distance from the shore and in so doing, although they did not know the reason, avoided yellow fever. In *Roderick Random* there is a description of an appalling outbreak of yellow fever in the British Navy at Cartagena in 1740, due to neglecting this precaution.

There was an outbreak of yellow fever in Philadelphia in 1793. The fever first appeared in July near the docks. As it spread towards the end of August Mathew Carey described how 'the streets and roads leading from the city were crowded with families flying in every direction for safety to the country', strangely reminiscent of the Plague of London. Oliver Wolcott, Secretary of the Treasury, wrote: 'business is in a great measure abandoned; the true character of man is disclosed, and he shows himself a weak, timid, desponding and selfish being.'

The College of Physicians met and offered advice. They suggested isolation of cases, the marking of doors and windows where the sick lay, cleaning the streets, and the setting-up of special hospitals. The tolling of bells was prohibited. The burning of gunpowder and the smoking of tobacco were recommended as preventive measures. Even women and children had cigars in their mouths; others relied on garlic and chewed it the whole day. The panic spread to New York and the militia was brought out to control the

4

passage of travellers. These efforts are strangely reminiscent of the recommendations made in Exeter for the control of cholera. With the coming of the cold weather the number of cases decreased. Out of a population of 50,000 one-third left the city, and of the remaining 34,000, 4000 died between August and November from yellow fever. This disease, then, is similar in many respects to plague, typhus, and cholera, breaking out with explosive violence, with many deaths and ensuing panic, and then quite suddenly disappearing. No wonder that many thought of these outbreaks of pestilence as visitations from God.

We know that they were due to various factors, such as climatic conditions, which affected the breeding cycle of the intermediate hosts or made it difficult for the organism to survive, or in other cases to the exhaustion of a sufficiency of susceptible persons. In a remarkable series of experiments with mice it has been shown that the rise and fall of epidemics in human populations can be reproduced in animal experiments under controlled laboratory conditions. In any population at a given time there will be some more susceptible than others to any particular disease. If it is a new disease there will be relatively little immunity and the disease will sweep through the herd, attacking a high percentage; many will die but others will survive, having gained an added immunity as a result of contact with the disease. After a few months there will no longer be any susceptible people left and the disease will disappear as quickly as it came. For several years the community will enjoy a freedom from attack until gradually a young susceptible population is built up again from new births, and then when a certain level is reached, the community will be ripe for an epidemic which will only occur when the necessary conditions prevail. In this way do the rise and fall of epidemics occur, depending in their frequency and severity on a whole host of things such as climate, presence of suitable vectors and intermediate hosts, the virulence and dosage of the infection, opportunities for its introduction from centres where it is already present, and the percentage of susceptible persons in the community.

Yellow fever had much to do with the defeat of the French in Haiti in 1803, most of the negroes being immune whilst the French suffered a high mortality. There were frequent outbreaks at Gibraltar, for example in 1804 and 1828, and in Spain and Cuba.

In 1878 yellow fever followed a similar pattern in the Mississippi valley. In July a new tow-boat, the *John D. Porter*, set out for Pittsburg. When she reached her destination 23 men had died, and she had transmitted the disease through a thousand miles of river, until 20,000 people had died and 100,000 people had caught the disease. New Orleans, Vicksburg, and Memphis suffered the most. Refugees crowded the trains to the north and trade was brought to a standstill. Money was raised in the north to provide for the sick and a special commission of the American Public Health Association was appointed to investigate the cause. Many people still thought that it could arise spontaneously from filth.

The United Kingdom did not escape and several cases were recorded from Swansea in 1865, caused by infection from a ship which had called in Cuba.

The first suggestion that yellow fever might be spread by mosquitoes was made by Dr. J. C. Nott, of Mobile, Alabama, in 1848, but the first really serious proponent of this theory was Dr. Carlos Finlay in Havana in 1881. Nobody felt very convinced, until the matter was proved by Dr. Walter Reed, who was sent to Cuba as president of a commission to study the disease. The first successful experiment was carried out on a member of the commission, Dr. James Carroll, on 27 August, 1900; he allowed himself to be bitten by a mosquito which had previously fed upon 4 yellow fever patients. He was taken ill four days later and for three days he was extremely ill. Dr. J. W. Lazear contracted the disease from an accidental bite and died a week later. Nevertheless, convincing proof of the method of spread required an adequate number of human volunteers and a further series of experiments. There was no dearth of volunteer subjects from the United States Army, their only stipulation being that they should receive no monetary gain. Camp Lazear was set up for the prime purpose of testing the method of spread of yellow fever by bringing susceptible persons into contact with yellow fever patients. Thus it was shown that susceptible persons living in close contact with the disease escaped infection so long as they were protected from the bites of the mosquito. In September, 1900, Dr. Reed produced yellow fever in 3 volunteers who allowed themselves to be bitten by mosquitoes which had previously fed on patients ill with the disease. On 15 October, 1901, he injected filtered serum from an experimentally infected patient into 3 human volunteers; 2 of these developed yellow fever. These experiments proved that the organism which caused yellow fever could pass through a fine filter; it was, in fact, called an ultra-filterable or ultra-microscopic virus. This was the first time that a filterable virus had been proved to be the cause of a specific human disease. These experimenters could only use human volunteers for this research as no experimental animal was known at that time which was susceptible to the disease. The same difficulties beset research workers in malaria. As we shall see in later chapters, there have been many examples since of medical research which could only be carried out in this way, but there have been few examples of men who have willingly allowed themselves to be given a deadly disease, knowing that there was a good chance of dying from it. Many scientists working with yellow fever died as a result of their experiments. The list includes, in addition to Dr. J. W. Lazear: Dr. Howard B. Cross, died 1921, aged 33 years; Dr. Adrian Stokes, died 1927, aged 40 years; Dr. Hideyo Noguchi, died 1928, aged 52 years; Dr. Paul A. Lewis, died 1929, aged 50 years; Dr. William A. Young, died 1929, aged 40 years; Dr. Theodore B. Hayne, died 1930, aged 32 years. In Johns Hopkins Hospital, Baltimore, there is a memorial tablet to Dr. Lazear inscribed with the following words: 'With more than the courage of the soldier, he risked and lost his life to show how a fearful pestilence is communicated and how its ravages may be prevented.'

General Gorgas applied the acquired knowledge in Havana where he was able in 1901 to eradicate yellow fever and to reduce the incidence of malaria by applying antimosquito measures. This led to the elimination of yellow fever from Panama and it was only then that it was possible to cut the Panama Canal. Previous attempts under the Frenchman, de Lesseps, had failed because of the enormous mortality from the disease. Success had been achieved in a remarkably short space of time.

In 1928 a great advance was made when it was found that the Indian monkey was highly susceptible and could be used as an experimental animal. This greatly facilitated experimental research. An interesting story was told by Dr. Andrew Balfour in 1914. He records how, when crossing on a boat to the West Indies, he met a Mrs. Randolph Rust, long resident in Trinidad. She informed him that the old negroes always knew when there was going to be an outbreak of yellow fever because the red howler monkeys were found dead in large numbers in the woods. These stories had been ignored by earlier investigators. A further step forward took place in 1930 when the virus was cultivated by inoculation into the brain of mice. This resulted in the discovery of a test for the presence of immunity to yellow fever, the mouse protection test. In this way it has been possible to map out the areas of the world where yellow fever occurs. Extension of this work resulted in the production of a vaccine which afforded a high degree of protection.

During World War II an enormous outbreak of the jungle type of yellow fever broke out in 1940 in the Nuba mountains in the south-west of the Sudan, there being 30,000 recorded cases. This stimulated Kenya to undertake a widespread attack on the insect vectors of the disease. These outbreaks are of particular importance because they bring the disease nearer to India where, so far, the disease has not occurred. In 1946 there was an epidemic of urban yellow fever in southern Nigeria.

The geographical distribution of yellow fever has been accurately mapped out by the mouse protection test.

Many parts of Brazil have now been rendered free from the disease and so do not come under the endemic area as defined in quarantine regulations. The main areas are now in Central Africa between 15° N. parallel of latitude to 10° S. and in South America between 5° N. and 20° S.

The use of the special test has thrown an entirely new light on the spread of the disease. As first described in human populations it occurred in urban communities and was spread by a domestic mosquito which entered houses freely. Control of this mosquito eliminated the disease from most of the towns and cities where it occurred. It has now become primarily a disease of animals living in the jungle and cases of so-called rural yellow fever are seen in men who work in the forest by day and return home at night. The rest of the family are not infected unless the tiger mosquito is present. These men are usually woodcutters and the particular mosquitoes responsible live in the forest trees. They are day-feeding and have acquired their infection from forest monkeys.

In some areas, for example Ecuador, it was a great puzzle to know how these men became infected because there seemed to be very few mosquitoes at ground level, most of them living in the tops of the trees where they could feed on monkey blood, until one day a doctor working in the forest watched a woodman cutting down a tall tree. It fell to the ground with a crash and disturbed large numbers of mosquitoes of the genus *Haemagogus* and others, which immediately proceeded to bite the men viciously. This explained why it was found impossible in many areas to entirely eliminate the disease. It is kept going in monkeys and other animals and spread from animal to animal by mosquitoes which frequent the tree-tops. Only when man interferes with the jungle and begins to cut down trees is it spread to him. He can in turn spread it to other humans if the appropriate insect vector is present.

Jungle fever is especially common in the headwaters of the Amazon and Orinoco rivers. Wherever there are outposts of civilization in the jungle, there has the disease flared up. The deaths of many of the early Spanish explorers up the Amazon must have been due to this.

In Africa, the method of spread is somewhat different. The reservoir of infection is still found in the monkey, but it is spread to domestic mosquitoes when marauding monkeys play around human habitations. These mosquitoes can then infect human beings. Once more, then, we can see how the spread of the disease is determined by the personal habits of various species of insects.

The yellow fever of cities and in areas spread by the trade routes has been virtually eliminated, and as in typhus and plague the disease is now found in rural areas where it occurs in people whose occupations carry them into forests. This explains why it occurs much more frequently in men than in women and children. This is in marked contrast to urban or domestic yellow fever which attacks women and children as often as the adult male. Outbreaks of jungle yellow fever are preceded by widespread mortality in monkeys, a fact, as already mentioned, observed many years ago by the negroes of Trinidad.

There has been much controversy over the origin of yellow fever. Was it brought from West Africa to South and Central America by the old slave traders ? There is good reason to believe that the tiger mosquito (*Aëdes aegyptii* or *Stegomyia fasciata*), a highly domesticated species which can live and multiply on board ship, first came from West Africa and so probably brought yellow fever to the New World.

One question which is very difficult to answer is why has yellow fever never been imported into India ? There are large populations of susceptible human beings and monkeys are abundant. The *Rhesus* monkey of India is one of the most susceptible to the disease. The tiger mosquito is widely distributed. Moreover, the climatic factors are ideal and the habits of the people especially favourable for contact with mosquitoes. Malaria, as we have seen, is one of the greatest scourges.

Today very extensive precautions are taken to prevent the entrance of yellow fever into India by ship and particularly by air. There is, for example, regular spraying of the inside of aircraft with insecticidal sprays, such as DDT, and strict regulations regarding inoculation and quarantine, before entry is allowed. For some unknown reason yellow fever has always been rare on the East African coast and so there was not much chance of the spread by the direct sea route. The longer route from West Africa around the Cape probably was so long and the climatic conditions were so varied (i.e., low temperatures) that the infection could not survive. The sea voyage West Africa to Central and South America was shorter and took place in tropical heat all the time and so favoured the persistence of the infection.

Yellow fever has occurred in the Sudan and Kenya, but for some reason has never spread down to the Malabar coast which is not far away. Once there it could have been easily transported by the Arab dhows trading with India. The answer to this mystery has yet to be found, but whatever it is, it must have saved many millions of lives in that vastly populated country. What seemingly small events determine the fate of the peoples of the world and of generations as yet unborn!

Experimentally there are a number of animals which can be infected apart from monkeys, but the only other animal which shows a similar type of disease to that in man is the hedgehog.

As in the case of cholera and small-pox the treatment of this disease is virtually the same as it was fifty years ago. The new antibiotics have no action on the virus.

Preventive measures are therefore particularly important. The mosquito can be eradicated by the provision of piped water supplies and the destruction of breeding places. This has been particularly successful in large areas of Brazil. Excellent results have been obtained by adding DDT to the bilge water and water containers of boats on the Amazon, and the towns of Iquique and Antofagasta in Chile have actually added DDT 1 part per million to the drinking water. But non-domestic mosquitoes cannot be controlled in this way. Inoculation is the best means of protection in rural areas where eradication of mosquitoes is more difficult. In French Equatorial Africa 16,000,000 inhabitants have been immunized with a yellow fever vaccine.

Under international sanitary agreements all persons leaving by air areas declared as yellow fever zones must carry a certificate of immunization declaring that they have been inoculated at least ten days and not longer than four years before the date of flying. Mosquito control round airfields is of the greatest importance. Before leaving the subject of yellow fever, mention should be made of the remarkable efforts which have been made to control the disease by the Rockefeller Foundation, which has spent over £4,000,000 on research between 1916 and 1949 and up to 1948 had shipped 30,000,000 doses of vaccine. In Brazil, drastic steps have been taken to investigate the incidence of the disease and keep track of its spread. This can be very difficult as there are many cases occurring between epidemics which are not easy to diagnose.

Indeed, yellow fever may continue silently in a native population for long periods, and deaths are put down to other diseases, such as malaria, enteric fever, etc. In order to overcome this the Brazilian Government organized a scheme for the collection of specimens of liver from persons who had died of fever. By examination of the specimen it was possible to say whether or not the disease was yellow fever. There was considerable opposition to this and some simple means of taking a liver specimen had to be devised. Dr. E. R. Rickard designed an instrument which could take a small plug of liver without causing any external disfigurement to the body apart from a small puncture hole. This was called a viscerotome. This scheme grew so rapidly that by the end of 1949 nearly half a million liver specimens had been examined and a large area of Brazil was covered by the service, which had 1349 posts functioning. Serious attempts to carry out similar surveys in West Africa have been quite futile because of racial taboos.

The amount of money, time, and effort which has been expended on the control of yellow fever is probably greater than for any other disease, but complete success is still not assured. (*See* Strode (1951) for a full account of yellow fever.)

We have still not exhausted the number of diseases spread by mosquitoes; in recent years a number of new virus diseases of the brain have been described from all parts of the world. Many of these are spread by the bite of the mosquito from reservoirs of infection in animals and birds. Apparently these viruses can be modified for transmission also by mites and ticks. Flies are also important carriers of disease particularly African sleeping sickness, river blindness, trachoma, and dysentery.

SLEEPING SICKNESS
(Trypanosomiasis)

The African sleeping sickness has a wide distribution in tropical Africa, particularly along the Congo river. Infection is spread from infected animals, either wild or domestic, by the bite of the tsetse fly; this, like the bite of the vampire bat in the spread of rabies, may be so painless that the victim is quite unaware of the attack. In the dense woods flies will follow a potential blood-meal for miles, so that when the weary traveller rests he is easily and quietly attacked.

An area half as large again as Australia, from the Sahara to Zululand, is affected by the deadly fly. In these regions men as well as cattle are attacked by the disease and as a result the whole economy of Africa is affected. Cattle cannot be reared, thus depriving the African of much-needed animal protein. Not only this, agricultural activities suffer from lack of draught animals and their manure. These vast areas, 4,500,000 square miles in extent, are forsaken by the African and he crowds into the small areas free from tsetse flies; here the land is overworked and overstocked.

The most useful form of control is by regulated burning of the breeding grounds of the fly, but unfortunately only small areas at a time can be treated and unless they are properly developed for agriculture, the cover soon grows up again and the flies once more invade the area from those still unreclaimed.

The World Health Organization is also helping to control sleeping sickness by carrying out periodic surveys and schemes for mass treatment. (*Fig.* 11.) The French and Belgian authorities have used the drug pentamidine on a large scale to prevent infection, in the same way that mepacrine has been used to prevent malaria. These results have borne fruit; before the war something like one-tenth of the people of Nigeria were infected; today the infection rate is down to 1–300. The answer lies with the African himself; he can break

55

the vicious circle of sleeping sickness and under-nourishment, if he will 'occupy productively the vast empty spaces of Africa'.

RIVER BLINDNESS
(Onchocerciasis)

The recent independence of Nigeria should serve to remind us that nearly half a million people in the West African countries of the Commonwealth are blind. Most of these cases are due to infestation with a small worm transmitted by a certain river breeding fly. The disease, known as river blindness, is common in many parts of Africa and Central America causing, in addition to blindness, lethargy and abortion, which in turn lead to poverty and depopulation.

Treatment is not very effective; the greatest hope of lifting the scourge from Africa lies in control of the fly responsible for spreading the disease. Complete success has been achieved in eradicating this fly from certain parts of Kenya by spraying DDT from aeroplanes and by clearing the bush where flies breed. Adequate control will depend upon an accurate knowledge of fly breeding habits.

TRACHOMA

Before leaving this subject, let us consider for a moment a very common cause of blindness in the world today and known for thousands of years; this is trachoma. The spread of trachoma, like malaria and plague, can be traced back in history because it has such characteristic signs which can be recognized from the earliest writings on the subject. The most ancient medical treatise known is the Ebers Papyrus from Thebes. It dates from 1500 B.C. and was written a thousand years before the time of Hippocrates. It describes the typical symptoms of an eye disease which the Egyptians treated with copper. This must have been trachoma, which is still treated by copper sulphate today. In the days of the Pharaohs, however, Egypt was a country with high standards of cleanliness, and eye disease was not very common. It was well known in Greek and Roman times and was described in Biblical texts. It was probably common fifty centuries before Christ. This led Charles Nicole to describe it as 'one of the most widespread diseases in the world and probably one of the oldest'.

In the nineteenth century, the term 'Aegyptia ophthalmia' was used to describe a very common virulent infection of the eye, common in Egypt and the Middle East. French and British troops contracted the infection and it spread to the British Isles and the New World.

It is always a fascinating problem to try to discover where a disease first originated and a knowledge of ethnology can help us in this type of study. There is some evidence that the origin of trachoma may have been in the steppes of Central Asia. The peoples of Finnish and Mongol descent have been more susceptible to the disease than their neighbours. Thus the Finns, Estonians, the people of northern Siberia, and the Magyars have in the past experienced epidemics of this disease and the same applies to the people of

Mongol descent, the Tartars, Kalmuks, Chinese, and Japanese. On the other hand, the Slavs, Swedes, Danes, Norwegians, British, and Teutons are all relatively immune. The large-scale migrations of history may have been responsible for spasmodic trachoma in the same way that plague and typhus have been spread. The Crusades, the conquests of Islam, the Mongol invasions, the Napoleonic wars, and the civil war in Russia have all caused recrudescences of the infection in susceptible races, which have produced islets of infection within a sea of immune races around them.

The Arabs are very susceptible to the disease and wherever they have spread to colonize the world, so have they taken trachoma with them. It is now widespread on the coasts of Spain and North Africa where the Arabs settled for 700 years and inter-married with the native population. They even spread infection as far as Java and the Sunda Islands in the Indian Ocean.

Before the Tartar invasion of Russia in the thirteenth century, trachoma had been present only in the Finnish races living in the Volga basin, but the Tartar invasion spread infection to Kazan, Astrakhan, and the Crimea.

The importance of wars in the spread of trachoma can be seen today in Greece. The highest incidence is found in the Peloponnese which was occupied by Egyptian troops in the Greek War of Independence (1821–7). It is also very high in the island of Zante where many of the inhabitants of the Peloponnese fled during the war, living in overcrowded and wretched conditions. But in parts of Greece where there have not been these large-scale movements of populations the incidence of the disease is definitely much lower.

Some parts of the world have been invaded in recent years because of economic reasons; thus in 1930 it became common in the Belgian Congo when the railway line linked up the country with Mozambique, where the disease was prevalent. Like so many other diseases, trachoma flourishes where living standards are low, where there is poor personal hygiene, and malnutrition. In such conditions flies are very common and by their habits spread the infection from case to case, not only of trachoma but also of intestinal diseases, like dysentery.

This latter disease can be prevented by improving living standards and destroying flies. Instruction in personal hygiene is very important. Trachoma can be cured with sulphonamides or antibiotics if it is caught in the early stage, but the chief problem in many of these countries is bringing adequate treatment to the sufferer, because of lack of health services. (*Fig.* 12.)

Before concluding this chapter on mosquitoes and flies we must repeat a warning which has already been voiced in relation to the control of fleas and lice—all over the world vectors of disease are becoming resistant to DDT and other insecticides. In Trinidad the yellow fever mosquito is now highly resistant and in all countries where insecticides have been used on any scale it is now impossible to control flies by this means. The search for new weapons of attack continues in the never-ending struggle to be always one step ahead of the enemy. We shall now consider a group of diseases which are spread by direct contact from person to person, and which should serve to remind us that 'the greatest pathogen of man is man himself'.

CHAPTER VI

THE GREATEST PATHOGEN OF MAN IS MAN HIMSELF

In the Middle Ages there were three great disfiguring diseases all spread by personal contact—small-pox, the great pox (or syphilis), and leprosy. Their ravages are depicted in many of the paintings and sculptures of the times. The destruction of skin and other tissue produced the most hideous effects on the face, and many a sufferer shunned society and suffered the agonies of the social outcast as a result.

One of the worst oaths a man could utter in those days was 'The pox upon you!' Today it has disappeared from our language because it has lost its meaning. For various reasons the three horror diseases have almost disappeared, certainly in the form that our ancestors knew them. They still produce their ghastly effects in certain parts of the world, but there is sufficient knowledge to bring them under control in those countries where they occur. The main need is for sufficient technical and financial aid. However, widespread ignorance hampers the work of controlling them.

SMALL-POX

One of the earliest accounts of small-pox was written in China in 1122 B.C. and the disease was well known in ancient India. It has occurred for many centuries in central Africa and was especially common during the Middle Ages in Europe and the Middle East. The Crusades caused a widespread dissemination of the disease in Europe. It was introduced into the Americas by the Spaniards and 3,500,000 people in Mexico died in a short time. It has been stated that small-pox was responsible for killing half the North American Indians when the disease first became rampant. They had little immunity and died like flies. The African-slave trade kept small-pox alive in North America. In Iceland in 1707 out of a population of 50,000, 18,000 died within the year. Up to the end of the nineteenth century small-pox was usually an extremely virulent disease with a high mortality, a great deal depending on the numbers who had been attacked before, an attack of the disease conferring a very high degree of immunity, but in a population which was highly susceptible to the disease the mortality would be as high as 40–50 per cent. Many of those who recovered were often disfigured for life by the hideous pock marks; others were left blind or affected mentally. The virulent form of small-pox is still prevalent in India, China, and Mexico. At the beginning of the twentieth century a milder form of small-pox appeared due to the prevalence of vaccination. As we shall see later, outbreaks occur in

England from time to time, usually due to the importation of cases from India, which are characterized by a high mortality.

The disease is spread mainly by personal contact; the secretions from nose and mouth and the skin lesions are all highly infective. Transmission has been reported from contaminated bed-clothes, by dust from a patient's room, and from infected cotton; the infecting organism is known to be a virus.

Geddes Smith tells the story of the small island of St. Kilda which was attacked by small-pox in 1724. Sheep-shearers who left the main island to visit a smaller island for the sheep-shearing were marooned for several months by storms. On their return all but a few of the adults left on the main island had died from small-pox. A community which has not experienced a disease for many years is highly susceptible to it. Thus measles killed about 25 per cent of the population of the Sandwich Islands in 1775, and in both World Wars it was a commonplace to see men from the Hebrides coming to Glasgow for the first time struck down by a severe attack of measles; it was a new disease to them and they had no resistance.

THE STORY OF VACCINATION*

Our story begins with Lady Mary Wortley Montagu. As the precocious Lady Mary Pierrepont, she eloped at the age of 19 years with a Mr. Wortley Montagu, who became Ambassador to Turkey and lived in Constantinople. Her life was affected by her marriage to a man she did not love and she lost her beauty through small-pox. She was a firm friend of King George I. She had numerous love affairs, including one with Alexander Pope, who had fallen in love with her; unfortunately he was later spurned and from writing some of the loveliest poetry about her, he turned to penning some of the nastiest literature ever written. He accused her of lesbianism and of having venereal disease amongst other unfortunate things. His lines written about her are famous:—

> From furious Sappho scarce a milder fate,
> Pox'd by her love, or libell'd by her hate.

Lady Mary was one of our great natural historians, taking an active interest in everything around her and making shrewd observations in the letters she wrote home. She loved the East and its ways and ventured into the bazaar and the Great Mosque of Solomon the First in her search for information. In one letter written in April, 1717, she described the Turkish practice of 'engrafting to prevent smallpox'.

An old woman would perform the 'operation' by scratching the 'venom' (small-pox) into the child's skin; a week later there developed a temperature and a pustular rash, leaving behind scars known as pocks. Lady Mary had her own children 'engrafted' and on her return to England persuaded Princess Caroline of Wales to use the method in the Royal nursery. For fifty years it was the standard method for the control of small-pox. It was a very bad method because it was highly contagious, although rarely fatal in

---

* From the Latin *vacca*, a cow.

the person inoculated. It endangered the community because it kept the disease alive by spreading small-pox from case to case. That it was used at all is an indication of the widespread prevalence of the disease. Most families felt that they were going to get the disease anyway so the children might as well have it when they were young and get it over with.

The importance of the discovery, however, was in the fact that at last someone was prepared to experiment with methods of inoculation to try to prevent infectious disease, and was the forerunner of much experimental work which achieved its greatest success in the control of diphtheria by immunization. In 1774, nearly sixty years after Lady Mary's letter had been written, a Dorset farmer called Benjamin Jesty performed the first vaccination; with a needle he scratched material from cow-pox, a disease of cows, into the skin of his wife and two children. He followed this with an engrafting of small-pox material and showed that they did not catch the disease. Unfortunately, Benjamin Jesty was not a medical man and he did not record the observations which led to his action, and when he claimed priority over Jenner for the discovery of vaccination, the fashionable London doctors laughed him to scorn. There can be little doubt that his observations must have shown him that those who had been in contact with cows infected with cow-pox were immune from small-pox.

Jenner was a much milder and less venturesome person than Lady Mary, but he had been brought up in the Hunterian tradition of medicine which said 'Experiment!' The fact that cow-pox protected against small-pox had been known as a tradition for a long time amongst West country farmers. Jenner, whilst a medical student, had heard a milkmaid say, 'I cannot take small-pox, I have had cow-pox.'

Jenner made his experiment on 14 May, 1796, when he vaccinated an 8-year-old boy, James Phipps. He obtained the vaccine from a blister on the hand of a dairymaid, Sarah Nelmes, who was infected with the cow-pox from one of her master's cows. A typical local reaction followed and the boy suffered on further ill-effects. He had, in fact, been given the harmless disease cow-pox.

The next step was to test the efficacy of his method. Jenner therefore inoculated the boy on two separate occasions with material taken from the pustule of a case of true small-pox. The boy remained quite healthy. In addition he inoculated small-pox matter into 10 people who had contracted cow-pox previously; they were all resistant to small-pox.

In 1796 Jenner presented his results to the Royal Society but the paper was refused. In fact, at that time he was best known for his work on the migration of birds and for his observations on the cuckoo, which had shown how that bird lays its eggs in the nests of other birds. He eventually published his observations on vaccination in 1798 in a book with the grandiloquent title of *An Inquiry into the Causes and Effects of the Variolae Vaccinae, a Disease discovered in some of the Western Counties of England, particularly Gloucestershire, and known by the Name of the Cowpox.* Jenner was a true natural historian in the tradition of Hippocrates and Gilbert White of Selborne. (*Fig.* 13.)

His fame was now firmly established; in 1802 he was voted £10,000 by the House of Commons, a very large sum in those days, and later another grant of £20,000. He became one of the best-known men of his time. As a result of his work vaccination became compulsory in Britain and the success of his method was demonstrated all over the world.

In America the first Professor of Medicine in the Harvard Medical School, Benjamin Waterhouse, was convinced of its value and on 8 July, 1800, vaccinated his son Daniel Oliver Waterhouse, aged 5 years. This was the first vaccination to be carried out in America.

The protective value of vaccination was demonstrated in a classic experiment in Boston in 1802; 119 boys were vaccinated with cow-pox on 16 August, and on 9 November were inoculated with small-pox. They all remained healthy. Two unvaccinated boys were used in a control experiment; when they were inoculated with the same small-pox material they both contracted the disease.

Thomas Jefferson in 1806 wrote to Jenner the following words: 'Future nations will know by history only that the loathsome small-pox has existed and by you has been extirpated.'

Among 13,686 patients suffering from small-pox in London between 1928 and 1934, only 7 showed evidence of vaccination performed within the previous ten years.

The story of vaccination is remarkable because it demonstrates the value of critical observation of naturally occurring phenomena, and also because it is the only example known whereby the giving of a mild disease produces immunity from a severe one. It led to an intensification of research into the causes of immunity which was carried out with success by Louis Pasteur.

We know that for vaccination to be really effective it should be repeated every five years at least as the immunity does wane a little; however, even one vaccination in infancy confers added immunity.

There has always been considerable controversy about vaccination on the part of the public because vaccine lymph had to be prepared from animals, usually the sheep or calf (*Fig.* 14), but today strains can be cultured on chicken embryos growing in eggs. This may produce sensitivity reactions in egg-sensitive persons. The best time for vaccination is in early infancy because reactions are less and because it is essential to confer immunity as soon as possible. Today most young people have to be vaccinated when they enter the Services. Primary vaccination at this age is more likely to produce complications, and particularly the complication known as post-vaccinial encephalitis. This is very rare indeed, but is more likely to occur if primary vaccination is carried out in adult life. This is another important reason why vaccination should be carried out in infancy (at the age of 2–3 months).

In the late nineteenth century over 95 per cent of people were protected by vaccination and as a result small-pox gradually disappeared. Today the percentage has fallen to under 30 now that vaccination is no longer compulsory. As we shall see in the next few pages, vaccination is the most important means of protection against small-pox and there are disturbing signs that in recent

61

years virulent small-pox has been entering Britain. Fortunately so far, the efforts of our public health departments have prevented any large-scale outbreaks, but, nevertheless, in 1962 there were more than 100 cases in Europe.

SMALL-POX IN SHEFFIELD

One of the most fascinating accounts of small-pox and its effect upon the life of a large city is to be found in a report by Dr. F. W. Barry, Medical Officer of Health for Sheffield in 1887, entitled *Report on an Epidemic of Small-pox at Sheffield during 1887-1888*. It is a remarkable document for many reasons and is one of the most detailed accounts of an isolated epidemic ever written. There are 39 large-scale street maps giving the details of the spread of small-pox house by house, and a detailed description of a vaccination census in which 275,878 persons living in 60,000 houses were personally interviewed by house-to-house visits. This enabled a unique experiment to be carried out in which it was possible to compare the death-rates and attack-rates in relation to the state of vaccination, and so made it possible to measure the protective value of vaccination. It was the most important performance of its kind ever attempted.

The report of the epidemic takes account of 6088 cases and 590 small-pox deaths and refers to the period from March, 1887, when the first case occurred, to 31 March, 1888. The detailed personal observations on every death do not include the 90 deaths which occurred in the rest of 1888. The population of the city was just over 300,000. Dr. Barry divided Sheffield into eight separate districts and reported very thoroughly on each.

There had been small-pox before, but not on such a grand scale as occurred in the year 1887-8. The first case occurred in a man who worked in an office in the Wicker and he subsequently infected several of his fellow employees; another man was a tram conductor and was an important means of spreading infection. It was difficult to trace the origin of infection because there was no systematic means of getting information about cases. There was a system of voluntary notification of cases by doctors who were paid 2s. for each case notified, but not all cases were notified and there were many mild missed cases.

It was only when house-to-house inquiries were made that it was possible to elicit information on all cases. This method was invaluable in providing accurate statistics which could not possibly be provided by notification alone. Thus by May, 1887, only 8 cases had been notified whereas subsequent inquiries showed that there were actually 32 cases during this period.

The first cases were admitted to Winter Street Hospital and from that time the hospital operated as a centre of infection and the houses around were attacked at a rate twelve times greater than the rest of the borough. Many thought this was due to aerial spread of infection, but it was probably due to inadequate control of staff and visitors to the hospital.

The effect of the epidemic upon the vaccination state of the children of school ages was remarkable; in 1862, 13–14 per cent were found unvaccinated;

in 1888, less than 1 per cent were in this state. Of 307,966 vaccinated persons, 1·62 per cent were attacked and of 6556 unvaccinated persons, 15·68 per cent were attacked by small-pox. Dr Barry estimated that of the total population 98 per cent had been vaccinated. The death-rates per thousand at various age-groups and in various stages of vaccination are shown as follows:—

Age	Vaccinated Twice	Vaccinated Once	Unvaccinated
Under 10 years	—	0·09	44
Over 10 years	0·08	0·1	51

In other words, in those unvaccinated the death-rate was about 500 times greater than in those properly protected by vaccination. Moreover, these figures of crude death-rates are no measure of the vastly greater amount of pitting and scarring of the skin and of blindness amongst those who survived the attack and had not been vaccinated.

Of those at special risk were 161 persons who were employed in hospitals; 6 developed the disease, and 1 died. Of 830 troops, all vaccinated, 12 developed the disease and 1 died, of 373 men in the police force, 10 contracted small-pox, but not one of 290 postmen contracted the disease. All those in these special groups who contracted the disease had not been successfully vaccinated a second time. Dr. George Buchanan, in commenting on the outbreak, considered that if there had been no vaccination there would have been at least another 13,000 deaths.

The local authority had to provide further hospital accommodation and altogether 1741 patients were treated in hospital. Special burial facilities were arranged and public libraries were closed. A most interesting development was the formation of small-pox associations by the employees of many of the large firms in Sheffield. They had one principle in common: that all members should pay weekly a certain sum to the fund which was to be applied to (1) the maintenance of those families who contracted small-pox, and (2) the payment of money to healthy members living in small-pox houses on condition that they remained away from work. This latter provision was often abused, as some men who had been paid out of the fund were found to be attending public houses and theatres. This is a remarkable example of lay persons joining together to form an association for the benefit of its members during adversity and to protect the community as a whole from the danger of epidemic disease. The payment of healthy contacts to remain away from work has always been a difficult matter, and was carried out in a recent small-pox outbreak in the West Riding of Yorkshire.

The rules of the James Dixon & Sons Mutual Assistance Fund laid down that a levy of 2½ per cent of the earnings should be paid weekly, and the benefits to be paid weekly should be the same as the weekly wages. The scheme covered scarlet fever and cholera as well as small-pox. This provision was made by the workpeople on their own initiative.

Rules of other associations varied slightly; one laid down that any workmen in receipt of pay from the small-pox fund who were known to go into any public place of amusement should at once have their pay stopped. I am not aware of any other voluntary associations which had a fund for this purpose, although there were many funds for sickness benefits. By the end of March, 1888, there were 142 associations with 33,477 members.

There were many ways in which the spread of small-pox was facilitated, at funerals, by visiting hospitals and workhouses, by children playing in the streets, and at banks and shops.

One interesting influence was the purveyor of quack medicines and cures. In January, 1888, a Mr. Herring of Leeds wrote a letter to the Health Committee of Sheffield saying that he could cure small-pox in half an hour and offering his services to the town. A petition signed by 2000 persons forced the mayor to call a public meeting to hear the claims of Mr. Herring. A full account of this remarkable meeting appears in the *Sheffield Daily Telegraph* of 9 February, 1888. It must have been one of the most remarkable meetings ever held in a large city. The man was obviously an ignorant charlatan, but had a great following. The mayor, who took the chair, had great difficulty in controlling the meeting, and there were frequent stormy interruptions. What type of man it was who was claiming to cure the disease can be gathered from the following dialogue. Mr. Herring was being asked about a patient who had died under his treatment, which consisted of giving potassium permanganate baths. His reply was as follows: 'I did not say he was lifeless; I said he were dead. His flesh were dead. He was simply breathing in and out of his mouth and that was nearly closed. His flesh were all gone, no life in it. Of course if there is no life in your flesh you are dead, are you not? I did not mean to say the man were lifeless, I said he were dead.' (A voice: 'You ain't had a board school education.') The meeting finally broke up in some disorder and there were many exclamations of wrath against the mayor.

Mr. Herring soon had a large following as a result of the publicity, and the belief of the people in an easy cure resulted in a remarkable and immediate decrease in those coming forward for vaccination. During the week of this meeting there were 2322 vaccinations and the week after only 359. The statements that Mr. Herring made as to the freedom from infectiveness which his treatment conferred had a widespread effect in making people careless about the disease.

Mr. Herring of Leeds was not the only possessor of an infallible remedy; there were at least forty others. The following advertisement taken from a Sheffield newspaper is typical of many which appeared during the epidemic:—

GOOD NEWS FOR SHEFFIELD

How to stamp the Small-pox out in 28 days, never to return

Everybody take the Champion of Medicines. £5 reward and all funeral expenses for the first case it fails to cure. Also £1 reward for the first case it fails to prevent. Over 4,000 cases cured, and not one single failure. Warranted to cure 19 cases out of every 20 of consumption, bronchitis, and rheumatic. It is the Champion for fevers, measles, whooping cough, colds, scurvy, breakings out and children's teething. May be obtained through any chemist, or patent medicine vendor, Mr. Askew, Charlotte Tavern, Charlotte Street; Mr. J. Fishburn, 17, Walker Street; or from the proprietors, W. Edwards and Sons, Medical Dispensaries, 40, Wicker, Sheffield, and

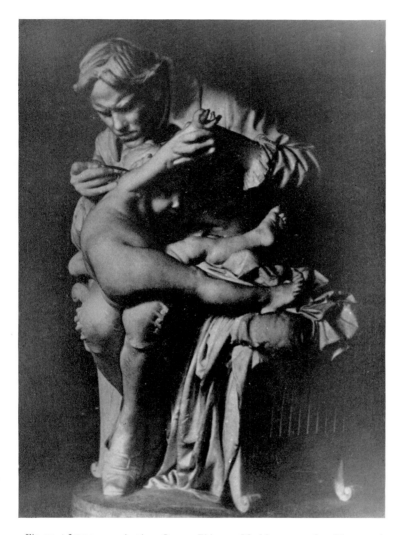

Fig. 13.—Jenner vaccinating James Phipps. Marble group by Monteverde (1837–1917). The original bronze by the artist is in the Wellcome Museum. Jenner discovered the principle of vaccination against small-pox in 1796. Although more than 150 years have elapsed this lethal disease continues to rage today in many parts of the world, a manifest anachronism.

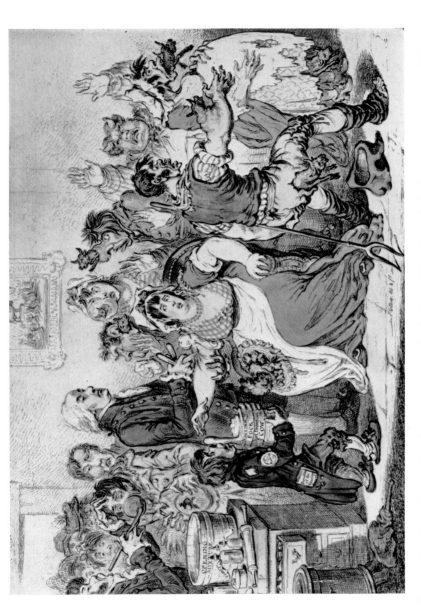

Fig. 14.—The effects of vaccination. From a coloured etching by James Gillray (1757–1815). From an impression in the Wellcome Historical Medical Museum.

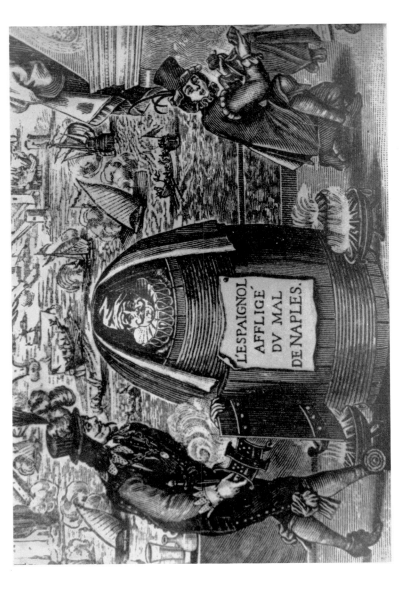

Fig. 15.—The Renaissance helped in spreading syphilis, which Europeans at war mutually accused each other of originating. Here it is called Naples sickness by the French. Treatment: mercury, sweating.

L'ESPAIGNOL
AFFLIGÉ
DV MAL
DE NAPLES.

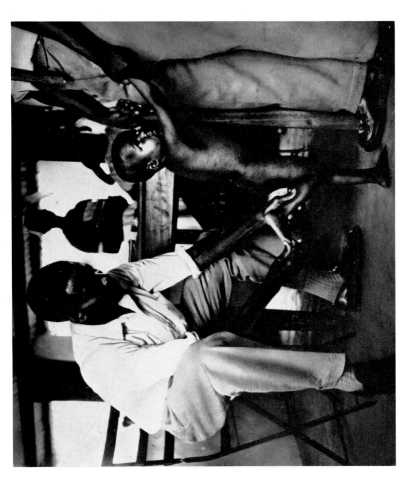

Fig. 16.—Yaws in Nigeria. Every member of the community has to be examined for yaws sores which are likely to appear first on the soles of the feet or the insides of hands.

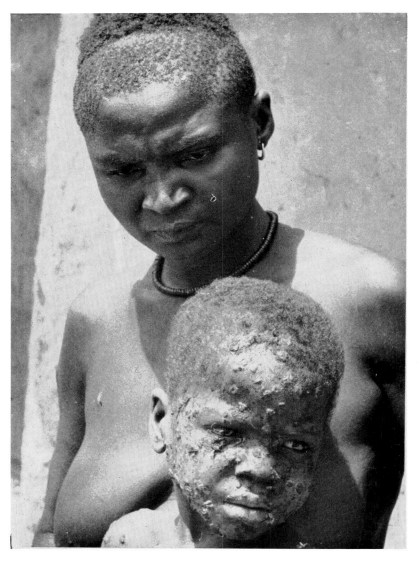

Fig. 17.—These ugly sores can mean a lifetime of pain. This little boy is 5 years old. He lives in a bush village in Nigeria. A victim of yaws, he rarely smiled. Neither did his mother. That was before the visit of a W.H.O.-assisted yaws team.

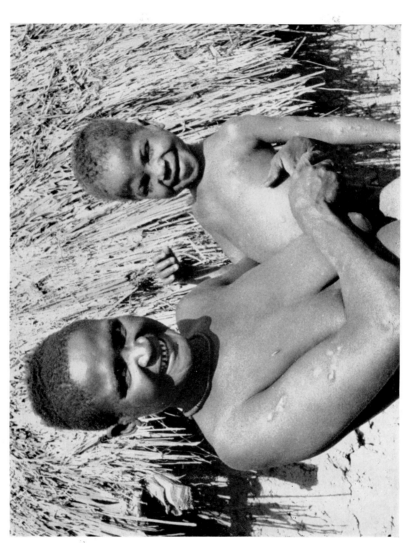

Fig. 18.—The miracle of one shot of penicillin. Cost? Less than 80 U.S. cents. Ten days after receiving a single injection of penicillin the boy's sores have almost disappeared. W.H.O.-assisted yaws teams, using penicillin provided by the U.N. Children's Fund, have examined, up to 1957, more than 60 million people in tropical regions and treated some 15 million.

Peel Square, Barnsley. In bottles, 1s. 1½d. each. Hours of attendance, 10 and 12 a.m.; 2, 4 and 6 p.m. Visits free, except in the night and Sundays.

Apparently the £5 and funeral expenses were paid up in more than one instance. Another remedy in great vogue at the time was a string of onions hung in the chimney, there being a current belief that they absorbed the 'miasma' of small-pox infection.

There can be no doubt that advertising of these remedies did a great deal of harm.

The total amount expended by the Corporation, the Boards of Guardians, and the Small-pox Associations was £32,257. This is, of course, but a fraction of the total loss caused to the inhabitants. In addition, there were loss of wages, expenses of doctors, caring for the sick at home, and cost of funerals. But probably even greater in its importance was the loss in trade. For a long time Sheffield was avoided by all outsiders and the hotels were empty. It was stated that during the year of the epidemic the trams carried 200,000 less people than usual. No account can be rendered, however, of the disfigurement, blindness, and permanent ill health, especially in those houses inhabited by the unvaccinated.

This detailed account gives a fascinating picture of the impact of small-pox on a large industrial city during the nineteenth century, but comparing it with the cholera epidemic at Exeter earlier in the century (see Chapter VII) it is clear that we had made rapid improvements in our arrangements for dealing with such matters. There was now an efficient system of local government with adequate financial resources, a whole-time Medical Officer of Health in charge, with a large staff, and adequate hospital accommodation. Fortunately, Sheffield had a high percentage of its inhabitants vaccinated, probably 98 per cent, and the death-roll was kept down. But for that there must have been many thousands of deaths, something like 13,000 in fact. Compare this vaccination percentage with today, when about one-quarter of the population is vaccinated.

OUTBREAKS OF SMALL-POX SINCE WORLD WAR II IN BRITAIN

A fundamental change occurred when in 1935 major small-pox ceased to be an endemic disease in Britain. Since the end of World War II, however, there is evidence that the disease has been occurring with increasing frequency.

In 1942 there were 5 cases, in 1944 there were 14 cases with 3 deaths, in 1945, 4 cases; then in 1946 there were 47 cases with 14 deaths, resulting from no less than 15 separate importations of the disease. Vaccination and careful watch on the contacts brought each outbreak under control with remarkable speed. This sharp increase was due to the increased homeward-bound traffic from the East, and to the fact that small-pox was prevalent in Bombay in the early part of 1946.

Between January and June, 1946, seven large ships crowded with passengers arrived at English ports with cases of small-pox on board and 14 other ships arrived with small-pox contacts on board. The passengers were

5

returning service personnel or civilians who had for many years been separated from their families and who were anxious to get home as quickly as possible. The difficulties of control were enormous and scattered outbreaks occurred, mostly in Liverpool and Birkenhead. Many cases were mild ones occurring in vaccinated persons, but in these cases diagnosis of the disease is more difficult. Fortunately, there is now available a suitable laboratory test.

In 1947 there was an even larger number of cases, 79 in all, from two separate importations. The first from Grimsby spread to Scunthorpe, Doncaster, Barnsley, and Sheffield; the second was from a sergeant in the Army who had been flown home from India, and this spread to centres in the Black Country. In these two outbreaks 6 persons connected with the control of the disease were affected and none had been vaccinated recently. They included a doctor, a medical student, and a nurse; this shows how important it is that those whose duties involve the handling of small-pox cases should be recently vaccinated; it is a clear indication of our state of unpreparedness. Outbreaks occurred in other parts of the world where they are not normally expected. In New York there were 13 cases. As a result of the scare, 5,000,000 people were vaccinated in two weeks. The danger of importing small-pox has been greatly increased with the rapidity of air travel. The incubation period is usually 12 days, so that a person can be in contact with small-pox in India, fly to this country, and not develop the disease until 12 days have elapsed from the first contact, by which time he may have infected others.

The acceptance of vaccination between the years 1942 and 1946 was about 40 per cent of children born and before that it had been less. After July, 1948, the Vaccination Acts were repealed and the acceptance rate fell. At the moment only about one-quarter of infants born are being vaccinated.

Fortunately, there were no cases in 1948, but in 1949 there was another small outbreak with 19 cases, and a very high mortality-rate resulting in 5 deaths. The disease was imported by a man and his wife who went ashore from a liner *en route* for this country at Bombay on 10 March, 1949. They were only ashore a few hours. Both died from small-pox, the man on 1 April and his wife on 6 April. The passengers and crew numbered 1394 and the contacts were vaccinated. The majority were allowed to go home, and their addresses were notified to the local Medical Officer of Health for surveillance for 16 days. None of those who died had been recently vaccinated before the outbreak.

An outbreak which occurred in March, 1950, in Glasgow illustrates once more how easy it is for infection to gain entrance into this country despite strict precautions at airports. On 11 February, 1950, the S.S. *Chitral* sailed from Bombay, calling at Aden and Port Said and docking at the Port of London on 5 March. One of the passengers was Mooser Ali, a Laccadive Islander who was travelling from Bombay to join a new ship at Greenock as part of her crew. On the night of 8 March he complained of headache. He was admitted on 10 March to an infectious fever hospital with pneumonia. On 14 March he developed a rash. He was diagnosed as a case of chicken-pox by experienced consultants who were aware that he had just arrived from

India. On 26 March small-pox was diagnosed in one of the hospital staff and eventually there were 18 confirmed cases; 6 had no vaccination scars. All these patients died; they included 3 nurses and a doctor. The usual methods of control were immediately carried out with great vigour, all contacts were traced and vaccinated and kept under close supervision. This meant the daily visiting of 2000 persons in Glasgow alone. The fact that the Easter week-end came within the period of observation made matters extremely difficult. Five medical-student contacts had already disappeared into the Highlands without leaving any address. Needless to say, there was, to put it lightly, considerable trepidation within the city, and a great public demand for vaccination. Some 162,000 persons were vaccinated. The services of the Press and the B.B.C. were most valuable in tracing contacts.

This outbreak once more shows the importance of vaccination as a preventive measure and the need to protect hospital staffs especially. If the vaccinated person contracts small-pox it is of a mild atypical type. The diagnosis of these mild cases is often extremely difficult, especially in coloured people. Nevertheless, when the disease spreads to the unvaccinated it is still as virulent as ever.

In December, 1950, an epidemic of small-pox broke out in Brighton lasting until the third week of January, 1951. A well-vaccinated officer in the Royal Air Force had flown from India whilst incubating the disease. Because of the mild nature of the attack the diagnosis was never made and he recovered uneventfully. This infection caused 28 cases of a highly fatal form of small-pox with 10 deaths. Of these, 7 had never been vaccinated and 3 only in infancy. Nearly 90,000 persons were vaccinated in Brighton out of a population of 156,000. Thirteen hospital staff and patients contracted the disease; 3 had been vaccinated in infancy, and of the other 10, all unvaccinated, 7 were nurses, 3 of whom died. In fact, a large percentage of the nursing and domestic staffs had never been vaccinated. The lesson had still not been learnt, and brings to light in a vivid fashion the neglected state of vaccination of our hospital staffs. That the outbreak was not more wide-spread and severe was only due to the efficient, energetic, and prompt manner in which it was handled by the Medical Officer of Health of Brighton, Dr. R. Cramb. He was not aware of the presence of the disease in the district until the third crop of cases had occurred. By this time there were many contacts in the town, including the patients and staff of a large hospital, the employees at a local laundry, a large number of people who had ridden in a certain taxi, and workers in the Post Office Telephone Exchange. In addition, there had been many Christmas visitors at the hospital. The Press and the B.B.C. co-operated in warning these contacts to report to their local Medical Officer of Health.

In 1952 there was another outbreak, this time in Rochdale, spreading to other towns in south-east Lancashire. Fortunately, the 135 cases notified were all of the mild type of small-pox. There is some possibility that in-fection may have originated from cotton, and the same suggestion was made to account for the origin of an outbreak in 1953 in Lancashire and the West

Riding of Yorkshire. This suggestion, however, has never been confirmed and the origin of the infection in both outbreaks was never traced. It was traced back on both occasions to workers in cotton mills, but there the quest reached a dead end. In the 1953 outbreak there were 40 cases reported with 8 deaths, so that the infection was much more violent than in 1952 and points to a different source. Infection was spread from the first cases in Todmorden by lorry drivers into the West Riding and it may have originated from a missed case from Merseyside

Today outbreaks still occur in Europe; in 1961, for example, there were cases in Germany, England, and Spain, imported as a result of international travel by air, and in 1962 there were 36 cases in Germany, 65 cases in the United Kingdom, and 29 cases in Poland.

The highest levels of small-pox are now to be found in India, Pakistan, Burma, Indo-China, South America, Mexico, and parts of Africa. As far as individual ports are concerned, Calcutta, Delhi, and Bombay show the highest rates. India and Pakistan have about 50,000 deaths each year from the disease.

As I pen these words in the heat of an Indian summer (1957) I am reminded that small-pox is still a common disease in India; a great epidemic flourishes in Calcutta and cases are being admitted every day to the infectious diseases hospital. I have fifty doses of vaccine lymph in my refrigerator and tomorrow I shall try to persuade the two hundred-odd mothers who will attend the well-baby clinic to have their infants vaccinated. I shall indeed consider myself lucky if I use up all my lymph. I know, too, that in many of those who are vaccinated there will be secondary infection, and the inoculation will not take because many mothers will smear the site with cow-dung. They believe that small-pox is due to the anger of the Badi Mata, goddess of small-pox, and she must be placated by worship at her shrine. In West Africa the worship of the small-pox god is prohibited by law because it is an active means of spreading the disease from person to person. When a case occurs in a native village the practice is to call in the witch-doctor, who placates the small-pox god by sprinkling on the other members of the family the dried and powdered dust collected from the small-pox pustules.

The public vaccinators in India are paid very low salaries, their conditions of service are very poor, and there is little supervision of their work. Mothers tend to shirk vaccination because small-pox is not considered to be preventable, despite the fact that vaccination is compulsory in 81 per cent of the towns and 62 per cent of the rural areas, and the incidence of protection in some villages is still very low.

Small-pox, then, is still a serious menace and can have a mortality as high as 50 per cent, even with all our knowledge and skill. Whilst the new antibiotics can prevent secondary infection they are of little value in mitigating the serious results of the disease itself.

As far as the future is concerned W.H.O. is now planning a concerted attack upon the disease, in the hope that it will be eradicated from the areas where it is now endemic and eventually from the whole world. Only by united efforts on a global scale can this be achieved. (*See* Dixon (1962) for a full account of small-pox.)

THE GREAT POX

The great pox, known today as syphilis, was the most malignant of all the venereal diseases found in Europe in the Middle Ages.

Examination of the bones of Egyptian mummies has failed to reveal any evidence of this disease. It is not mentioned in the literature of Greek and Roman times, although there are frequent references to other venereal diseases which were common in those days as a result of the loose morals which prevailed. The question of the origin of syphilis is one of the classic controversies of medical history. Bones from all over the world have been examined to try to determine the geographical cradle of this disease. Some have considered this to be in the Americas, the most commonly held view, whilst other theories point to Europe, the Near East, or Africa as the original home of the infection. In 1939 a skull was discovered in Iraq which showed evidence of syphilitic disease. It was believed to date from the first half of the first millennium A.D. In the Bible the plague of Moab has been identified as syphilis, and a similar type of infection was known in the Chinese coastal towns as 'seamen's jealousy'! Despite the fact that a virulent form of infection was brought back from America by Columbus to Europe it would appear that a milder form of syphilis had occurred in Europe and Asia for many centuries before. In 1493 a Spanish surgeon in Barcelona described 'a disease previously unknown, unseen and undescribed'. It ran through the susceptible populations with great rapidity and virulence. It has been established that it existed in the Americas before this, because syphilis has been found in the bones of Indians buried in A.D. 1000. The scourge quickly spread over the rest of Europe, carried by the camp followers of the armies of Charles VIII of France when Italy was invaded, and by the hordes of Jews expelled from Spain and forced to migrate all over Europe. By 1497 it had spread as far north as Scotland, and the town councils of Aberdeen and Edinburgh tried to stamp out the disease by the isolation of patients on islands off the coast. The 'sibbens', or Scottish disease, was prevalent in the seventeenth century after the time of Cromwell. It was transmitted by communal drinking bowls. A similar type of disease occurred amongst the Red Indian tribes and is common today in many parts of the world. The disease was very destructive in its effects and often pursued a rapid course resulting in death. There was gross destruction of bones, joints, and lungs with foul suppurating ulcers of the skin. Such a disease gave rise to much literature and supposition as to its causes. It was named 'French disease' by the Spanish and 'Spanish disease' by the French (*Fig.* 15).

Unfortunately, as in yellow fever, one of the greatest difficulties in the experimental study of this disease was the lack of any suitable experimental animal. John Hunter decided that the only way to learn more about this disease was to experiment on himself, and in 1767 he inoculated himself with infective material from a person suffering from the disease. He developed signs of both gonorrhoea and syphilis, so showing that the disease could be spread by inoculation from one person to another. He eventually died from the effects of the disease in 1793, after describing a virus which he thought caused it. It was not until 1905, however, that the delicate filamentous organism responsible, the spirochaete, was finally demonstrated under the microscope, and later there followed the discovery of certain blood-tests which could detect the disease even in its latent phases. The organism is very difficult to culture outside the human body and quickly dies. The commonest method of transmission is undoubtedly by sexual intercourse and it can be contracted by blood transfusion from an infected person. Surgeons and pathologists have been known to acquire the disease after cutting themselves when performing operations or post mortems on infected patients, so inoculating themselves with the organism. Midwives, physicians, and wet nurses have spread infection to others by lack of personal cleanliness in themselves, particularly in the early days of vaccination and 'cupping'. Tattooing and various inoculation procedures have all caused a spread of the disease. The most tragic mode of infection is of a wife by an infected husband, sometimes resulting in the birth of a child with congenital syphilis. In many cases the wife is quite unaware of the origin of the disease.

In some parts of the world, however, a milder type of disease prevails, especially amongst children. It is a family disease spread by direct contact from one member of the household to another. This type is known as 'endemic syphilis' and was common in Bosnia. Syphilis was brought there by repeated invasions, first by the Romans, then by the Slavs, Turks, and Austrians, and finally by the migration of refugees in the Second World War. The disease was spread in small closely packed villages by the use of communal drinking bowls, such as the 'ibrik'. A similar non-venereal disease is common in the Middle East and North Africa, where it is known as 'bejel' and in the New World where it is known as 'pinta', the blue staining disease. In parts of Latin America one in fifty of the population is said to be affected.

Naturally enough, the history of the treatment of this dread disease is not without interest. In the early days, like most diseases it was treated by bleeding, but it was not of course very efficacious. The Arabs used mercury with some success, but unfortunately it is itself toxic, causing ulcers in the mouth and loosening of the teeth, severe abdominal pain, and diarrhoea.

It was much in favour during the nineteenth century, but many patients suffered more from mercury poisoning than from the disease itself. One of the most popular of all the remedies, which could be bought openly in the streets of London, was sarsaparilla; it was sold as a 'blood purifier' opposite Westminster Abbey and near to Westminster Hospital in tumblerfuls from a cart. In India, textbooks of Ayurvedic medicine still recommend sarsaparilla for syphilis.

The greatest advance, however, was made when Paul Ehrlich carried out the first important experiments on the effect of chemicals on the spirochaete in the laboratory. He tried a large number of substances and at last in 1909 found one which worked. This was an organic compound of mercury which he called '606' because it was the 606th substance which he had tried out in his experiments. This discovery revolutionized the treatment of the dread disease and heralded the age of chemotherapy—the treatment of disease by specific chemicals.

Unfortunately the drug was extremely toxic when injected into human beings, and despite the discovery of better and safer chemicals closely allied to '606', e.g., '914', it was still necessary to have many courses of injections and, moreover, the most important thing of all, the injections did not render the patient non-infective for several months. There was a high default rate after the first few injections because they usually cleared up the lesions from which the patient suffered, but they did not cure, and they lulled infective patients into a sense of false security so that they once more spread infection abroad. From a public health point of view, then, the discovery did not do a great deal to prevent the spread of the disease and syphilis still remained common. By the twentieth century, however, it was no longer the acute fulminating disease which our ancestors had seen.

As people lived longer with the disease it was now more common to see its late stages which affected the brain, producing paralysis and insanity. Moreover, the earlier symptoms were often quite slight, so that a person could become infected and show very few symptoms for twenty or thirty years, when suddenly the late manifestations would appear. It is remarkable that general paralysis of the insane (G.P.I.), which is a late manifestation of syphilis, is practically unknown in China and India where syphilis is common; this is probably due to the widespread incidence of malaria which seems to suppress G.P.I.

One form of treatment that has been used effectively in this disease is the giving of malaria to the patient, following the discovery that persons in the tropics infected by malaria showed remarkable improvement. It is not the first time we have witnessed the giving of one disease to cure another.

Many of the world's most brilliant men have suffered from general paralysis of the insane. The most typical signs of the early stages are delusions of grandeur when the sufferer embarks upon all sorts of grandiose schemes, and it is possible that many of the greatest achievements were conceived in brains stimulated by the cerebral irritation of the early stages of the disease.

The greatest advance in the treatment of syphilis has been the discovery of penicillin by Sir Alexander Fleming. The importance from the public health point of view is that one injection renders the patient non-infective. As a result there has been a great decrease in the incidence of the disease. Moreover, the diseases of skin, bones, heart, and brain which were formerly caused by it are becoming extremely rare. The patient is much more likely to come in the early stages for treatment now that he knows an effective cure can be given with very few injections. Some of the later cases may still be resistant to complete cure, but as the foci of infection become fewer and fewer, so will these later stages disappear.

In the nineteenth century the only diseases for which free treatment was provided in Britain were the acute infectious fevers, such as scarlet fever, diphtheria, typhoid fever, cholera, and small-pox. In 1917, however, special arrangements were made to provide free confidential treatment for those suffering from venereal disease, but it was never made a notifiable disease as the more acute infectious diseases were, because it was thought that such a scheme might drive the victims of the disease to seek treatment from patent medicines. It is now illegal for anyone to advertise treatment for venereal disease.

In many of the under-developed countries syphilis is spread by close personal contact, as, for example, between mother and child and amongst children. In this respect it is very much like yaws, a tropical disease also caused by a spirochaete which is extremely sensitive to penicillin. This disease begins in childhood and destroys the skin and bones. (*Fig.* 16.) Because of the frequency with which it attacks the palms of the hands and soles of the feet it is of great economic importance, because it destroys a person's ability to carry out agricultural work. Children who are affected with the disease are a most pathetic sight, and before the use of penicillin it was estimated that there were 50,000,000 victims in the world. The long-acting penicillins make it possible to cure yaws and early syphilis with one injection, and effective mass campaigns have been organized by the World Health Organization. By the middle of 1955, 40,000,000 people had been examined and about 10,000,000 treated with penicillin. The effect is magical (*Figs.* 17, 18) and it is possible to eradicate the disease as a public health problem in a short time. In Haiti, for example, which had 1,500,000 cases of yaws out of a rural population of 3,000,000, the disease was eradicated within three years. There are also great centres of infection in South-east Asia, and particularly in Indonesia, Thailand, India, and the western Pacific, and already 2,500,000 cases have been treated in these areas. The greatest reservoir of infection left at the moment is in Africa, where there are something like 25,000,000 cases. Africa is the original home of yaws and it was carried to Haiti and other countries in Central America by the slave-trade. Work is now starting on a large scale in Africa, giving hope for millions of people now crippled and deformed by this painful disease. There are few important diseases that can be cured so quickly and so cheaply. The cost is from 2*s.* to 5*s.* per person treated, including all the costs of administration.

Some measure of the incidence of venereal disease in England today can be obtained from figures supplied by the Reports of the Chief Medical Officer of the Ministry of Health. The number of new cases attending at treatment centres in England and Wales for syphilis rose during the war, reaching a peak in 1946. In that year, 17,675 patients with acquired syphilis with infections of less than one year's duration attended at treatment centres in England and Wales. In 1953 the corresponding number was 1074. In the same period the number of cases of congenital syphilis under one year, dealt with for the first time, fell from 363 to 95. Deaths from general paralysis of the insane fell from 441 in 1946 to 117 in 1953.

Our seaport cities are the main reservoirs of infection which would rapidly fill in the event of a national emergency. The most important measure in the further control of the disease is the tracing of contacts, to find those hidden latent sources of infection, a difficult and often disappointing task. This question of undiscovered cases was investigated by the United States Public Health Service in 1949. They estimated that in 48 States there were 150,000 fresh syphilitic infections, 80,000 of which remained undiscovered. The number of cases existing in an area has been studied in great detail in the U.S.A. by special surveys. Thus in 39 States, a premarital examination is required by law. This involves a special test for the presence of venereal disease. In Virginia, 15 per cent of negro applicants for marriage certificates were found to be suffering from the disease and roughly 50 per cent amongst negro males in a private practice in Alabama. One of the most significant analyses of the prevalence of syphilis was carried out by the U.S. Public Health Service in 1941. It showed that the percentage of people with the disease increased with age and was greater age for age in negroes than in whites. Thus the lowest incidence was found in whites aged 21–25 years, i.e., 1 per cent, and highest in non-whites aged 31–35, i.e., 36 per cent. These figures are an amazing revelation and show that a quarter of the young adult blacks in the United States were infected with syphilis.

The other important venereal disease in the Western world is gonorrhoea, once important as a cause of blindness in young babies who were infected from their mothers at birth. Since the introduction of the routine use of silver nitrate instillation in the eyes of newborn babies this cause of blindness has now become very rare. Gonorrhoea, like syphilis, can be cured by penicillin, but unfortunately the disease is often so mild and hidden that people, especially females, do not bother to seek treatment. There has been an increase in the disease in most countries of the world in the last few years, especially in teen-agers.

Syphilis is a disease which sailors and soldiers spread wherever they go. The white man has given it to the Eskimo and like all new diseases it has spread amongst them with devastating consequences. Wherever there are large comings and goings of people, as in war-time, there will be an increase in the disease. The great seaports of the world are the hotbeds of vice and disease, and syphilis is there with them in London, New York, Shanghai, Singapore, and Hong Kong. And let us not imagine that it is the professional prostitute who is only to blame; her sister, the enthusiastic amateur, is probably more dangerous. The answer to the prevention of this group of diseases is simple as far as the individual person is concerned—avoid promiscuous intercourse. Unfortunately, the knowledge that penicillin can cure does nothing to prevent promiscuous behaviour. Once more we must utter a note of warning: penicillin, like DDT, is losing its killing power on various strains of organisms. On no account can we afford to rest on our laurels, and so the search for new and better antibiotics must go on. Since the original discovery of penicillin other new antibiotics have been discovered, many of them hailed as new 'miracle cures' by the popular press. In point of fact penicillin still remains the best all-round antibiotic for general use.

LEPROSY

In the Middle Ages this much feared disease was epidemic in Europe, having been introduced by the returning Crusaders from the Middle East. At one time it was estimated that there were 19,000 lazarettos in Europe, France alone having 2000. It has practically disappeared from Europe for reasons unknown and occurs now only in Rumania, the Baltic States, Spain, Turkey, and the U.S.S.R. There has been a remarkable rise and fall in Norway.

It was at one time very common in England, and in 1346 Edward II tried to control the disease in the City of London by ordering that diligent search should be made for lepers in order that they might be expelled. In 1375 the entry of lepers into the City of London was forbidden and severe penalties were inflicted on all those who allowed their entry. Today there are about 200 cases of leprosy in England and Wales, all of which have been contracted abroad.

The disease was probably brought to America by slaves and was first recognized in Louisiana. In 1950 there were 390 patients in the National Leprosarium at Carville, Louisiana, and Dr. James Doull considers that there are probably at least twice as many outside the institution. This would make a total of about 1200 in the U.S.A. today.

It occurs now most commonly in Africa, Burma, China, India, Japan, Korea, Oceania, and South America, particularly Brazil and Colombia. During the past century most of the islands of Oceania have become infected. The disease became a serious public health problem on Hawaii, and the government established a settlement on the island of Molokai, where Father Damien, working amongst the lepers, contracted the disease and died from it.

It is difficult to say with any accuracy how many lepers there are in the world, but expert estimates have put the figure at between 10,000,000 and 12,000,000.

The fear of leprosy is almost certainly due to the influence of the Bible, but our views on lepers have changed a great deal since those times. They were formerly regarded as unclean and kept in strict segregation; the danger of contracting infection from a leper struck terror into the hearts of people. That attitude is still prevalent in many parts of the world; it makes life for the leper doubly difficult. Leprosy is only mildly infectious and is only transmitted by very close contact. It is therefore mainly caught during childhood and like tuberculosis it is a familial disease, spread from one member of a family to the next. Adults are relatively immune and a person can live with safety in a leper colony without fear of contracting the disease, provided he does not come into close personal contact with an infected leper. In 1956, when Queen Elizabeth II visited a leper colony in Nigeria she walked amongst the patients and talked to many of them. Photographs of her in this colony were circulated in many newspapers. This must have done a great deal of good in helping to dispel the prejudice and fear which many people have for lepers. The disease is very common in Nigeria and there are probably one or more cases in almost every school. The river settlement is one of the biggest colonies which in 1947 had 14,000 patients; there are now only 8000. There has been a remarkable change in outlook due to the new sulphone drugs, sulphetrone and promin, which can cure the disease in many cases provided they are given in the early stages. But as in so many other conditions other aspects of the disease are important. Attention must be paid to the general nutrition of the patient and the psychological aspect of the disease. Leprosy causes severe disfigurement because of the extensive destruction of skin, bone, muscle, and nerve tissue, particularly in long-standing cases. For these cases, physiotherapy, skin-grafting, and specialized surgery may be necessary. Today many patients are being discharged home as cured, but as in all diseases, prevention is better than cure. General improvement in standards of housing and nutrition will no doubt cause the disease to become rarer in the future. Propaganda is of enormous importance in educating the masses of the people to the knowledge that cure is possible in the early cases. BCG inoculation is one way of increasing immunity to the disease, but what is needed is an effective immunizing agent. In underdeveloped countries with relatively small financial resources the tendency nowadays is to treat the disease at home and to reserve hospital treatment for those patients who require special forms of treatment such as surgery. There is some evidence that treatment of family contacts with dapsone (D.D.S.) will prevent them developing the disease.

In the past, missionaries have been particularly active in caring for sufferers from this disease and a number of doctors and nurses who have been in close contact with patients have sometimes contracted it. Well-known examples are Sir George Turner in Pretoria, Mary Reed in India, Father Damien in Hawaii, and Father Bagliolo in New Orleans.

There are still many things we do not know about leprosy. In China and Japan it is believed that the disease is spread by sexual contact, whilst in Norway it has been stated that a fish diet predisposes to the disease. Rats suffer from leprosy, but the role of these animals in the spread of the disease has never been demonstrated. Many people have considered the possible role of parasitic insects as vectors, but so far no satisfactory proof has been forthcoming; we are not even sure of the causative agent.

It is a remarkable fact that plague, which we know is spread by the rat, disappeared from Britain in the seventeenth century. Why did leprosy disappear also about this time? Can it also have had something to do with some alterations in the equilibrium of the rat population? No doubt further research work will clear up many of these questions and we may eventually be able to say why leprosy, like plague, finally disappeared from Britain.

These disfiguring diseases—small-pox, syphilis, and leprosy—spread by direct personal contact, are now well under control.* There are other diseases spread from man to man by more indirect means which we must consider. Such are the important group of infections spread by drinking and eating; of these Asiatic cholera is still the most terrible.

---

* Rugby footballers will be familiar with yet one more form of pox, that known as 'scrum pox'. This disease is familiar to most mothers of young children under another name—impetigo. It is a weeping contagious skin eruption confined to the face, caused by poor hygiene and spread by the use of communal towels and baths.

CHAPTER VII

DR. SNOW IN SOHO

It is easier to destroy our villages than to change our customs.—BOSNIAN PROVERB

THE IMPACT OF CHOLERA ON THE SOCIAL LIFE OF NINETEENTH-CENTURY ENGLAND

THERE is considerable evidence that cholera has existed in India for many centuries. The people in Lower Bengal have for a long time worshipped the Goddess of Cholera, and in a temple at Gujrat in western India there is a monolith dating back to the time of Alexander the Great with the following inscription relating to cholera: 'The lips blue, the face haggard, the eyes hollow, the stomach sunk in, the limbs contracted and crumpled as if by fire, those are the signs of the great illness which, invoked by a malediction of the priests, comes down to slay the braves.'

The first authentic account of this terrible disease, however, was published by a European, one Gaspar Correa, in a book entitled *Lendas da India* (Legends of India). He observed that the army on the Malabar coast was struck by a disease which came 'suddenlike, which struck with pain in the belly, so that a man did not last out but eight hours time'. This was in 1503. Since that time many descriptions of epidemics have been given by European settlers. It does not appear that there had been any extensive spread westwards of true epidemic cholera before the nineteenth century. During the eighteenth century it spread to China, Burma, and Ceylon, as well as to other parts of India. The early descriptions of the disease leave no doubt in one's mind about the role of pilgrimages and military operations in propagating it.

At the beginning of the nineteenth century cholera suddenly became of world-wide importance. The disease which had formerly been localized in India now spread to all parts of the world, the great pandemic of 1817.

The start of the epidemic was probably associated with abnormal climatic conditions. The years 1815 and 1817 were marked by terrible floods due to the heavy rainfall, and famine and disease followed in their wake. In the words of Macnamara, 'within three months from its appearance the disease had been generated throughout the province of Bengal, including some 195,935 square miles and within this vast area the inhabitants of hardly a single village or town had escaped its deadly influence'.

The epidemic continued to rage in India until 1821 when it became more localized. In the meantime the disease had spread to Burma, Ceylon, Siam,

Java, Borneo, and the Philippines. The infection spread both by the old overland trade routes to inland cities and by the sea routes to the ports. It spread to Canton and Peking, up the Yangtze Valley, and entered Russia by the old caravan routes.

The disease first appeared in Japan in 1822, having been imported into Nagasaki by a ship from Java. It spread rapidly throughout Japan, taking a terrible toll in lives.

The disease also spread westward to Arabia, Persia, and Russia, infection spreading rapidly along the great river valleys of the Tigris and Euphrates, reaching the Caspian and Black Seas. Fortunately because of the severe winter of 1823–4 the disease did not reach Europe. Africa itself was only slightly affected, no doubt because of the low density of the population. It was limited to the Zanzibar coast, carried there by the Arab dhows which trafficked between Arabia and East Africa.

The island of Mauritius had a severe outbreak in 1819, with 6000 deaths, mostly African slaves, when a ship from Ceylon called at Port Louis and landed patients there who had contracted the disease during the voyage.

Finally the pandemic subsided into Lower Bengal—the home of cholera—leaving a terrible trail of death in China, Ceylon, Burma, and Persia.

The second and greatest pandemic of cholera occurred in 1829. Already in 1826 there had been a flare-up of the smouldering fire of cholera along the Ganges. It advanced rapidly through the Punjab, and thence through Afganistan and Persia to south-east Europe and soon it had spread to all parts of the Western world. It had reached Moscow by 1830, spreading as far as Archangel and Finland, then westwards into Poland, Austria, and Hungary. In August, 1831, the wave of infection reached Berlin and in October of that year it reached Hamburg. In England the spread of the epidemic westwards across Europe had been witnessed with fear and trepidation and its occurrence at Hamburg stirred the population to take some action. The towns of England were in a filthy state; there was gross overcrowding, impure water supplies, and inadequate means for the disposal of sewage; in fact, many people drank out of the same streams into which was thrown the refuse and which drained the sewage from the houses. For the first time in England's history, cholera spread throughout the land, attacking many large towns including London, Newcastle, Hull, York, Leeds, and Sheffield. It lasted into 1833 and there were 14,796 cases with 5432 deaths recorded.

Cholera spread to other parts of Europe and it was not long before it had entered North America (in June, 1832), spreading to the north, south, and west. The disease smouldered on in Europe throughout the rest of the nineteenth century, breaking out into great conflagrations whenever conditions were especially favourable.

The dire effects of Asiatic cholera on the Continent had already stimulated the British Government to take action before it reached these shores. Central and Local Boards of Health were set up, in a consultative capacity only, and rules were drawn up to try to prevent the entry of the disease into the country and to deal with any outbreak which might occur.

The cholera epidemic reached the shores of Britain at Sunderland in October of 1831. Unfortunately, the Boards had no authority and suffered from financial difficulties. In order to combat cholera money was needed, and this had to be provided by public subscription; this was readily forthcoming whilst the epidemic raged, but after it was over people lapsed into the old *laissez-faire* attitude.

In 1831 the Boards of Health had recommended that towns should be divided into districts with a Medical Officer in charge of each, but the first permanent Medical Officer of Health in this country was Dr. Duncan, who was appointed in 1847 by the City of Liverpool. London followed in 1848 by appointing John Simon as its first Medical Officer of Health.

By compiling voluntary statistics from certain areas it was possible to arrive at some measure of the mortality caused by cholera. In William Farr's *Report on the Cholera Mortality in England 1848–9* there were 31,376 deaths in certain places in Great Britain with less than 5,250,000 inhabitants. The ravages of the disease were aptly described by Farr:—

If a foreign army had landed on the coast of England, seized all the seaports, sent detachments over the surrounding districts, ravaged the population through the summer, after having destroyed more than a thousand lives a day, for several days in succession, and in the year it held possession of the country, slain 53,293 men, women and children, the task of registering the dead would be unimpressibly painful, and the pain is not greatly diminished by the circumstance, that in the calamity to be described, the minister of destruction was a pestilence that spread over the face of the island and found in so many cities quick poisonous matter ready at hand to destroy the inhabitants.

However, these bare statistics do not tell us much about the great impact which cholera had on the lives of our ancestors. Let us remember that it was an unknown disease and had never before occurred in these islands, but there were plenty of stories of the horrors of the disease in the East. Gradually, as the dread pestilence spread westwards and the various reports of its progress reached these shores, a feeling of terror and panic must have been gradually rising in every town and village. Although frantic efforts were made to try to control the disease, unfortunately nobody knew the real cause. At first during the winter of 1831 the outbreaks were limited, due to the cold weather, but with the warm weather of the summer of 1832 cholera once more gained the ascendancy. Once it entered a town it burst out with explosive violence like a visitation from God, creating panic, terror, and despair. Since no one had experienced it before there was no natural immunity, and it spread through the people like fire through a field of corn.

Cholera in Exeter and Sheffield

There have been left to posterity several eyewitness accounts of the epidemic as it affected local towns. These are far more revealing than the dry statistics of William Farr.* The Rev. W. Leigh described the outbreaks at

---

* Dr. T. Mollison described the ravages of the disease as it occurred in Newcastle, Dr. J. Lizars added his observations relating to Edinburgh and the neighbouring district, and Dr. T. Acland did the same for Oxford.

Bilston in the Black Country where, out of a population of 14,700, 742 died in a few months in 1832. Dr. John Stokes, in a much later publication, delved into old parish records and produced an interesting account of cholera in Sheffield. The most remarkable of these local histories is a rare book written in 1849 by Dr. Thomas Shapter entitled *The History of the Cholera in Exeter, 1832*. Dr. Shapter was physician to the Devon and Exeter Hospital, the St. Thomas Hospital for Lunatics, and the Lying-in Charity Hospital. He played a prominent part in fighting the outbreak and wrote from first-hand experience. His account gives a vivid picture of the effect of an epidemic upon the life of a city. It could apply equally well to many diseases or to any other English town of the nineteenth century. Dr. Stokes's book, written in 1921, suffers from a lack of first-hand knowledge, and seems dry and uninteresting by the side of Dr. Shapter's, but, nevertheless, it enables one to draw some interesting comparisons between the two towns.

In 1832 Exeter had a population of 28,242. As in all English towns the sewerage and drainage were quite inadequate for the rapid growth of population which had taken place during the Industrial Revolution. The waterworks, though much improved, afforded an amount of water totally inadequate to the requirements of the people, while that from the wells and pumps was inapplicable to many domestic purposes. (*Figs.* 19, 20.) Much of the water used was, therefore, laboriously obtained by dipping it from the river or adjacent streams. This was an occupation which engaged, and was regularly pursued by, a large number of persons. The water was usually carried about in buckets, with a square or round piece of flat wood floating in each to prevent the water from splashing over; these buckets were suspended from a broad belt or strap across the shoulders by means of iron hooks at the ends, and kept apart by a hoop resting upon the upper rims, and against which the inner portions of the handles pressed. Water was carried to the more distant parts of the city in casks fixed upon small carts drawn by hand or by a donkey. The price paid by the consumer was one halfpenny a bucket-full. In the words of Dr. Shapter:—

This inadequate water supply, combined with the deficiency of drainage, is of itself sufficient evidence, that the necessary accommodation for the daily usages of the population must have been very limited. The fact is, that though in the houses of the wealthier this stain was removed, or in the process of removal, amongst the poorer population conveniences of this nature were almost entirely wanting. Doubtless, much of the filth of the lower parts of the City was thus rendered inevitable, but much was also voluntary and immediately remediable. The extent to which it obtained, and the mischief produced thereby, could now scarcely be credited, and such as was not supposed, even at that time, to exist. The Reports of the District Committees detail a state of things beyond all belief—to enter upon these would be tedious, if not disgusting —suffice it is to say, they speak of dwellings occupied by from five to fifteen families, huddled together in dirty rooms with every offensive accompaniment; of slaughter-houses in the Butcher Row, with their putrid heaps of offal; of pigs in large numbers kept throughout the City; the note appended to the description of one house states, 'thirty-one pigstyes kept in such a state as would beggar description', and similar notes are frequent; of poultry kept in confined cellars and outhouses; of dung-heaps every-where—one courtlage was visited in which the accumulated filth and soil of thirteen

79

years was deposited, and esteemed so valuable a property, that its removal was strenuously resisted. To add to all this, in many parts, the visits of the scavengers took place but once a week. While the general characteristics of the City were those of health and pleasantness, such was the prevailing condition of the lower and neglected portions.

Sheffield, with a population of 91,692, was in a similar state; such sewers as existed were leaky and inefficient, so that the soil had been choked for years with sewage. In the thickly populated areas the people lived mostly in back-to-back houses. Sheffield was more fortunate than Exeter in that it had an abundant supply of water from the many streams which flowed from the Pennines, and with the growth of the cutlery trade adequate reservoirs had been provided to supply the needs of the industry. Many houses in the better parts of the city were provided with standpipes, but there were still many householders drawing their water from shallow wells liable to contamination from the sewage-soaked soil. Others drew their water direct from the Don and other small rivers. During the seventeenth century a small reservoir was formed at Barker's Pool. This is now in the centre of the town, with a taxi rank and two large cinemas. The state of the town can be judged from an amusing account taken from the autobiography of Samuel Roberts in 1849:—

> About once every quarter, the water was let out of Barker's Pool, to run down all those streets into which it could be turned, for the purpose of cleansing them. The bellman gave notice of the exact time, and the favoured streets were all bustle, with a row of men, women, and children, on each side of the channel, anxiously and joyfully awaiting, with mops, brooms, and pails, the arrival of the cleansing flood, whose first appearance was announced by a loud continuous shout: all below was anxious expectation—all above a most amusing scene of bustling animation. Some people were throwing the water up against their houses and windows; some raking the garbage out of the kennels; some washing their pigs; some sweeping the pavement; youngsters throwing the waters over their companions, or pushing them into the widespread torrent. Meanwhile a constant Babel-like uproar, mixed with the barking of dogs and the grunting of pigs, was heard above and below, till the waters, after about half an hour, had become exhausted. Such was the mode in which the town was in those days kept clean.
>
> There was a supply of water brought for about a mile to the town, but the quantity was small, pipes being laid in only a few of the principal streets. A receptacle was made for this in Townhead Street from which it was the business of a number of men to take it in casks, fixed on the body of a wheelbarrow, holding about fifty gallons, to all parts of the town to sell.

There seems to have been little to choose between Sheffield and Exeter, except that the former had a more abundant and certainly purer water-supply. Such then were the sanitary circumstances of two great cities, one an ancient county capital, the other a growing and prosperous northern manufacturing town.

After the first cases of cholera had been reported in Sunderland, the Central Board of Health drew up certain rules and regulations for the control of the disease. They indicate the general opinions prevailing at the time. The chief items were as follows:—

1. After stating that the approach of the disease to neighbouring shores involved increased caution, it recommended that all persons should aid in carrying out most strictly the quarantine regulations, and that every persuasion

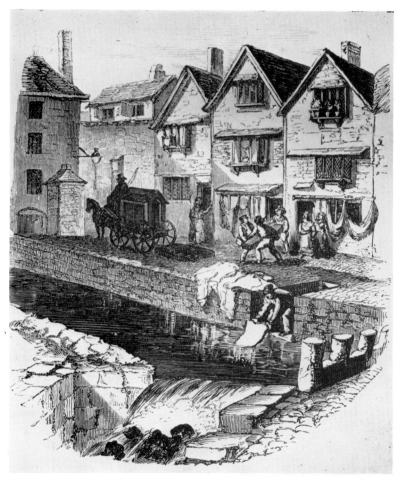

Fig. 19.—A patient has just died of cholera. As his body is carried out, infected bed linen is washed in the stream which supplies water to the town (Exeter).

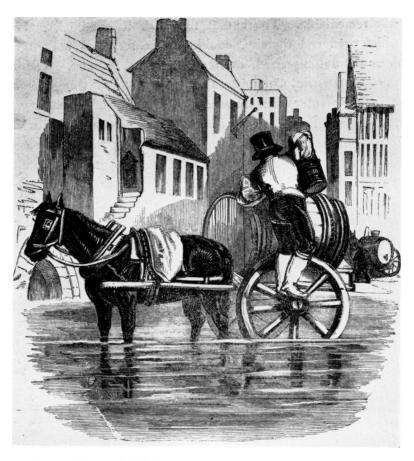

Fig. 20.—The spread of cholera. Drawing polluted water for drinking (Exeter).

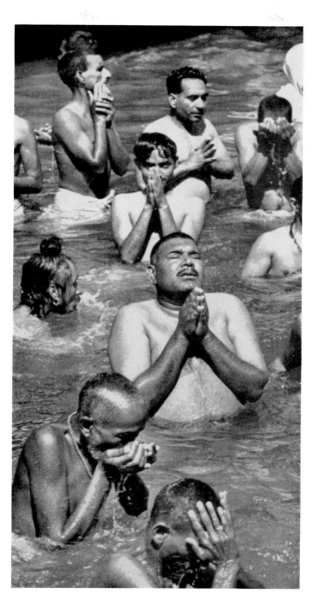

Fig. 21.—The spread of cholera. Men bathing at Kumbh festival, India, and drinking polluted water.

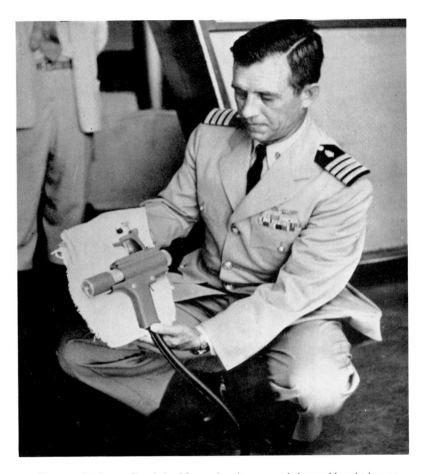

Fig. 22.—Cholera at Bangkok. Men and nations around the world rushed emergency aid to the people of Thailand as an epidemic of cholera threatened that nation in May, 1958. Millions of doses of vaccine, modern medical equipment, and technical advisers were airlifted to Thailand until the emergency was under control. A new hypospray jet injector flown to Thailand to fight the cholera epidemic inoculates painlessly twenty times faster than by the usual hypodermic needle.

should be used to induce those living near the coast to forgo intercourse with smugglers.

2. That in every town and village local Boards of Health should be formed, of which 'one of the medical members should be appointed to correspond with the Board of Health in London'.

3. That early information of the occurrence of the disease should be given.

4. That in order to effect the separation of the sick, houses for their reception should be procured, but that in case they should refuse to be removed, 'a conspicuous mark ("Sick") should be placed in front of the house, to warn persons that it is in quarantine; and even when persons with the disease shall have been removed, and the house shall have been purified, the word "Caution" should be substituted, as denoting suspicions of the disease; and the inhabitants of such house should not be at liberty to move out or communicate with other persons until by the authority of the local Board the mark shall have been removed'.

5. That houses where the disease had occurred should be purified, as also the goods, for the effecting of which the means were detailed; some of these latter were directed to be burnt. General cleanliness was much inculcated.

6. Detached burying-grounds were to be provided, and the 'nurses should live apart from the rest of the community'.

7. Where removal of the sick from the healthy cannot be effected, all unnecessary communication should be avoided with the public out of doors; all articles of food, or other necessaries required by the family, should be placed in front of the house, and received by one of the inhabitants of the house, after the person delivering them shall have retired.

8. Convalescents, and those who had had any communication with the sick, should be kept 'under observation' at least for twenty days; and the reporting of the occurrence of the disease was enjoined.

9. All intercourse with any infected town was to be prevented.

10. And if necessary, 'troops, or a strong body of police', might be used for this purpose.

The order then stated that the dissipated, ill-fed, and badly lodged were the principal victims of cholera, and that ill-drained, ill-ventilated places were its chief seats, and recommended attention to those subjects. To this was appended a very graphic description of the disease, with some short suggestions on its medical management.

These rules were displayed in public places in the city of Exeter on 23 Oct., 1831. They were printed in the *Sheffield Courant* on 28 Oct., 1831. The Mayor of Exeter called a meeting of magistrates and physicians at the Guildhall on 27 Oct. From then on there were numerous meetings and conferences, and by 1 Nov., 1831, Exeter had already formed a Local Board of Health as recommended by the Central Board.

These Local Boards were set up all over the country, but as there was no system of Local Government as we know it today and no organized means of carrying out the measures advised, their effectiveness was limited. Local Government was a chaos of area, a chaos of authorities, and a chaos of rates.

Moreover, there was no knowledge of how cholera was spread and the most fantastic hypotheses were advanced. In Exeter, for example, 7695 flannel belts were made to ward off the evil. Needless to say, they were not of the slightest value. Despite these seemingly unsurmountable difficulties, however, it was remarkable what was achieved by voluntary effort.

In Exeter a sum of £4082 14s. 9d. was raised by voluntary subscriptions, a sum larger than that raised in any other city. In addition, the Corporations of the Poor and the Guardians of the Poor paid out £1833 for the relief of persons rendered destitute by the epidemic. Sheffield raised the paltry sum of £34 16s. 1½d. from collections at churches and chapels, but it was the Overseers of the Poor who had to bear the brunt of the cost (£2662).

In Exeter general directions were given for cleansing the city, but it was difficult to achieve very much without widespread structural alterations and improvements involving the expenditure of large sums of money. Arrangements were made for watering the streets and for the removal of refuse, but the facilities available were quite inadequate for the purpose. There were numerous meetings involving many acrimonious disputes throughout the winter of 1831–2 and local feeling ran high.

On 13 July, 1832, cases of cholera were reported from Plymouth and on 19 July it became generally known throughout the city that cases of cholera had occurred during the previous night and morning. The weather had been fine and sunny and very little sickness prevailed, but in this last respect how sudden was the change. From this time the disease spread rapidly, reaching a peak in August and rapidly declining in September. The last cases were recorded on 27 Oct., by which time there had been some 400 deaths from the disease. At first there was panic and many people left the city. This is aptly described by Dr. Shapter:—

> The general silence of the city, save when broken by the tolling of the funeral bell, and which, as mentioned in a former page, was eventually silenced, was most remarkable; the streets were deserted, the hurried steps of the medical men and their assistants, or of those running to seek their aid, alone were heard, while the one-horse hearse, occasionally passing on its duty, was almost the only carriage to be seen in the usually busy streets. The desolation which reigned has always been most strongly marked on my mind, by the astonishment and singular feeling which engrossed me on witnessing, as the disease was subsiding, two gaily-dressed females emerge from one of the principal shops in the Highstreet; so foreign and unusual were they to the scene, and distracting to the train of thought that had so long absorbed one, that I found myself unconsciously pondering over and speculating upon what they could be doing, or why they should be there.
>
> Amid this desolation, the profligacy and drunkenness of the lower orders increased to such an alarming extent, as to become a matter of public remark and censure. Much of this vice was induced, not only by the general excitement prevailing, but by an idea that brandy was a preventive and panacea for the Cholera; and amongst the lower orders nothing was undertaken without previously resorting to it.

The outbreak in Sheffield was of a much shorter duration; it was probably brought to the town by a visitor from Thorne who died from the disease, and the epidemic started on 8 July, 1832; it reached its peak in July and was over by 3 Aug. During this time there were about 400 deaths from the disease.

In Exeter in the first instance additional medical assistants were appointed to deal with the disease. There were 1135 cases reported and probably many more minor cases. A special cholera house was eventually acquired, not without some difficulty, but was later abandoned because of strong opposition from those living in the vicinity. A house was also procured for receiving relatives of those who had died from the disease.

Two members of the medical profession were on duty throughout the night at the Guildhall to answer emergency calls. They were provided with two carriages and a man to attend them. The Corporation of the Poor hired twenty-four extra nurses but this was quite inadequate and they had to advertise for more by means of the town criers. This involved the city in the expense of 3s., as shown by the following bill:—

Exeter, August 11, 1832.

ISAAC SPRATT, City Crier.

	s.	d.
Cried for the gentlemen of the Board of Health to obtain Nurses for the Cholera patients	1	6
Ditto second time	1	6
	3	0

Nurses were paid the sum of 2s. 6d. weekly, the total cost to the city for the services of nurses being £270 8s. 6d.

The provision of separate burial grounds was rendered necessary from the situations and crowded states of the existing ones. There was considerable difficulty, as the following quotation shows:—

A Committee of the Corporation of the Poor immediately proceeded to Little Bury Meadow, and having there staked out a piece of ground, . . . for the purpose of a burial-ground for persons dying of Cholera, deputed their Chairman to wait on the Mayor of Exeter as chairman of the Board of Health, and inform him thereof.

On this, some circumstances worthy of passing note occurred: under the impression that the above portion of ground was now dedicated to the purpose of a Cholera burial-ground, an order was given that the body of a person then lying dead of Cholera, should be there interred, and the grave-digger was accordingly directed to proceed with the necessary arrangements. The parishioners of St. David's, having felt generally aggrieved at this appropriation of ground in their parish, rose in tumult, and somewhat of a riot ensued—the grave-digger's webs were cut to pieces, his tools scattered abroad, he himself assaulted, and eventually obliged to fly; while the warden of the parish retained many persons in his own house during the night, in order to prevent any further attempt at the interment. It was however evident, on consideration, that this was not yet a legally constituted burial-ground, and the interment of this body therein was consequently abandoned. It took place early the following morning in the Bartholomew-yard, but it was with the greatest difficulty the men employed to assist could be prevailed on to enter upon their duty. On the coffin appearing in the street supported by webs 'underhand', great indignation arose, and the procession proceeded followed by a large concourse of turbulent persons, and attended, amidst swearing, hooting, and abuse, with much confusion and excitement.

There was also considerable local opposition over the method of burial. The usual mode in which the bodies of the poorer classes of persons had been carried to the grave was on the shoulders of bearers. The opinions and feelings entertained of the nature of the disease rendered this course objectionable, and the first few that died were carried 'underhand'. This gave great offence to the people, not only as being contrary to custom, but from their esteeming it a mark of ignominy and disrespect. The Corporation of the Poor were therefore induced to procure a hearse to be specially devoted to those dying of cholera, and on 24 July, in somewhat quaint and characteristic terms, they resolved 'that a close conveyance, properly pitched, be provided at the expense of this Corporation, and placed on a carriage to be drawn by one horse, for the purpose of conveying paupers dying of Cholera to the burial-ground, and that the Assistant Treasurer do provide proper persons to assist at such burials, and that such conveyance be deposited (when not in use) at the burial-ground'. A shed for this purpose was then erected in the Bartholomew-yard. (In Sheffield the same difficulties arose; they called their hearse the cholera basket.) Unfortunately one hearse was insufficient; the question of a second hearse was discussed.

This second hearse formed a topic of much discussion and of many resolutions. It was eventually procured by and at the expense of the Board of Health, but then arose the question, who was to maintain it, i.e., provide the horse and the driver, and where was it to be kept? On 27 Aug., at a meeting of the Ward Committee, it was reported 'that the Board of Health have this day undertaken to pay every expense of the second hearse on every Monday morning through their treasurer', and a communication from the said Board of Health having been read requesting this Committee to appoint where the said hearse should be kept, it was resolved 'that the said Board be respectfully informed that this Committee are of opinion the second hearse should be kept in a place to be provided by the Board of Health in the second Cholera burial ground'. This was accordingly done, and the shed erected in the Bartholomew-yard was removed thence to the Pester-lane ground.

The graves of those dying of cholera were dug to an extra depth of not less than 6 feet. An order was at the same time given that, when filled in, the surface mound should be covered over with a layer of lime. The effect of this on passing by the burial-grounds was very startling; the white lime conspicuously pointed out the numerous deaths that had occurred, the more so as none was buried in the same grave, except in the case of husband and wife or children. Seeing how much people were shocked at this, the practice was abandoned, and it was subsequently ordered (2 Aug.) that the graves should be dug from 8 to 10 feet, and that the lime should be placed over the coffin. The resolution of the Corporation of the Poor on this point runs thus: 'that the Assistant Treasurer be directed from time to time to purchase such quantities of lime as may be required for putting into graves, with the bodies of Cholera patients who may be interred at the expense of the Corporation of the Poor, in order the better to prevent infection arising from the interment of such bodies'.

Because of the frequency of the funerals the grave-digger and his usual assistant were obliged to procure extra aid. The men hired for this purpose could only be kept at work by high bribes and the persuasion of frequent draughts of beer and brandy, and then, when half drunk, would rarely do more than assist in digging the graves; they almost invariably refused to touch the coffins, or even to go near to them; the two sextons were for the most part themselves obliged to do all that was necessary towards placing them in the graves. A not unusual scene in the burial-ground, at this season, was two men without coats, their shirt sleeves turned up to the elbows, with short tobacco pipes in their mouths, carrying a coffin 'underhand' towards the grave; at a good distance off from the grave was the surpliced clergyman performing the last solemn duty of religion. If this were by night, as frequently was the case, there was also the flickering light of one or two lanterns. Such was the scene on 16 Aug. when the last burial of a person dying of cholera took place in the Bartholomew-yard. The circumstances accompanying this funeral are not devoid of interest; it took place at midnight, the moon shone bright and calm, and when the grave was filled in the old grave-digger placed over it the oldest tombstone in the yard; it was a blue stone, and had for two centuries covered, near where was situated the lower seat in the town wall, the last resting place of one 'Salathiel Jennings', whose remains were amongst the earliest in this burial-ground, having been there interred shortly after its consecration by Bishop Hall, on 24 Aug., 1637.

The sum of £117 19s. 10d. is stated to have been expended in making the graves of an increased depth; the price paid appears to have been after the following rate: for a grave of 6 feet deep, 5s.; for one of 8 feet, 11s. 2d.; and for one of 10 feet, 15s.

The general aspect of the city of Exeter, as may well be supposed, was gloomy in the extreme, and it was much heightened by the discordant tolling of the different church bells, which incessantly broke upon the silence that otherwise reigned in the deserted streets. This was felt to be so great and unnecessary an evil, and was so much complained of, that at length the Board of Health interfered, and on 16 Aug. 'recommended to the clergy that the tolling of the bells in the different churches for deaths or funerals be discontinued for the present'. This request was to a great extent complied with.

With a view to preventing the spread of the disease, various means had been suggested by the Orders in Council, such as fumigations, the use of chloride of lime, whitewashing, general cleansing, the destruction of the clothes of those who had died, etc., many of which were very fully adopted. In compliance with the Order of 13 Dec., 1831, the bodies of those who died of cholera were, on its first occurrence, directed to be enveloped in cotton or linen saturated with pitch or coal-tar. This proved, however, so serious an annoyance to the other inmates of the house, especially to those who might be then ill, that it was immediately abandoned.

Fumigations of different kinds were freely used, and by a resolution of 3 Aug. the Corporation of the Poor recommended to the Mayor and the Board of Health 'the lighting of fires with tar, and tar barrels broken to pieces, in the most confined parts of the City, in order to purify the air during the present diseased state of the City'. On the first signs of the disease the burning of a tar barrel was not unusually to be met with. Vinegar was also burnt. Chloride of lime was very freely resorted to, at times inconveniently, if not injudiciously, so. Some idea of the extent to which this material was used may be appreciated from the fact that in one day (3 Aug.) the Corporation of the Poor stated that 'they have distributed it to 500 persons, and that they have a large quantity ready for delivery at their station-house', while nearly 8 cwt. was distributed by the Board of Health, besides that which was procured and consumed by private persons, and which, as its use was universal, must have been a very large amount.

The mode in which the clothes, etc., were destroyed was by burning during the first fortnight or so, and afterwards by burying them in pits with quicklime. On receiving proper directions the inspectors resorted to the houses indicated to them, and examined, condemned, valued, and removed such of the clothes as they thought should be destroyed. For the latter purpose a hand-cart, covered over with canvas, in order not to alarm passers-by, was chiefly used; but at the lower part of the town, and contiguous to the river, a boat, purchased specifically for this object, was also employed. The goods at first destroyed consisted of bedsteads, bedding, and wearing apparel. The compensation paid for them amounted to a very large sum. The following shows the nature and character of the bills rendered on this account:—

4 Sept., 1833.

Goods destroyed belonging to Mr. Coombs, whose two children died:

	£.	s.	d.
1 Sheet	0	4	0
1 Quilt	0	7	0
2 Blankets	0	8	0
1 Bed (down)	0	6	6
2 Pillows, bolster, and cases	0	7	6
To a crate and stand	0	3	6
To three men for taking the corpses to the burial ground	0	7	6
To destroying goods	0	5	0
	2	9	0

Clothes were also washed in the river and this was of course a very sure way of spreading the infection (*see Fig.* 19).

A special Provision Committee was appointed to distribute bread and meat, 1 lb. of beef or mutton and 2 lb. of bread to each person. Food tickets were provided with the following instructions:—

Directions to Distributors

No person or family to be supplied with more than one ticket in the same day.

Any person or family having received relief through the tickets of the Board of Health, cannot receive any further relief except from the hands of the gentleman who originally supplied them—or by the transfer of his authority.

The following trades-people are appointed under the authority of the Committee to supply provisions:-

Butchers	Bakers
Mr. G. C. Brown, Butcher Row	Mr. Flood, St. Sidwell's.
G. Taverner, ditto.	Horwill, ditto.
Allen, North Street.	Cuthbertson, South Street.
Manley, St. Sidwell's.	Ocock, High Street.
Batten, ditto.	Woodman, North Street.
	Ratcliffe, Fore Street Hill.

This charity was, however, most grossly abused by the indiscriminate and injudicious distribution of the bread and meat tickets. It was ascertained, amongst other instances of a like kind, that upwards of 40 lb. of meat had in one day been given to the inhabitants of one small lodging-house. The amount of food thus distributed may be appreciated by the cost incurred on this account between 11 and 31 Aug., amounting to £721 4s.

Soup kitchens were also set up. At the height of the epidemic about £20 in bread and £40 in soup were being expended weekly, and in one month 13,120 quarts of soup and 10,300 provision tickets were distributed. The cost amounted to £1831 10s. 6d.

There was, of course, a great deal of unemployment and poverty as a result of the almost complete stoppage of trade; as a result a system of district visiting was introduced giving a complete history of poverty and need in the city.

The return of the destitute poor in Exeter gives some interesting facts about the effect of the cholera on the domestic life of the family. The following is one extract:—

No. 16. Schoolmaster, age 41, and wife and 5 children. Average earnings of the family, weekly 4/-; rent 5/- per week; parochial relief 4/-. Industrious people, their goods seized for rent, having lost their school during the Cholera.

The disease sometimes killed with extreme rapidity as the following quotations show:—

A large, tall, powerful man, a bargeman (J. D., 1 Aug.), left his home early in the morning apparently in good health; while at work on the river he was taken ill, came home, died that evening, and on the following morning was buried in the clothes he had worn at the time he left home, and which had never been removed from him. A little lad (H. H., 7 Aug.), led by idle curiosity, followed the hearse to a house where it stopped, and then crept into it: he was taken home and died within seven hours. An undertaker (J. B., 12 Aug.) made a coffin for a person who died at Westgate, and put the body into it: he himself died the same day. A respectable tradesman (J. N., 6 Sept.) was taken ill while out shooting, was brought home and died. As an illustration of mere rapidity, the instance of a man (T. H., 13 Aug.) may be quoted, who was taken ill, died, and was buried on the same day. Another occurred in a man (E. M., 14 Aug.) who was taken ill early in the morning when preparing to go to work, and died in the course of the day; the rapidity of this man's death was strongly marked by the firkins, which he had that morning filled with cider to supply the anticipated wants of the day, standing as he had filled them by the side of his coffin.

Many similar examples of the extreme rapidity of the disease might be mentioned, but its appalling character was more strongly marked by the numbers lying dead in the same houses at one time. On 7 Aug. there were five so lying dead in Sun-lane; on 19 Aug. there were three in the building then known as Russell's Barracks, and on 20 Aug. four in a house in Gandy-street.

The consideration and kindness of the poor towards each other at this period was, as is usually the case in illness and difficulty, most marked and praiseworthy; they were generally willing to render to each other every assistance. A few examples to the contrary, however, occurred amongst them, some which are most affecting to contemplate. The death of one poor woman (J. W., 28 Aug.), who was in an advanced state of pregnancy, was much contributed to, if not caused, by the most wilful neglect. Another poor female (A. C., 11 Aug.) died with her nameless offspring at her breast, unassisted by her mother and sister, who, regardless of her safety, and seeking solely their own, were rendering the air unbreathable by burning tar in the room; this sister was a violent and loose character, and had been a chief promoter and agent in the disturbances of the season. But the most lamentable and unnatural instance of neglect which happened was that of some children by their father: this man, who resided in St. Sidwell's, having bedding and ample accommodation, placed his two dying children (H. and S. L., 22 Aug.) on the landing of the staircase upon straw and there they both died; his sole reason for this inhumanity being the saving of his goods.

In Sheffield, the burial ground was marked by the building of a cholera memorial, where it still stands at Claywood, near Norfolk Park, to commemorate the 400 who died from cholera, amongst them the then Master Cutler, the late John Blake.

Sheffield came in for some rough treatment from the *Leeds Mercury*, which printed the following:—

> The disease, which was very mild here at first, has, we are sorry to say, become very alarming and extensive in its ravages. There is, we understand, nothing strange in this, for Sheffield is a town in which there is generally great intemperance; the first two days of the week being by very many of the workmen spent in idleness and dissipation. We trust this vice will receive a check by the awful disease now prevailing there.

The impact of the disease was greater in Exeter (400 deaths in a population of 28,242, as against 400 in Sheffield with a much larger population of 91,692).

Such, then, were the scenes which were witnessed in many of our towns and villages little more than a hundred years ago. The same story had no doubt been repeated many times before, but men were now beginning to do more than accept things as an Act of God. Dr. Shapter, who has written such an excellent account of the impact of a new disease on a small city, did not really contribute anything to our knowledge on its mode of spread. His account has been dealt with in some detail because it illustrates so vividly the widespread effects of epidemics on public and family life and the frantic attempts which were made to deal with the problem. The description refers to cholera, but it might well have applied to plague, typhus, yellow fever, or small-pox.

The chief recommendation resulting from the outbreak was that a better supply of water should be found to cleanse the dirty streets. Exeter suffered more than Sheffield in this respect. But it was many years before a pure water-supply was provided, and further outbreaks of cholera occurred.

Dr. Shapter studied the causes of the outbreak in Exeter in great detail and after taking everything into consideration finally came to the conclusion that 'Asiatic cholera is essentially an epidemic chiefly due to aerial influences'. He was way off the track and yet, strangely enough, two delightful little sketches which he himself drew and which illustrate his book provide the answer. They are shown in *Figs.* 19 and 20. One illustrates a coffin being carried from a house where an occupant has died from cholera; soiled sheets are being washed in the stream. The second illustration shows water being drawn from the same stream for distribution as drinking water. Here is a clear demonstration of one way in which infection is spread.

THE CAUSE OF CHOLERA

There were pandemics of cholera in 1852, 1863, 1881, and 1899 which spread throughout most of the world, but the great centre of cholera was still India along the banks of the mighty Ganges river. The pilgrimages to Mecca were the occasion for great outbreaks of the disease, as in 1831, in 1846, and in 1865; the last great outbreak occurred in Mecca in 1912.

In 1892 cholera broke out in Hamburg from the distribution of unfiltered water from the Elbe. This was the last great epidemic in western Europe and by the turn of the century cholera had virtually disappeared from the western world, although there have been outbreaks in eastern Europe, particularly in Russia, the last great epidemic there being in 1921–2.

In general, cholera has attacked all parts of the world, with the exception of the most northerly and most southerly places, such as Northern Siberia, Lapland, Iceland, Norway, the Faroes, Shetland, the Orkneys, the Hebrides, Newfoundland, Northern Canada, Greenland, South Africa, Chile, Argentina, the Falkland Islands, and also some isolated islands such as St. Helena, Ascension, and Bermuda.

India is still the home of cholera and the disease now causes many more deaths there than plague. The most important centre is Bengal, but there are other important centres in Madras and also in the Yangtse valley in China. There have been over 14,000,000 deaths from cholera recorded during the present century.* In the period 1939–48 there were 200,000 deaths from cholera as against 22,000 from plague. Obviously plague is coming under effective control in India, but not cholera. So far there have been no signs of a satisfactory decrease and there is required urgently an easy and efficient method of control.

We have seen that each world pandemic of cholera from 1817 onwards has originated in India. The great focus of infection, the home of cholera, has been and still is in the delta region of the two great rivers, the Ganges and Brahmaputra. These are densely populated low-lying areas near the coast.

The great danger in India is caused by the annual religious pilgrimages to the numerous shrines. Each year something like 20,000,000 people make long journeys of this kind, and in so doing spread the disease over large areas. The sanitary arrangements along the routes and at the shrines are appalling, the ritual often demanding that the pilgrims should bathe in the waters of some river. These rivers are running sewers taking the excreta and filth of millions of human beings. Many rivers also supply the communal drinking water. Small wonder, then, that infection can be spread so easily and so quickly.

There is a marked seasonal incidence, the disease being most common during the hot summer months. It is clearly transmitted by human beings. Thus it has travelled through Persia along the caravan routes by the great rivers of India and the Middle East, the Ganges, Brahmaputra, Euphrates, and Tigris. Pilgrims travelling by sea carried it eastwards and westwards to Mecca, Arabia, and Syria, and along the Volga through Russia. In islands the disease first appeared at a seaport, introduced by an infected patient or his soiled linen. One of the marked features of the disease is the copious watery

---

* We can begin to understand what these figures mean in terms of human misery and suffering when we compare them with the 400 deaths in the Exeter epidemic.

diarrhoea, so that the bed linen is always soiled. In this way it has been very easy for the hands of an attendant to become contaminated, and if he does not wash them, and then prepares food, the infection can be easily spread by the eating of this food. More often, however, the infection has been spread by the drinking of water which has been contaminated with the excreta from a cholera patient. The death-rate in epidemics was very high and death often occurred quickly, in some cases within twenty-four hours of infection.

DR. SNOW IN SOHO

Dr. John Snow first proved this method of spread in the Broad Street Pump epidemic of 1854 and a description of his investigations gives a revealing picture of the conditions prevalent in London at that time.* This outbreak of cholera was most prevalent in the part of London we now call Soho; the chief localities affected were Golden Square, Berwick Street, Wardour Street, Dean Street, Marylebone Street, Tickfield Street, Great Windmill Street, and Brewer Street. The number of people in this 'cholera area' was 14,000 and during the epidemic 618 died from the disease. Broad Street (now Broadwick Street) was in the centre of this area and consisted of 49 houses. There was considerable overcrowding, most houses holding several families, and in one house there were 54 persons. The outbreak began in earnest on the night of Thursday, 31 Aug., 1854, although there had been a few cases recorded before that. Within a 250-yards' radius of the junction of Cambridge Street and Broadwick Street there were 500 deaths in 10 days. The havoc was greatest in the most overcrowded areas; in one house, a whole family was wiped out, father, mother, and 4 children, and in others, only a single child survived. Panic seized the inhabitants and within a week of the beginning of the outbreak 80 per cent of the inhabitants had left. This certainly limited the mortality locally. There were 79 deaths in the first two days of September, all in people drawing water from the Broad Street Pump. The water was used in the local coffee shops, eating houses, and public houses for washing crockery and preparing food; it was also used in neighbouring shops for making sherbet drinks. The keeper of one local coffee shop told Dr. Snow that she knew of 9 of her regular customers who were dead from the disease. Many of those who had fled the district also died later from the disease in other parts of the country.

Out of 97 persons who escaped the cholera, 87 did not drink the communal well water at all; the other 10 only took it in small amounts, as, for example, in spirits. Further evidence was provided by the experience of two factories; one had its own well and none of its employees drank the Broad Street water; there were no deaths here; the other factory, which employed 9 men, drew its drinking water from the Broad Street well; 7 died from cholera and 2 had

---

* John Snow was born in 1813. A Yorkshire man, he became an articled pupil to a Newcastle surgeon at the age of 14 years, and in 1836 he went to study at the Westminster Hospital; he qualified in medicine in 1838. He was well known as an anaesthetist and attended in this role at the birth of some of Queen Victoria's children.

diarrhoea. One stranger to the district in good health had dinner in a Wardour Street restaurant and died from cholera within a few hours after drinking water from the well with his meal. Another visitor from Brighton visited No. 6 Poland Street to see his brother, who died shortly afterwards from cholera. The visitor stayed twenty minutes, drinking a glass of brandy diluted with water from the pump. He was dead the next evening. The following story is most revealing.

A lady at Hampstead used to have water from the Broad Street well brought daily to her in a bottle, because she thought it was very good for her. She drank this water on 31 Aug. and 1 Sept. and died on 2 Sept. There was no cholera at all in Hampstead at the time. Her niece who was on a visit from Islington also drank the water and died from cholera.

Dr. Snow found that there were 70 employees in a brewery in Broad Street. They all drank beer in preference to water, but the teetotallers got their water from a well in the brewery. Not one of these men suffered from the disease. He plotted the location of each case and showed that the incidence fell as the distance from the pump decreased. By his painstaking inquiries and logical deductions he had collected an impressive weight of evidence implicating the pump as the cause of the outbreak. On 8 Sept., on the advice of Dr. Snow, the pump handle was removed at a time when the number of cases of cholera was already falling rapidly. There was considerable opposition to this at the time, since the water had a very high reputation locally, as evidenced by 'the lady from Hampstead'. Some thought the cause was due to smells from bad drains (it is strange that even today people have the same idea). Others put it down to the old Plague Pit in Little Marlborough Street, where plague victims had been buried 200 years before.

Now to a consideration of the well itself; it was a shallow well, 30 ft. deep, in gravelly soil which was pervious to water and sewage, situated close to No. 40 Broad Street. The main drain of No. 40 Broad Street was defective and the sewage from the house was percolating through the soil. This led to further excavations, and a defective cesspool was found, also leaking into the porous soil all around the well. It was clear that sewage from No. 40 Broad Street had been contaminating the well for years. The side of the defective drain was only 32 in. from the brickwork of the well. The brickwork of the cesspool, drain, and well was decayed and leaking like a sieve. Chemical analysis of the water showed it to be highly contaminated. It had a great reputation because it was cold and sparkling, but it soon lost its sparkle and developed a film, and if left for two or three days became quite offensive; this is a characteristic feature of sewage-contaminated water. Cesspools existed in large numbers in the area; thus when Derby Court, Piccadilly, was demolished, no less than thirty-two cesspools were found. They were usually forgotten and the brickwork in various stages of decay; the slightest blockage of flow caused overflow and contamination of cellar and subsoil with sewage. There were many shallow wells in the area, all liable to pollution in the same way. The people of Soho had been drinking sewage-contaminated water for years. It was obvious that sewage alone did not cause cholera; how then was the specific infection introduced ? Dr. Snow's inquiries gave the answer; he found that on 28 Aug. a 5-month-old baby living in No. 40 Broad Street was attacked with disease; the soiled napkins were washed in a bucket, the contents of which were poured into the privy and thence into the cesspool. Where the baby acquired the infection is not known, but there had been odd cases in the district for several weeks. The massive contamination of the well with the specific organism of the disease was the cause of the sudden explosive outbreak.

The Committee of Inquiry appointed to investigate the outbreak recommended that shallow wells should be abolished altogether and that water should be provided by main supplies. Although it was many years before this ideal state of affairs was universal, it was the first time that the spread of water-borne disease had been shown to be due to specific contamination of a water-supply by an agent present in the excreta of people suffering from the disease. It was many years afterwards (in 1886) that Robert Koch demonstrated the live vibrio of cholera as the infective agent responsible.

As a result of this inquiry towns all over the country gradually improved the quality of their water-supply until today we can say with confidence that water-borne epidemics have been wiped out in our cities.* Our story is not yet finished, however, because as soon as cholera disappeared, men forgot and lapsed into their old careless attitude, exemplified in a leader in *The Times*, commenting on a debate in the House of Commons, 31 July, 1854, which said that 'the English people would prefer to take the chance of cholera and the rest rather than be bullied into health'.

CHOLERA IN INDIA

The people of India still have epidemics of cholera as a result of religious rituals which provide opportunities for the specific contamination of their drinking water with the cholera vibrio. Their shrines have been set up to their own gods. In London we can visit a shrine which immortalizes Dr. John Snow and his fundamental discovery which was responsible for the elimination of cholera in England: where the famous pump once stood there is now a public house called the 'Dr. John Snow' in Broadwick Street, Soho. The inn sign is a painting of the famous man and inside there are some relics of his life. As you examine them you can quench your thirst with a glass of best bitter, and know that your health will not suffer as a result!

Recent work has added to our knowledge of cholera but has not really changed the original concept of its mode of spread. The commonest mode of infection is by ingesting contaminated water; uncooked fruit and vegetables are potent sources of infection in the East, as they may have been washed in infected water. Flies are certainly important carriers of the disease from infected faeces to food, as they are of dysentery and other intestinal infection.

---

* This is not necessarily true of country districts where attacks of 'tummy' trouble in the summer are often put down to eating green apples. These are usually due to drinking infected water from unsafe shallow wells.

Personal susceptibility plays an important part. Everard Napier described an incident in a children's hospital which demonstrated this in a remarkable manner; 6 children were infected, 2 died from cholera, 2 had diarrhoea, and 2 remained healthy, but all passed cholera organisms in their excreta. Clearly such cases can play their part in keeping the infection spreading throughout the people of the world. No doubt the dosage of organisms has something to do with it, in addition to such factors as starvation and debility from other causes. In the 1831 epidemic it was noticed frequently that the highest mortality occurred in the poor. The organism survives on clothes from 1 to 3 days and will survive for some days in water, particularly in the warmer months of summer.

Cholera is found in the poor and malnourished, not only because they are less resistant to infection but also because they search for food everywhere, in filthy rubbish heaps and garbage bins. If there is only one well in a village, which is often safer than the river water, then the depressed classes are not allowed to use it, nor can they afford the bucket and rope which are necessary to draw water from the well. Consequently the weak, the sick, the poor, and the elderly must drink from the heavily polluted river. The river is particularly liable to give infection because it is here that the soiled clothes and linen of sick persons are washed; also people go to the edge of the river to defaecate and use the sludge from the river bank for cleansing and polishing their brass drinking vessels. I remember one village in India where I was told that the villagers preferred the taste of the river water which they had drunk from time immemorial to that of the clean water from the new well that had been provided for them. It is remarkable that in India people have little knowledge concerning the cause of cholera; they think that the disease is due to the wrath of the gods and that it can be prevented by prayer and by offerings at the temple. Their age-old customs decree that persons who have died from cholera should be immersed in the river at dead of night and not burnt as is the usual custom; the body remains in the river and is consumed by the fish; in fact, infection may be maintained by fish in this way. In the morning people come to collect water from the same river. Pilgrimages to holy places are a marked feature of life in the East; one essential of many of the rituals is to drink and bathe in water from the holy river or lake (*Fig.* 21); under such conditions, cholera can easily become epidemic. Thus, because of the social habits of a community a preventable disease is not prevented. The proverb from Bosnia and the comment by *The Times* apply equally well in India.

Because it threatens world health the eradication of this focus of cholera is not just a problem for India. Accordingly the World Health Organization is giving all the help it can. (*Fig.* 22.) A cholera vaccine is available and has been widely used for protecting pilgrims journeying to Mecca and is compulsory for persons entering a cholera area. Unfortunately, immunity wanes after six months and the inoculation has to be repeated. In Egypt in the 1947 epidemic an attempt was made to inoculate the whole population of the country, about 20,000,000. Health education and propaganda can play their part by teaching all people in these areas to boil water* and to pay strict attention to personal cleanliness and hygiene, particularly when attending the sick. The most important measures are to frequently wash the hands, to protect all foods from flies, and never to eat uncooked food.

There have been no advances in the treatment of cholera in the last forty years; none of the new antibiotics seems to be of any value, and the death-rate can still be high (50–60 per cent) in severe clinical cases. In 1960, 12,500 deaths were recorded from the disease in the whole world. The main efforts at control must be directed to providing pure water-supplies in the villages in India, a costly and difficult business. Let us not forget that there are still unsafe water-supplies in many parts of Europe, especially in rural areas. It seems clear that gross contamination is really necessary for an epidemic of cholera; in the case of other water-borne diseases, however, even slight contamination can cause disaster. (*See* Pollitzer (1960) for a full account of cholera.)

---

* It is difficult to get villagers in India to boil water because fuel is scarce and expensive.

CHAPTER VIII

FOOD, FLIES, AND FILTH

TYPHOID fever has occurred from the earliest times when clinical cases of disease were first described by medical writers. Hippocrates evidently knew the disease and describes typical examples in his writings. It was often confused, however, with other continued fevers, such as the prevalent famine or jail fever which we now call typhus. Certain differences in behaviour had been noted by writers in the Middle Ages, but it was not until the nineteenth century that typhoid fever was first accurately described as a distinct clinical disease. This was due to the detailed analysis of the symptoms of these different fevers by Sir William Jenner in 1850.

We have already seen how the natural history of cholera was studied by Dr. John Snow and so led to his discovery of the cause of its spread. In the same way, Dr. William Budd of Bristol described the way in which typhoid fever was transmitted from person to person by the pollution of drinking water with the excreta of persons suffering from the disease. Dr. Budd's investigations were carried out in the country districts around Bristol. In those days water-borne typhoid fever was a very common disease, especially in the summer months.

The following is an extract from William Budd's treatise on typhoid fever; it is so revealing that I repeat it in full:—

On October 24, 1866, my friend, Dr. H. Grace, who I had met on other business, told me that if I had half an hour to spare he would show me a striking illustration of my views on the spread of typhoid fever.

The temptation was too great to be resisted; so, jumping into his dog-cart, we presently pulled up in front of two labourers' cottages built in a single block, by the roadside. These cottages may be called, for convenience' sake, Nos. 1 and 2. In the form of a lean-to against the gable end of No. 2 was a privy, which served in common for the inmates of both dwellings. Through this privy there flowed, with very feeble current at that time, a small stream, named the Wayne-brook, which formed a natural drain for it. Having already performed the same office for some twenty or thirty other houses, higher up its course, this stream had acquired, as was patent to more than one sense, all the characters of a common sewer, before reaching the cottages in question. From this point, after skirting the high road for about 40 or 50 yards, it passed into a field, and crossing, now as an uncovered drain, some three or four meadows, the stream came into the open again in a large court occupied by two other labourers' cottages and some farm buildings. These two cottages may be conveniently called Nos. 3 and 4. The sanitary relations which the stream held to their inmates was an exact repetition of that which obtained in regard to Nos. 1 and 2 already described. Passing through the court uncovered, it acted as a drain to a small privy, common, as before, to both cottages. I did not measure the distance which separated these two little homesteads, but I judge it to be somewhere about a quarter of a mile, as the crow flies. The four cottages thus situated were the scene of the series of events which Dr. Grace was anxious to bring before me.

The outbreak began in the person of the father of the family living in No. 1. There were two circumstances attaching to this man which made his case different from that of any member of his own or his neighbour's household.

1st. He was the only one of the group whose way of living took him away to the neighbouring city: and

2nd. He was the only one who was known to have been exposed to the infection of typhoid fever.

Having a horse and cart, he plied a small trade with Bristol, partly as a hawker and partly as a huckster. His chief business in the city lay in the filthy back-slums of St. Philip's, where, for some time immediately before his illness, typhoid fever—as I can affirm from my own observations—was epidemic. Whether he got his fever here, it is, of course, impossible to say with absolute certainty, but that in the course of his business he must have been largely exposed to its specific infection there was no doubt. That his disease was contracted away from home was further indicated by the fact that when he was stricken all the other inmates of the two cottages were, and, indeed, continued for some time after, to be, in their usual health.

His attack proved to be severe and protracted, and for a considerable time was attended by a profuse diarrhoea. As a matter of course, all the discharges were thrown into the common privy. In this way, for more than a fortnight, the stream which passed through it continued to be daily and largely fed with the specific excreta from the diseased intestine of the patient.

Some weeks passed away thus, without any fresh incident; but, in the latter end of the third, or beginning of the fourth week—which as M. Piedvache has justly observed, is about the time when the contagion of this fever generally begins to show itself in fresh crops of the disease—a new order of events occurred.

Several persons were simultaneously attacked with the same fever in all the four cottages. Not, be it observed, in Nos. 1 and 2 merely, whose inmates might be described as living in more or less contiguity to the already infected man, but in Nos. 3 and 4 also, nearly a quarter of a mile away.

Within the space of a few days Dr. Grace was attending quite a cluster of cases in each of the four, and before long the majority of the persons living in them were in bed with the fever. One fact must be recorded to render the history complete. From first to last, the outbreak was confined to these four cottages, and there was no other cases of typhoid fever at the time in that neighbourhood.

These facts speak for themselves. If we look at them by the light of what has gone before—if, especially, we bear in mind the established fact that, in some way or other, this fever has the power to propagate itself, there can be no reasonable doubt that the second crop of cases was the offspring of seed cast off by the first sufferer. But if this be so, the circumstances of the outbreak in the two lower cottages, Nos. 3 and 4, show by the most striking evidence what was the particular form under which this seed was liberated. The significance of these circumstances will be appreciated at once when it is added that those who were attacked in this particular outbreak had not only held no intercourse of any kind with the inmates of Nos. 1 and 2, but had not the remotest suspicion of the origin of the deadly pest which had appeared thus silently in their midst.

The little stream laden with the fever-poison cast off by the intestinal disease of the man who had been stricken with the same fever some weeks before, was the only bond between them.

We have already learnt to see in this disease of the intestine the specific eruption of a contagious fever; we here see, as in small pox, and other contagious fevers, the poison shed by this eruption producing fresh fruit.

But if the remarkable history here related shows with the utmost clearness that sewage when charged with the specific excreta of typhoid fever is all-potent in the propagation of that disease, it appears to me to show with equal clearness that sewage not so charged has no power of the kind.

While Dr. Grace was seeing his patients in Nos. 1 and 2 and I was standing outside, a gentleman on horse-back drew up, and addressed me in these words: 'Ah, I see what you are upon. The only wonder is, that all these poor people have not died of fever long ago. For, any time, these last six years, but in summer especially, to anyone coming down this lane, the stink has been enough to knock a man down.'

But although—so to speak—strong enough to knock a man down, it had failed all these long years to cause a single case of fever.

How, if sewage emanations be as potent to cause typhoid fever as many teach, can this possibly be explained ?

This failure, to recur to an argument used once before, could not have been because the seasons had not been favourable to the development of the pest, for within this period this fever had more than once committed great havoc in the same parish. It could not have been that the little community who were now suffering so severely from it were proof against it, for as the event proved they were only too susceptible. The very magnitude of the contrast between these many years of past entire immunity from fever, and present great prevalence of it is, surely, in itself, decisive of the question.

I have already stated that before reaching cottages Nos. 1 and 2 the stream served the office of common sewer to some twenty or thirty houses higher up. But while in Nos. 1 and 2, and in the two cottages *below* them, nearly every inmate was stricken with fever, in not one of the thirty houses above these, was there, from first to last, a single case.

It was down the stream that the seeds of the plague flowed. Higher up, the stream was common sewage only; lower down, it was sewage *plus* the specific excreta of the fever patient. Hence the cardinal difference in the fate of those who were exposed to its emanations in the two situations.

The only inference that it seems possible to draw from these facts is, that while sewage charged with the specific fever-poison is all-potent in breeding fever, sewage not so charged has no power to breed it at all.

The typhoid bacillus can live twelve days in crude sewage and several weeks in ice-cream, butter, and cheese, so that infection of food is now a common method of spread. Food and drink which are taken raw are the most dangerous, for example, water, ice, milk, ice-cream, and oysters. Freezing does not kill the organism, but boiling or cooking does.

In the nineteenth century incidence of the disease was highest in the cities where the population was the greatest. There have been several outbreaks of water-borne typhoid which have been studied in great detail. Thus at Blackburn in 1881 there were 258 cases due to the pollution of the town's water-supply from house privies. At Worthing in 1893 there were 1411 cases with 186 deaths. The outbreak was probably due to the fact that one of the workmen laying the water mains was a carrier.

In 1897 Maidstone suffered a severe epidemic from the contamination of spring water by hop-pickers. The population of the Maidstone area was almost doubled each autumn by the immigration of 60,000 persons from the East End of London. They were housed in small huts with gross overcrowding; thus in some instances 15 persons were crowded together in huts measuring 9 ft. by 10 ft. The sanitation was extremely primitive and there was widespread fouling of the ground. In this outbreak there were 1847 cases and 132 deaths. Chloride of lime was used for the first time to sterilize the water mains.

7

In Lincoln in 1905 there were 1008 cases with 119 deaths. The outbreak was due to defective drains and sewers leading to contamination of the water-supply.

In 1921 Bolton-upon-Dearne suffered an outbreak with 397 cases and 45 deaths due to contamination of water-supplies.

In 1932 the Malton epidemic was due to pollution of a well from a broken sewer from the isolation hospital.

In 1937 there was the famous Croydon outbreak resulting in 310 cases with 43 deaths. This outbreak was due to the fact that a workman who had gone down a deep well to effect repairs was a carrier. There were 36,000 people at risk here.

These outbreaks are but a few of the many which have occurred in this country, and all civilized countries can repeat the same stories. They show that an unprotected water-supply liable to contamination may be used without any ill-effects, until it becomes infected with specific infection. Then sudden disaster may follow. Gradually, however, with the improvement in water-supplies, including chlorination, water-borne typhoid has virtually disappeared from the towns and cities of Western countries. It is still a very common disease in tropical and semi-tropical countries.

The way in which oysters can spread infection is aptly illustrated by two outbreaks, one at Winchester and the other at Southampton in 1902. Oysters live in the estuaries of large rivers, which are usually heavily polluted. The Thames, for example, takes the sewage from several millions of inhabitants, and there are many famous oyster beds at its mouth. Oysters and mussels filter water through their gills and any solid matter is left behind. They can in this way filter off typhoid bacilli from infected water.

On 10 Nov., 1902, a sumptuous feast was given to the ex-mayor of Winchester. Of the 134 guests, 62 were taken ill. Not all were cases of typhoid fever, some were probably due to sheer excess; for example, one man had turtle soup, turbot and lobster salad, sweetbreads, roast mutton, braised tongue, roast turkey, Sir Watkin Wynn pudding, liqueur jelly, maraschino cream, ice-cream, and cheese. Ten guests and one waiter developed true clinical typhoid fever. On the same day a banquet was held at Southampton with 132 guests; 53 were taken ill; 10 of these were definitely typhoid and one waiter also developed the disease. The experience seems to have been remarkably similar in the two outbreaks. The only article of food taken by all was the oysters, although there were a number who ate oysters and did not become ill. The oysters in both cases were of French origin, stored in ponds at Emsworth until needed. Other outbreaks were reported from eating Emsworth oysters in Portsmouth, Brighton, Hove, Bermondsey, and Wandsworth. The meal at Southampton seems also to have been a gargantuan one. Nine persons ate the following: oysters, turtle soup, boiled turbot, Dover sole, sweetbreads, roast lamb, beans and potatoes, sorbet, roast pheasant, quail, potatoes, salad, Burgomeister pudding, Charlotte à la Prince de Galles, Bouche au Chocolat, Riz à la Mirabeau, ice-cream pudding, and dessert. Seven suffered no immediate ill-effects; what it did to their livers is anyone's guess.

Sir Arthur Newsholme describes an amusing incident which occurred when he was Medical Officer of Health at Brighton. He had warned the town council of the dangers of oysters and as a result he became extremely unpopular with the fishermen of Southwick, but his warnings were unheeded and matters came to a head when one of the town councillors gave a champagne and oyster supper. Within the next sixteen days three cases of typhoid were notified from guests at the party. One of them was the chairman of the Health Committee and was the patient of Dr. Newsholme in the Fever Hospital. Fortunately he recovered, but there was no more opposition to suggestions made for rendering shellfish safe.

Readers will be relieved to know that these days there is little to fear from oysters and mussels in the British Isles. The well-known oyster-beds in the Thames estuary and most of the mussels are stored before distribution to the public in chlorinated water so that the shellfish can free themselves of any infection which may be present. In some cases ultra-violet light is used for sterilization.

Milk can be contaminated at the farm by carrier, but outbreaks from milk are now rare because it is usually boiled or pasteurized. A cup of tea or coffee taken with infected milk can spread the disease as the temperature is usually not sufficient to kill the organism.*

THE CASE OF THE CARRIER AND THE COUNTRY HOUSE

The outbreak at Bournemouth in 1936 illustrates the importance of milk in the spread of typhoid. The Medical Officer of Health of Poole telegraphed the Ministry of Health on 21 Aug., 1936, that he had received a notification of typhoid fever. An hour later the deputy M.O.H. of Bournemouth reported that he too had received some notifications.† It soon became apparent that there were many cases scattered throughout Bournemouth, Christchurch, and Poole. Water was an unlikely source as it would have meant the simultaneous infection of three separate supplies. The only factor common to all patients was the drinking of raw milk from one distributor supplying about 10,000 people. The milk was supplied in bottles from a central depot in Poole to private houses and hotels by twelve roundsmen. All their supplies were involved. The first cases had occurred on 21 Aug.; after the morning round on 22 Aug. all milk from this depot was pasteurized and so rendered safe within thirty-six hours of the first cases being notified.

The preventive services of a modern city had swung into action with remarkable speed and efficiency, and what were the important features of this attack? First of all, prompt notification by general practitioners of cases of typhoid fever, then immediate action by the public health authorities to

---

* In many parts of China typhoid is less common than one might expect because of the practice of boiling water to make tea. The boiling of milk is universally practised in India, otherwise it would soon go sour in the hot climate; at the same time it prevents an enormous amount of milk-borne disease.

† Dr. Shaw from the Ministry of Health held a conference at Poole on 22 Aug.

investigate the cause, and finally vigorous action to put into effect the measures advocated. Despite this action, however, there occurred in this outbreak 718 cases of the disease, with 70 deaths; 200 cases occurred in holiday-makers visiting the town. Bournemouth, like many other seaside resorts, was over-crowded with visitors. If prompt action had not been taken who knows what the death-roll might have been ? The loss to the town was enormous; many visitors left and others cancelled their reservations. Unfortunately, typhoid fever takes some time to develop; thus after drinking infected fluids it takes about two weeks (it may be as long as three weeks) before the first symptoms appear. The onset of the disease is slow and many patients do not seek medical attention until a further week has elapsed. Moreover, the first few cases may not be correctly diagnosed immediately, and it may take the doctor some days before he notifies the disease. Probably then the milk had been infective for at least three weeks before 21 Aug. Some patients had only paid fleeting visits to the town, and from their history it was clear that the milk was first infective on 20 July. From that date to 22 Aug., then, many people, something like 10,000, were drinking infected milk; new cases could be expected to occur for two to three weeks following 22 Aug., and in fact this is what happened. An analysis of the number of cases occurring showed that the milk was most highly infective about 6 Aug. and that its infectivity declined rapidly after 10 Aug. This date is extremely significant, as we shall see later.

The next step was to trace the source of infection of the milk. This was carried out with great perseverance and ingenuity by Dr. Vernon Shaw.

The milk for the depot was supplied by 37 producers in farms scattered throughout a large part of Dorset. It was collected twice daily in churns by three motor lorries. The milk was mixed at the depot into one bulk supply, so that infected milk from one of the 37 producers would infect the whole supply. All the employees at the milk depot appeared to be above suspicion and an investigation of the milk producers was therefore instituted. In all, 192 persons were examined and suspicion was finally centred on one farm.

Mrs. A. from this farm had become ill on 10 Aug. and died on 7 Sept. from typhoid fever. She was the only person who had *not* drunk the common supply. She was the wife of a milk producer who produced about 20 gallons of milk a day. In the meantime, her only son, aged 12 years, also developed the disease. She continued to do her housework until 17 Aug. and was nursed by her husband at home until 24 Aug. Both Mr. and Mrs. A. were therefore doing housework, preparing food, etc., and Mrs. A. was doing all the work in the dairy for two weeks whilst there was a case of typhoid fever in the house which had severe diarrhoea. It should be noted that the first cases were not notified in the general epidemic until 21 Aug. The arrangements on the farm for cleaning were very primitive; for example, water had to be heated on the kitchen range for cleaning the milk utensils and also for washing soiled linen. There can be little doubt that this poor woman was responsible for bringing the infection into Bournemouth, Poole, and Christchurch via the milk-supply.

It is of interest to note that a next-door neighbour had died from typhoid over two years previously in May, 1934. She used to eat watercress from a stream running near the house. We must still ask ourselves, how did Mrs. A. become infected ? Gradually the chain of evidence was being built up link by link, but still there were many painstaking inquiries to be made before success was assured. No stone could be left unturned until the culprit had been finally run to earth; somewhere lurking in the background there was a human carrier responsible for the outbreak.

About 40 ft. west of the cottage where Mr. A. lived there was a stream, 6–9 ft. wide, running into the river Stour. The cows from the farm grazed in a field adjoining and drank the water from this stream. Farther up the stream there was a 4-in. pipe discharging a dirty brown fluid into the water. Examination of this effluent on two occasions showed large numbers of typhoid bacilli present. They were also present in the stream. This effluent came from a small septic tank, a hundred yards east of the stream, built many years previously to take the sewage from a large house. One can imagine the excitement as Dr. Shaw made this momentous discovery.

The next step was to make inquiries at the house. When Dr. Shaw made his visit there were 16 occupants, but the numbers varied from time to time; usually at summer week-ends there were more people in the house-party and on these occasions there was gross overloading of the sewage system, with a profuse flow of sewage from the cesspool into the stream. Specimens of excreta were taken from 14 people and the tell-tale examinations began. The results were entirely negative in 13, but the other contained typhoid bacilli in large numbers. This person was unaware that he was a carrier, and was most distressed to learn of his role in the origin of the epidemic. There can be little doubt that he was the source of the infection. He had suffered from a severe illness many years ago, which was probably typhoid fever. He was in the house on that occasion two years before when Mr. A.'s neighbour had contracted typhoid fever. He was also present in the house during the summer of 1936 until 10 Aug. when he left. This date is of great importance, because a study of the cases had already shown that the infectivity of the milk had decreased very rapidly after 10 Aug.

A study of the particular organism found in this carrier showed that it was the same type of typhoid bacillus that was found in all the cases (716) in the outbreak.

It only remains to consider how the infected stream infected the milk. There were several ways in which this might have occurred. In summer the organism would remain alive for several days at least. There was no evidence that water from the stream could have been used for dairy purposes. The cows could have spread the infection by fouling of the udder and teats, as they often drank in the infected stream, or by excreting the organism in the milk or dung. Experiments carried out more recently have shown that this last hypothesis is extremely unlikely. Feeding of heavy cultures of typhoid bacilli leaves the milk and faeces quite free from infection; the cow is immune to typhoid fever. The most likely explanation then is that the cows carried the infection from the stream on their udders and teats and so infected the milk. Mrs. A. was probably infected from the stream in some way and not from the milk-supply. This is a remarkable epidemic for several reasons. A healthy innocent person on holiday in a country house spreads infection via the sewage of the house to a stream; the chain of infection is then carried on by the cow, causing infection of a small milk-supply; this is then carried to a large depot in a seaside town infecting a large supply and causing 716 cases of typhoid fever with 70 deaths. Probably at least one death had been caused in 1934 in a similar manner. What can we learn from this disaster? Prompt dealing with an outbreak is not enough; it is rather like shutting the stable door after the horse has bolted; infection had already been spreading for three weeks in the community. The lesson to be learned from this is the importance of pasteurized milk for the inhabitants of large cities drinking bulk supplies of milk.

The transmission of infection could have been interrupted at one of several points—a proper sewage disposal system in the country house, a clean water-supply for the cows and dairy, and pasteurization of the bulked supply.

As in the days of the cholera epidemic in 1831 there were sudden demands for hospital beds. At the beginning of the outbreak there were 98 beds available in the Bournemouth and Poole isolation hospitals. This was quite inadequate to cope with the number of cases and temporary hospitals had to be provided with all their ancillary facilities and staff.

In most large cities supplies of water and shellfish and milk* are now treated so that they are incapable of spreading infection. Unfortunately, typhoid fever has not disappeared entirely because carriers in our midst are still fairly common, and are increased in number when soldiers return from areas where typhoid is common. Moreover, carriers can spread infection when engaged in the handling of food.

The following is a typical story.

The Story of Typhoid Mary

This is a classic story of how typhoid fever can be spread by an infected carrier handling food.

Mary Mallon, who had been a cook in a family in New York for three years, developed typhoid fever in 1901, and about one month later a laundress in the same family developed the disease. In 1902 Mary left to take up a position as cook in another family; within a few weeks of her arrival there were 7 persons ill with the disease. In 1904 she went to Long Island; within three weeks of her arrival 4 servants were attacked. In 1906 she changed her job once again and 6 members of the new family were affected. She changed her position again on 21 Sept., 1906, and another case occurred in the new household. In 1907 she entered a home in New York City and further cases occurred. Between 1902 and 1907 she is known to have been the cause of 26 cases of

---

* Other diseases which can be spread by milk are tuberculosis, dysentery, scarlet fever, diphtheria, and undulant fever.

typhoid fever. From 19 March, 1907, she was kept under close control by the New York Department of Health in a hospital for three years. During this time she was continually excreting typhoid bacilli. Some days there would be none but on others there would be enormous numbers. She was christened 'Typhoid Mary'. She escaped from hospital, however, and was not heard of again until 1915. In January of that year there was an outbreak of typhoid fever amongst the staff of the Sloane Hospital for Women in New York. The cook was Mary Mallon. She left the hospital at short notice and did not return. She was eventually traced although living under a false name. She was given a handsome pension by the New York State Department of Health on condition that she reported at regular intervals and did not engage in any activities involving the handling of food.

Further investigation of her history showed that she had been responsible for many other outbreaks and that she was probably the cause of the famous outbreak in Ithaca, New York, in 1903, in which there were 1300 cases.

THE CASE OF THE STRASBOURG BAKER'S WIFE

On 20 May, 1904, an apprentice lodging with a master-baker's wife in Strasbourg developed typhoid fever and died. It had been noticed that every apprentice became ill shortly after taking up residence in this house. The baker's wife said it was due to a 'too good diet'. On 26 May, 1904, and on several subsequent occasions examination showed her to be a carrier. On 8 Aug. another tenant, aged 29 years, sickened and died from typhoid fever. She was persuaded, under police pressure, to have a more thorough investigation and was shown to be excreting large numbers of typhoid bacilli.

THE CASE OF THE CHINESE EGGS

In England and Wales during August and September of 1955 there was a sharp rise in the notification of enteric fever, mostly due to paratyphoid, the milder sort. There were several outbreaks, all caused by the same type of organism. This in itself was of great interest, indicating a common origin of infection. Most of the outbreaks of paratyphoid since the war have been due to artificial cream added to buns, sponges, and éclairs.* Evidence in these cases pointed once more to bakeries supplying confectionery of this nature. It pointed further to a batch of Chinese frozen eggs and on investigation the same type of organism (type 3A) was isolated from two tins. Egg is not a constituent of artificial cream, and the infection was probably passed to the cream by its being made up in a bowl which had been used for making up the egg and which had not been adequately cleansed and sterilized. It is clearly impossible to trace how the Chinese eggs became infected. To ban the import of all eggs would impose an unnecessary penalty on many firms with high standards of hygiene. Besides, they are imported in such large quantities that it would seriously affect the catering industry.

---

* The particular danger of artificial cream lies in the fact that it is uncooked.

One thing is clear, our standards of hygiene in bakeries and catering establishments are still lamentably low; adequate cleaning and sterilization of all kitchen utensils would prevent the contamination of uncooked foodstuffs.

Unfortunately, it is extremely difficult to cure the chronic carrier and the only answer is to prohibit him from preparing food for the public. The danger has increased in recent years because of the return of soldiers and refugees from countries where typhoid is common. There are probably 2 carriers for every 100,000 of the population in Britain, making a total for the country as a whole of something like 1000 carriers.*

Many of the outbreaks of food-borne typhoid are associated with synthetic cream because, being uncooked, it is an excellent medium for the multiplication of typhoid bacteria. Flour is also a good medium as the organisms can remain alive in it for nearly a year; moist flour sacks form an excellent culture medium, so that some outbreaks traced to bakeries and confectioners may not be due to the baker himself but to a carrier who handled the flour many months before. Another interesting possibility of infection is by butter; it has been shown that typhoid bacilli can remain alive in butter for several weeks. It is, of course, extremely difficult to prove because of the complex system of distribution and the fact that butter is stored for so long and once bought is usually eaten straightaway. There is some evidence, however, that an outbreak in Sheffield in 1946 involving 162 cases may have been due to imported butter.

The outbreak of typhoid at Aberystwyth in 1946 shows how ice-cream can spread infection. The normal population of Aberystwyth is nearly 10,000, but at this time it was something like 15,000. There were 209 cases recorded in the epidemic, 104 from Aberystwyth and 105 in other parts of England and Wales. All the persons affected had eaten ice-cream from one particular producer. He had suffered from typhoid fever in 1938 and when examined he was found to be an active carrier. The ice-cream was made in a shed and distributed on a barrow. Due to the hot weather during the period 2–12 July there had been a great demand for the ice-cream. Incidentally, it was the only period of good weather during the summer of 1946. The ice-cream mixture on this occasion was not heated and the infected vendor had transmitted his infection to the ice-cream. As a result of this outbreak legislation was introduced to make it compulsory to pasteurize ice-cream mixers, and to tighten up the regulations concerning its manufacture. As would be expected a high proportion of the victims were children.

Before leaving the question of typhoid fever we must mention something of the latest developments in the detection of the source of infection. It is possible to classify typhoid bacilli into a large number of different types, called 'phage' types. Many of them are very rare, and in these cases it is an extremely valuable method in associating cases occurring at widely different times and in different places.

---

* At the present time efforts are being made to compile a list of all persons who are carriers by examining all those who have suffered from the disease.

During the last war, just before D-day a number of people in London, some of them high-ranking officers, developed typhoid fever. Investigation showed that the cases were all due to the same phage-type of organism, a type not previously identified in this country. The sufferers had one thing in common: all had recently returned from a holiday at a fashionable hotel in Cornwall. Of those who enjoyed the holiday 5 died, including a high-ranking officer. Inquiry showed that other cases had occurred in 1941, 1942, and early in 1943 in people who had stayed at the hotel. Investigations carried out at the hotel incriminated a chronic carrier who was excreting the same rare type of organism. He remembered contracting typhoid during the South African War; moreover, he could remember the name of the stream from which he had drunk the water which had caused the infection. The facts were reported to the authorities in Johannesburg, and it was found that cases of typhoid were still occurring in the vicinity of the stream caused by the same phage-type which had remained with the Cornwall carrier for forty-three years. The outbreak was due to a primitive sanitary system which allowed seepage of sewage and polluted the water-supply. No one can say how much damage this man caused, but his wife had died of typhoid many years before and his two sons had both suffered from the disease. The hotel in Cornwall has now installed an up-to-date sewage disposal plant.

Another interesting use of phage-typing enabled investigators to trace the origin of a typhoid outbreak in a seaside resort in North Devon. Outbreaks had occurred in 1944, 1945, and 1946. Cases of typhoid had occurred in 1943, 1944, and 1945 in towns in different parts of England, but identification of the same phage-type of organism made it easy to associate them with the North Devon outbreak. Many thought that infection had occurred from bathing in water contaminated with crude sewage from a broken sewer. This particular seaside resort had normally a population of 1000 people, but during the season it grew to about 5000 and during this time the sewer which runs out on to the beach was overloaded with sewage. The same phage-type of organism was isolated from the sea water in 1945, and as a result the sewage was heavily chlorinated and the broken sewer repaired. At last everyone was sure that the town was safe, but, alas, in the summer of 1946 the sense of security was shattered by another outbreak from the same type of organism. The solution to the problem came much later, in 1948, following some very fine detective work by Dr. Moore of Exeter. He undertook a detailed bacteriological examination of the sewage by dangling in it pieces of gauze attached to long pieces of string passed through selected manholes, chosen so that he was able to trace the origin of the infection back from main sewers to drains and eventually to the individual home which was infecting the sewage. A start was made at the main sewer discharging into the sea; the sewage contained the special phage-type. He next began an examination of the sewage in the main branches; one only contained the tell-tale organism, the rest were negative, and so month after month as the work progressed, Dr. Moore and his colleagues were led slowly but surely to the one house in the town which was responsible. This was occupied by the attendant of an ice-cream van which had been suspected in 1946. The man's wife was a carrier and was excreting the same phage-type that had been responsible for the cases. There was no doubt that she was the cause. She must have been very surprised to learn that she had been detected by tracing back the sewage pipes from the beach to her house.

There is a very important lesson to be learned here. Every outbreak of typhoid must be investigated with the greatest vigour to find the carrier who is always responsible in the first place. Had the outbreak in 1943 been investigated with the same vigour, those of 1944, 1945, and 1946 could have been prevented.

This Devon resort has today a first-class sewage disposal plant and the manufacture of ice-cream is strictly controlled so that it is now a 'safe' food. You can bathe and eat ice-cream with complete safety thanks to Dr. Moore and others like him.

Before leaving intestinal infections we must make some mention of dysentery. One special form, amoebic dysentery, is usually a disease of tropical or subtropical countries and occurs fairly frequently in rural populations in the southern states of America. Food infected by chronic carriers or by flies is the usual method of spread, but water has been incriminated in a famous outbreak in Chicago.

THE CASE OF THE BEWILDERED PLUMBER

The World's Fair at Chicago in 1933 was attended by people from all over the United States. The hotels were full, and it became apparent that a large number of people staying at two of them, the Coliseum and the Atheneum, had been affected with dysentery. The outbreak was not discovered at first because so many persons left the hotels before the symptoms appeared. In this way infection was disseminated all over North America. A study of 1523 employees (they were large hotels) revealed 602 carriers, all apparently recently infected. Cases and carriers were reported from places as far away as Honolulu. Many of the patients had not eaten food at the hotel at all. One physician noticed that he had had no food, but had drunk the water. It was noticed that maids who worked above the second floor became heavily infected whilst maids on the first two floors remained free. The two hotels had a common water-supply. Obviously a common water-storage tank was the source of the infection, but the water was from a mains supply which was tested daily and heavily chlorinated. Eventually the infection was traced to a cross-connexion from the sewage system of one hotel with the water pipes from this tank. The plumbing in this maze of pipes had been a little complicated and some bewildered plumber had made the wrong connexion. In the morning when all the lavatories were being flushed there was a strong siphonage effect set up which forced sewage into the water. This polluted water was then pumped into the water tank which supplied certain bedrooms with tap water. Typhoid fever did not occur because any infection would have been killed by the chlorination, but the cysts of amoebic dysentery are resistant; they were probably introduced by some carrier from the tropics.

Over 1400 known cases of amoebic dysentery resulted, with many deaths, apart from the fact that infective carriers were disseminated over a wide area causing many unrecorded cases and foci of infection, and all this was due to the bewilderment of one plumber in the maze of plumbing to be found in a large modern hotel. It took over a million dollars and a mile of new pipe to put the plumbing right in these hotels; in the words of Geddes Smith, 'a hotel is no better than its plumbing'.

We are apt, then, to forget that chlorination does not destroy all organisms; thus the virus of poliomyelitis may not be killed and it can probably pass through the ordinary filters. But there is no doubt about the capacity of chlorination for destroying typhoid bacilli. I well remember when in the Army a convincing display which we used to give of providing safe water from a heavily polluted pond at the Army School of Hygiene. We used to filter the polluted water and then chlorinate it. We always invited the class to take a drink and I never heard of anyone suffering as a result.

Since dysentery is largely spread by flies it occurs wherever these pests are common. It was one of the greatest killers of infants in this country in the days of horse-drawn vehicles when horse manure formed a good medium for fly breeding. The fly carries infection from faecal matter to food. There has been a great decrease of dysentery with the better protection of food in shops and larders and with the disappearance of flies in our cities. Dysentery still occurs during wartime when there are many opportunities for fly breeding, and it is still common in rural areas where the dung of cows and horses forms a suitable nidus for fly breeding. The seasonal diarrhoea which occurs in many countries is not due to eating green apples; it is due to intestinal infection, which is largely seasonal, reaching its peak incidence in August and September. The worst years for dysentery were 1911 and 1921 because of the hot dry summers. For the same reason they were very good wine years, especially in the Rhineland.

Dysentery is a disease of armies, jails, mental hospitals, and nurseries.

Fly-borne dysentery was of major importance in the Middle East in the Second World War. The strict attention to hygiene practised by the British Army had a marked effect in reducing fly breeding to a minimum, but in the Italian and German armies the disease was rife and almost certainly contributed to their defeat. It has been estimated that at one time something like 50 per cent of the enemy were 'glued to the commode' by dysentery. Small wonder that they had little stomach for fighting. Lt.-Col. H. S. Gear, of the South African Medical Corps, has written a fascinating account of the hygiene aspects of the El Alamein victory of 1942, a battle which has been described as one of the most momentous in world history and certainly the turning point of World War II. But for the high standards of hygiene practised in the British Army the result might have been very different. Once again the course of world history has been shaped by ill health and disease; but let the reader judge for himself. The following are extracts from Lt.-Col. Gear's account in the *British Medical Journal* of 18 March, 1944.

The enemy lines and camps at El Alamein and the bases at Matruh, Tobruk, Derna, and Benghazi were revolting in the masses of human faeces and camp debris lying everywhere. One of our hygiene officers charged with the distasteful task of supervising the clearance of the previously enemy-occupied El Alamein area reported:

'That portion of the battlefield previously occupied by the enemy is just one huge fly farm, and has to be seen to be believed. Whilst both Germans and Italians order the use of shallow trench latrines (and no oil seal), this order is scarcely ever carried out. Enemy defensive localities are obvious from the amount of faeces lying on the surface of the ground.'

The enemy paid for his contempt of hygiene, as these insanitary conditions had the inevitable result of causing a heavy incidence of excremental disease. This became such a menace to the enemy as to effect from 40 to 50% of his front-line troops, as interrogation of captured medical officers revealed. To quote one of our hygiene reports:

'It has, however, been heartening to observe the difference between the enemy sanitation and dysentery/diarrhoea rate and our own. The enemy appears to have no conception of the most elementary measures, and has a dysentery/diarrhoea rate so very much higher than ours that it is believed that the poor physical condition of his troops played a great part in the recent victory of El Alamein.'

A front-line force with 40 to 50% of its strength affected by dysentery and diarrhoea can scarcely be called a vigorous army, and this was the incidence in Italian and German units.

In contrast, the Eighth Army in October and November was probably as fit mentally and physically as any army has ever been. The contribution of preventive medicine to this standard can be measured from the degree of success achieved in protecting our troops from infectious disease, in maintaining a high level of physical fitness, in ensuring adequate rations and water supply, and in adapting as far as possible the Army's clothes, fighting, and other equipment and camping conditions to accepted physiological standards. The hygiene officers and other ranks of the Eighth Army, by their heterogeneous force in a difficult environment, did good work. They—hygiene men recruited from the United Kingdom, New Zealand, South Africa, Australia, and India—may not have the glamour, glory, and excitement of their brothers in the clinical units, the field ambulances, and casualty clearing stations, of the medical services, but they have the satisfaction of knowing that the health of the Eighth Army, and hence in large measure its physical and mental capacity for forceful action, shown at El Alamein, owed much to them.

FOOD INJURY

Alas, although food is necessary for health and well-being there are still many other ways in which it can cause harm. Some people are sensitive to particular foodstuffs, such as milk, eggs, tomatoes, strawberries, or sea food, particularly mussels and oysters. One man's meat may well be another man's poison. Food is particularly liable to contamination by harmful organisms, as we have already seen producing such diseases as cholera and typhoid. It is also liable to be contaminated by deleterious chemical substances. Throughout history there have been many examples of the poisoning of cereals by the ergot fungus, called in medieval times St. Anthony's Fire, because of the agonizing pain which affects the limbs. Other types produce twitching, giddiness, delirium, and fits. When this attacks a whole village it may be due to poisoning of the village bread or it may be due to mass hysteria. Such an outbreak occurred in a French village recently from spoilt rye bread; the village baker was to blame.

There are many ways in which metallic poisoning can occur. Lead poisoning occurred when lead pipes were used to carry the soft peaty water from the Pennines to the industrial towns of Lancashire and Yorkshire. Sodium fluoride, used for killing cockroaches, can accidentally contaminate food. Arsenic-contaminated glucose has occurred in beer and sweets, and zinc, antimony, lead, or tin poisoning can occur from containers, wrappings, or vessels used in the preparation of food. The symptoms are very characteristic and the cause can usually be easily detected because the metals are easy to identify. But many bacteria can produce powerful toxins which produce similar symptoms. In these cases the cause is not always easy to identify because there are no known chemical tests for the toxin. In fact, in the early days of the investigation of these cases human volunteers were used to test for the presence of the poison. One of the most dramatic types of such poisoning is botulism, fortunately rare in this country, but becoming more common in the U.S.A. In the fifty years between 1899 and 1949, 483 different outbreaks have been recorded in the U.S.A. Of these, 183 occurred in California and 61 in Washington, followed by Colorado, Oregon, New York, New Mexico, and Montana in that order; in the rest of the States outbreaks are rare. This type of food poisoning is most unusual because it produces paralysis of nerves supplying the head, neck, heart, and lungs, and gastrointestinal symptoms do not occur. It is surprisingly lethal; two-thirds of those attacked die from its effects. There is no treatment of any avail. The organism itself is harmless and grows in soil. It only produces its powerful poison when grown under conditions where there is a shortage of air.

The organism contaminates fruit and vegetables and produces its poison when these foods are kept for a few days and then treated by preserving or processing in some way, such as canning, bottling, smoking, or pickling. Home-canned foods are often to blame and there is no danger from fresh foods. The toxin must be one of the most powerful it is possible to produce; thus one-millionth of a gramme (1 oz. is 28 g.) will kill a guinea-pig.

In Europe, sausages and ham have mainly been involved, but in the U.S.A. it has been mostly vegetables, such as peas, beans, asparagus, corn on the cob, spinach, and olives, and also canned fruits. Canned foods are much more popular in the U.S.A. and sausages popular in Germany. This is a clear warning of the importance of fresh food, important to the palate, but very important for health.

The most famous outbreak in Britain was at Loch Maree in 1922 when a fishing party of 8 ate for lunch some paste made from wild duck; they all died from botulism.

Commercial canning is now carried out in such a scientific way that there is no danger from this source. The reason why home canning can cause the trouble is the fact that the organism is very resistant to heat, for example, it may take six hours' continuous boiling to destroy the spores. It still remains a mystery why botulism is so much commoner in California than in Britain. No doubt the organism is rare in soil in this country; otherwise with all the inadequate home bottling of fruit and vegetables that goes on, the disease would have been more common.

'DON'T EAT PINK PORK'

Another remarkable type of food poisoning is produced by eating pork infested with the worm known as *Trichinella*; hence the name of the disease, trichinosis. The adult worm lives in the intestine of the pig and rat and the young worms enter the muscles of these animals and form tiny cysts where they may remain alive for many years. To complete the life cycle the flesh of the animal must be eaten raw, or imperfectly cooked, by another animal. The larvae are then liberated and enter the intestine where they grow to maturity. In a few days they produce a fresh batch of larvae which enter the muscles of the new host. Infestation is kept going in pigs by contamination of their food by rats, and also by pigs killing and eating rats, a pastime which they are adept at. Man becomes infested by eating raw or imperfectly cooked pork; hence the maxim 'don't eat pink pork', adequate cooking will destroy the larvae.

An interesting outbreak of this type of food poisoning occurred in Wolverhampton during the war between December, 1940, and March, 1941, from the consumption of raw sausage meat. Many cases occurred in the girls working in a particular factory who used raw sausage meat to make their midday sandwiches. Altogether 130 cases were found and further tests indicated that 500–600 persons had been infected, but their symptoms were mild in character. This is an important finding because it indicates that for every person affected clinically there are several not showing symptoms. The disease usually starts with a rising temperature, headache, and muscular pains; sometimes there is swelling of the face and eyelids; but these symptoms may occur in a wide variety of illnesses. No doubt the disease is often wrongly diagnosed and its epidemic nature is not always realized, cases occurring over a widespread area and each being treated by a different doctor. Infestation must be a good deal commoner than we think. A post-mortem examination of nearly 500 persons not known to have suffered from the disease showed that 10·5 per cent had been infected. If this applies to the country as a whole, these figures are remarkable. In the U.S.A. infestation rates are even higher, 15–20 per cent of the population harbouring the parasite, and it may be as high as 36 per cent. The disease is also common in Germany and in the Arctic where the raw flesh of the polar bear is eaten.

The preventive measures are as follows: (1) Thorough cooking of pork. (2) Prevention of rat infestation. (3) Great care in the feeding arrangements for pigs; for example, all pig-food must be thoroughly cooked.

Once more, then, the rat has been incriminated in a serious human disease, but this is not the only way they can infect food; both rats and mice often suffer from intestinal infections, known as salmonellae infections. The organism is passed in the droppings of the rodent. It is easy enough to see how in food stores and larders our food can become contaminated. The infection is then transmitted to human beings. Chickens, turkeys, ducks, and geese also suffer from similar conditions and can infect their eggs. White diarrhoea of chickens is common in the U.S.A. and 10 per cent of samples of dried egg in the war were infected with salmonellae. It can also occur in cats and dogs, but must be very rare in them, otherwise we should most certainly suffer from food poisoning more commonly than we do. It is perhaps fortunate that few of the bowel parasites of dogs are transmittable to man, since it was found in the War Dogs' Training School that 70 per cent of dogs were infested with some form of worm.

Tape-worms are also spread by eating raw or poorly cooked flesh. The fish tape-worm, which may be 18 ft. long, is common in Ireland, Russia, Siberia, Finland, Japan, Canada, the northern states of the U.S.A., and around the Great Lakes, in freshwater fish such as pike, perch, salmon, trout, and it can occur in caviare. In Finland it is probable that there are nearly 1,000,000 carriers of the worm, 25 per cent of the population. No doubt the last war has caused a spread of infestation to other countries where it was formerly absent. In Britain there are now over 30,000 nationals from the Baltic States who have come from heavily infested areas; there are certainly some carriers amongst them. As a result, since the war a few cases have occurred in this country and several freshwater fish have been found to be infested with the worm. There are a great many freshwater fishermen, and smoked freshwater fish is now a much commoner article of diet than it was, whilst caviare and trout are imported from the Continent. As with many of these worm infestations the majority of people affected remain symptom-free, but one of the effects of the fish tape-worm is a severe anaemia, very similar to pernicious anaemia. I wonder if in the future we shall see the disease becoming more common here. For my part, the fear of infection will not deter me from eating caviare or smoked trout when I get the chance.

Tape-worms occur also in the pig and cow, both transmitted by eating inadequately cooked meat.

The prevention of infestation by tape-worms depends on proper sanitation and adequate cooking of food.

The dog tape-worm is found commonly in sheep-raising areas where the intermediate stage is spent in the liver of the sheep. Both man and sheep are infected by ingesting the eggs of the worm found in the excreta of the dog. It can cause a serious disease in man, depending where the larvae settle. This may be in the liver, giving hydatid disease, or if it settles in the brain it can produce epilepsy. It is common in the great sheep-raising areas of the world, New Zealand, Australia, South America, Siberia, the Near East, and South Africa. It has not become established as a common disease in North America or Britain, although cases have occurred in the Welsh sheep-raising areas.

The control of dogs is an important preventive measure. As long as they are not allowed to eat raw offal from infected sheep they will remain free from infection. The disease in man is now much rarer than it was, due to this control. Thus in the city of Melbourne, stray dogs are destroyed and there is strict control at the abattoirs. The domestic dog does not suffer from the disease.

Before leaving the question of food poisoning we must mention man himself as a source of infection. The control of animals such as cattle, pigs, rats, and dogs has certainly done a great deal to reduce some forms of injury from food ingestion. The provision of better forms of sanitation has reduced some forms of food-borne disease, but unfortunately some forms of food poisoning are on the increase, namely, those in which man himself harbours or carries the infective agent. The staphylococcus is a very common organism which can be swallowed without harm. It is a common inhabitant of the nose, and of sores and burns, but if it is allowed to grow on the right kind of food it produces a powerful toxin. Unfortunately, subsequent cooking of the food does not render it harmless, because whilst the bacteria are killed the toxin is not. This form of food poisoning occurs where food is prepared some time before it is required and left for several hours in a warm place. If the cook is harbouring staphylococci in a sore hand, a burn, say, or in his nose, it is easy for the food to become infected. It occurs in restaurants and canteens which have bad hygienic arrangements. Of course, the most important thing is clean hands for the cook and on no account should he handle food if he has any sore places. Bad personal habits such as nose picking and infrequent washing of the hands predispose to the spread of infection. If food has to be prepared beforehand it should be stored in a refrigerator and never in a warm kitchen. Finally, there should be frequent sterilization of all crockery, cutlery, and food utensils.

There has been a considerable increase in food poisoning since the war. Many more people now have the habit of eating out in schools, canteens, and restaurants. Education of the food handler in the principles of health is the most important preventive measure because even with the most hygienic kitchen he can still spread disease. Almost as important is education of the general public. Until public opinion demands higher standards of cleanliness we shall never be completely successful. America has much higher standards than those that prevail in Britain. Perhaps we can conclude this chapter by telling an amusing story concerning a well-known food factory in this country. A visiting American Army doctor was being shown the wonderful hygienic lavatories provided for the workers, the latest and most up-to-date in design. As each person left the lavatory, an illuminated notice flashed in front of him reading 'Now wash your hands'. This was obeyed implicitly until one white-coated gentleman left the lavatory without washing his hands. The Army doctor remonstrated against this; 'That's all right,' said the attendant, 'he's not a food handler, he's only the dentist!'

CHAPTER IX

ONE MAN'S MEAT

VIRGINIA WOOLF has said, 'One cannot think well, love well, sleep well, if one has not dined well', echoing the words of the poet Schiller: 'Hunger and love hold the world together.' There can be little doubt that the need for food is the most fundamental of all biological urges; it certainly occurs more frequently than any other. Although food is necessary for life itself, it can also be one of the great pleasures which make life worth living. Unfortunately in Britain there is a general lack of appreciation of good cooking compared with, say, France or Italy. Of course, we do not need to be like the Romans, who set a ruinous standard in debauchery. Let us remember, however, that this was only for the aristocratic few and the proverbial excesses were rare occurrences; we only read of the highlights and forget that the civilization of Rome lasted nearly a thousand years. The gourmet, however, is not interested in quantity, but in tasty food which stimulates the appetite, as an aid to digestion, and a means to good health. The sensible gourmet is slim, a creed prescribed many years ago by that prince of gastronomes, Brillat Savarin, in his book *The Physiology of Taste*. It is very regrettable that such important sensations as taste and smell have for so long been largely ignored by the physiologists.

Sophistication in the art of eating reached its height in Roman times when Lucullus culled the corners of the known world for rare and exotic foods. We read of nightingales and flamingo tongues, peacocks from Persia, oysters from Colchester, whilst the ortolans, bunting, and edible harvest mice were bred in large numbers for the table. Gluttony reached its height when vomitoria were provided so that the replete diners could start again in their round of gorging. Today we are much more conservative about the food we eat, viewing with distrust many of the food habits of our neighbours.

This subject of food is so important that it seems worth while to review in some detail the amazing diversity of dietary habits amongst the different peoples of the world. A survey of the food habits of primitive peoples shows that almost any article of vegetable or animal origin has been used as food.

SEAWEED

Throughout the whole of the East, seaweed is used as an article of diet. The Chinese have used it as food from time immemorial and consider it a great delicacy, whilst in Japan even today it provides something like 25 per cent of the daily diet. The common type is the brown seaweed which is used to make noodles or it can be served with rice or in soup. The common

8 113

seaweed around the shores of Britain is also of this type. In Wales the red type is still eaten, where it is made into bread, or is eaten as a vegetable with vinegar and pepper. In Scotland this is called 'slack', in Ireland 'sloke', and in Wales 'laver'. It looks like spinach and is said to have the delicate flavour of the oyster. Research is being carried out at the Institute of Sea-weed Research at Midlothian in Scotland on the nutritive value of this food. The Institute has shown that around the shores of Britain there is something like 180,000 tons of seaweed between high and low water which could be easily gathered, whilst about 10,000,000 tons are available below low water. Seaweed contains carbohydrates, fats, proteins, vitamins, and a high mineral content, many of these showing marked seasonal variations. It would appear that seaweed contains all the mineral elements that are required by man, the most important being iodine. It is interesting to note that the iodine content of the air in Europe has fallen since the burning of kelp ceased, thus depriving man of a valuable source of this essential mineral. As far as vitamins are concerned, seaweed contains carotene, which is a precursor of vitamin A, vitamin B_1, and vitamin B_2, whilst the vitamin C content at one time provided the Eskimoes of west Greenland with their main supply of this vitamin. The red algae around our shores are also a valuable source of agar. Up to the beginning of the century China imported 1,000,000 lb. of agar annually, using it as a substitute for birds'-nest soup, and it is still used in Japan for making cakes. Seaweed is a valuable animal feeding stuff in some parts of the world; the sheep on some of the Orkney and Shetland islands use it as their staple diet.

MUSHROOMS AND TOADSTOOLS

People are, of course, familiar in Britain with the field mushroom, and nowadays mushrooms are cultivated on a large scale, although the flavour of these does not compare, in my opinion, with the natural field mushroom. Although many people are very wary about eating toadstools, the majority are edible and provide a welcome change in diet. The blewit is used in the north and sold in our markets, whilst the morel is used for flavouring soups and gravies. Ninety per cent of all poisonings are due to the death-cap and a very small amount will cause intense suffering often followed by death. The gills are always white or creamy-white, never pink or purple-brown as in the mushroom. The most characteristic feature is the cup-like volva with loose edges at the bottom of the stem. The fungus has a rather sweet, sickly odour and not the pleasant fragrant smell of the field mushroom. The death-cap is common in beech and oakwoods and may also be found in grass-land in late summer. Another poisonous variety is the fly agaric, which is easily recognizable by its bright red cap. In the two world wars fungi were much sought after by starving people on the Continent and refugees to this country are often amazed at our disregard of the large numbers of delicious fungi which grow in our woods and meadows. In some parts of the world they appear to be a staple diet. According to Darwin, the chief article of diet of the natives of Tierra del Fuego is a fungus which grows on beech trees, whilst in New Guinea there is a tribe of cave dwellers which exists mainly on fungi and palm sprouts supplemented by what rats and mice they can catch. In times of want people have turned to fungi for their natural diet. In the eighteenth century during a famine the people of Nuremberg subsisted entirely on fungi and black bread. The German forces in the French Cameroons during the First World War whilst they were on the run were compelled to live on fungi. Many animals such as rabbits and squirrels can be seen feeding on fungi which grow on trees. Slugs are particularly fond of them and will even thrive on the death-cap. Dogs, horses, cows, and sheep will all eat field mushrooms, and in France, Italy, and Spain pigs are used to root up truffles in the oakwoods. Dogs can also be trained to do this. The area around Périgord in the south of France is famous for truffles, where they are now becoming much scarcer. They can be bought in Spain in tins and are quite cheap. Brillat Savarin considered the truffle the diamond of the gastronome and truffled turkey the apotheosis of the gastronomic art. The cèpe or boletus is a great delicacy in Bordeaux; it also grows in the woods of Britain and in Norway and northern Finland; in these northern climes the cows have to be prevented from wandering into the woods during the fungus season since a diet of boletus will often make them go mad. When I was in Lapland some years ago I tasted the dry fungi which the Lapps use for feeding their reindeer during the winter; my verdict—most tasty, particularly when used in a soup. Mushrooms and fungi have, however, little nutritive value; they contain some potassium and phosphorus and small amounts of other mineral salts, but are very poor sources of vitamins. Despite this I am sure that people everywhere will continue to enjoy mushrooms and fungi for their delicate flavour and for their ability to convert an ordinary meal into a tasty one. This must surely have some effect in better digestion. Some of the best-known edible fungi in Britain are the horse mushroom, shaggy-caps, the blusher, tawny grizette, parasol mushroom, blewit, St. George's mushroom, oyster mushroom, fairy-ringed champignon, chanterelle, saffron milkcap, giant puffball, boletus, and morel.

INSECTS AS FOOD

In this country insects are hardly ever used as an article of diet, although spiders were used as a cure for malaria up to the close of the nineteenth century. I suppose that the eating of a caterpillar, an ant, beetle, or live spider would be nauseating to most Europeans. However, when I was in Nigeria I found that the natives there are particularly fond of the large queen ants which we used to dig out of the termite ant hills. They have a small head and a large body distended and glistening with eggs. The great delight of the natives was to take hold of the queen ant by the head and pop her writhing abdomen into their mouths and nip it off with their teeth. The subsequent crunching produced an obvious satisfaction to the partaker of this unusual meal. Sometimes they will fry the morsel on a hot stove. Throughout the East the eating of insects is a common habit; they are roasted and eaten with rice and salt. Locusts have been eaten in the East from Biblical times and the flavour is said to be quite pleasant, rather like a mild cheese. In Lao there are professional collectors who spend a lot of time and care collecting various insects in the forest and quite high prices are paid in the village markets for them. The wild honey bees are highly esteemed and the taking of their nests is apparently quite a dangerous procedure. A skilful collector may collect over two hundred nests in one night. A high price is paid for the honey and the wax, whilst the grubs are fried or eaten in curry. Nothing seems to come amiss to them; bees, wasps, ants, together with the eggs, larvae, and pupae, are all taken for eating purposes. In Mexico and in Bangkok, large water bugs, over 3 in. in length, are considered a special delicacy. The larvae of various kinds of beetles are also in great demand. They are soaked in coconut milk and then roasted. The Siamese are also fond of the giant fleshy spiders; the head is nipped between the thumb and forefinger and the fat succulent body nipped off with the teeth and eaten raw, or again they may be roasted, dipped in salt, used in a curry, or pounded up to make a sauce. It would appear that the diet of many of these peasants is very poor and they have to eat whatever they can get hold of. No doubt the eating of insects protects them from many nutritional deficiency diseases.

Some Foods of Primitive People

The food of the Australian aboriginal provides a very good example of the great variety of foodstuffs which can be eaten by man. They are, of course, nomads, just as the Eskimoes, the Red Indians, and the true Lapps are nomads, and wander, with their tents, following the animals they hunt. They make no attempt to cultivate the ground but live entirely off the land, staying where food is plentiful and moving on to new areas when the country has been denuded. Contact with civilization, however, has in many cases altered their habits, very often to their detriment. They then tend to settle down in settlements, eating the diet of the white man and developing all the diseases of Western civilization. This new type of food consists largely of adulterated white flour, soda, sugar, margarine, and tea. As a result they get vitamin and mineral deficiencies and many of them develop tuberculosis. Even today there are natives who still believe that half-castes are produced as a result of eating white flour. Compare this diet, then, with the natural diet which the true aboriginal of Australia enjoys. There are still many species of animals available for hunting such as the kangaroo, opossum, wallaby, echidna, dingo, rabbit, and buffalo. The sea cow is also used for food in the north, being hunted by the natives from canoes. Practically the whole of the animal is eaten, including blood, intestines, liver, and brain. Most of the animals are cooked by placing the body in hot ashes. Lizards, snakes, crocodiles, turtles, and their eggs are also eaten. One method of catching them is to set fire to patches of country and kill the reptiles as they flee from the fires. Some of the lizards are quite large, growing up to a length of 6 ft. The turtle is a particular delicacy and the female is considered the greater prize, particularly for the ovaries. As in France and in other parts of the world, frogs and snails are freely taken and are considered to be great delicacies. Fish, shellfish, and various kinds of insects are all collected and eaten wherever they can be found. In central Australia, the wild honey bee is replaced by the honey ant, which makes its nest in the ground, often at considerable depths. The natives have to dig down in search of these and regard the worker ant as a great delicacy. The first sensation is an acid flavour, due to formic acid. The honey is said to be very delicious. Birds are also in great demand, particularly the emu and its eggs, although this bird is very difficult to catch. They will even eat birds of prey which most people find unpleasant, whilst turkeys, ducks, pigeons, cockatoos, swans, geese, and doves are all much sought after. Every kind of wild vegetable appears in the diet and even the seeds and bark of some trees. It would appear that if you live in the wilds of Australia and are not very fussy about what you eat you can keep healthy and fit.

The diets of Eskimoes and North American Indians provide some most interesting examples of unusual food habits. They have been described by Amundsen, Perry, Ross, Rassmussen, Stephanson, and others. The food habits of these people change with the season of the year. In winter, for example, with low temperatures and long nights, the main food source is the seal. The Eskimoes congregate on the sea coast or perhaps on an ice-floe and sit at the breathing holes in the ice where the seal comes to get air. This is the so-called waiting hunting, which may be a very severe ordeal on a cold winter's day. The seal is one of the most difficult of all the northern animals to get; it provides everything for the use of the Eskimo and a very rich supply of fat, as nearly half the animal is blubber. The Eskimo eats almost everything, including the blood, whilst the sinews and the intestines are used for clothing.

In the spring the walrus becomes the staple article of diet; it is hunted by harpooning from kyaks. It is also a great time for stalking seals on the edge of the ice-floes, whilst the polar bear is sometimes hunted with dogs. The liver is not eaten because of its poisonous nature, due apparently to a very high content of vitamin A. In summer the Eskimo moves inland, hunting land animals such as the caribou. These animals, like the European reindeer, move north each year over the same route. The Eskimoes drive the caribou to wet or marshy ground where they can be easily caught. They are very fond of the fermented contents of the caribou paunch and eat the raw faeces either directly or in soup. This is a very rich source of vitamin C as the animal feeds mainly on lichen and berries. In the summer also, fishing for salmon is important. They are either speared or caught on hooks with ivory minnows; sometimes they are also netted. Eggs of birds are greatly favoured by the Alaskan Eskimoes, but they dislike fresh eggs, much preferring those that are highly incubated. Many of our rarer geese and waders are threatened with extinction because as they are colonial breeders it is very easy for the Eskimoes to catch the young birds and the adults in moult. The nesting colonies of the beautiful Ross's snow geese were discovered for the first time in 1938; they are threatened with extinction since the total world population is probably no more than 5000 and possibly much less. In 1949 Peter Scott went to these colonies on the Perry River in Northern Canada in order to study their habits. The Eskimoes do not realize that this is the last remaining colony in the world.

In summer also many kinds of berries are eaten, the black crowberry, cloudberry, and blueberry. They are very similar to those found in Lapland and when crushed the juice forms a delicious summer drink; thus in summer, as in winter, the Eskimo gets plenty of vitamin C. There are, of course, certain geographical variations in the diet; the Eskimoes in eastern Greenland hunt the whale, a very dangerous procedure, whilst the polar Eskimo lives almost exclusively on the narwhal. The skin is greatly relished and tastes like hazelnut. Some Eskimoes do not migrate to the coast in the winter, for example the caribou Eskimoes. They have to rely on caribou meat which is kept frozen during the winter months. Most Eskimoes eat their food raw, and much of the food is preferred when it is rotten; the caribou liver, for example, is allowed to ferment inside the caribou's stomach under the hot sun. The eating habits are communal and apparently very unhygienic.

The Eskimo diet provides enormous calorie value because of the large amount of fat which it contains. They consume huge quantities of vitamin A and vitamin D from the offal of the seal and narwhal, whilst the raw adrenal glands are rich in vitamin C. The protein content is also very high. The diet is, of course, very low in carbohydrate. Eskimoes seem to eat enormous quantities when food is plentiful. Simpson has described how two Siberian Eskimoes consumed 35 lb. of beef and 18 lb. of butter in less than three hours. This would provide over 100,000 calories, occupying a volume of something like 6 gal. Perry describes how the Eskimo thinks nothing of eating 8 or 9 lb. of meat and 3 or 4 lb. of blubber at one sitting. There must be something extraordinary about the digestion and metabolism of these people, as a European would be ill and unable to digest and absorb such large quantities. Diseases of civilization seem to be rare with them except when they come into contact with the white man. It would appear that the true Eskimo has adapted himself with extraordinary efficiency to life in the Arctic and provided he is allowed to live his own life remains happy and healthy; as in other parts of the world, however, contact with the white man has been his downfall, and life in settlements with its diet of adulterated food eventually produces the diseases of civilization—tuberculosis, venereal disease, diabetes, appendicitis, dental caries, and cancer.

Until recent times, cannibalism had been practised as a routine in a number of native tribes, and in times of starvation men will return to such habits. When I was in Belsen I saw many examples of cannibalism and the eating of human excreta. When a man is dying of starvation he will eat anything.

Perhaps in years to come our forebears will consider the Englishman's diet of the twentieth century the most unusual one in the world. We drink water to which chlorine and sometimes fluorides have been added, some people eat synthetic fats dosed with synthetic vitamins, our flour undergoes artificial ageing by exposure to nitrogen trichloride. Sir Edward Mellanby showed that hysteria in dogs was caused by feeding them on white bread doctored with nitrogen trichloride. In the confectionery and sweets industry there are a great range of chemical substances added to food, such as benzoic acid, sulphites, nitrites, dyestuffs, artificial fruit essences, sweeteners, synthetic fats, and so on. Considerable experimental work has been done on the role played by food and beverages in the causation of cancer. Of necessity the work has been done on animals and we do not know the precise effect of many substances on human beings when ingested over a number of years.

Many dyes which have been used for colouring sweets and confectionery have been shown to be capable of producing cancer, for example, oil orange E, orange I, nigrosine, benzopurpurine, Light Green SF Yellowish; dulcin should be prohibited as a sweetening agent because it induces liver cancer in animals. Diethyl stilboestrol is used for caponizing cockerels by hormone tablet implantation. Its use for this purpose and in cosmetics should be prohibited, as it can produce cancer.

There is some evidence that mineral oils like paraffin and over-heated vegetable oils and fats can be cancer producing.

There is a grave danger that many of the insecticides and weed-killers used on our crops can be carried over into our food. DDT, for example, can be recovered from the human body; there is a small but appreciable quantity of arsenic in cigarettes from its use on the tobacco crop, to say nothing of the cancer-producing tars. Let us take warning from the words of the late Sir Edward Mellanby: 'It is difficult to avoid the conclusion that at least some of the increases in disease are due to errors in living . . . one of these errors is the ingestion of food treated by unnatural chemical substances.' We should not forget also that the habitual taking of drugs, such as aspirin, dexedrine, luminal, and purgatives may have adverse effects in the long run.

We should try to ensure that our diet is as free from adulteration as possible, and as fresh as possible. In this way not only shall we remain healthier but we shall have tastier and more enjoyable food. In the U.S.A. today the greatest danger is of eating too much, particularly of the fatty foods.* In the past, however, our greatest danger was in not getting sufficient of certain essential foodstuffs. The history which follows of two typically English diseases, scurvy and rickets, illustrates this point.

SCURVY

WIDOWER'S DISEASE

One of the earliest known nutritional deficiency diseases was scurvy. We now know that it is due to an absence of vitamin C in the diet, but in the Middle Ages its cause was quite unknown and there were many conflicting theories. Probably many of the people of medieval England were on the

---

* Let us not forget, therefore, the old Latin tag, 'Gluttony kills more than the sword', nor the timely reminder by Oliver Wendell Holmes that 'we dig our graves with our teeth'.

verge of scurvy by the time the spring came, because the winter diet in those days contained very little in the way of fresh vegetables, consisting mainly of beer, bread, dried peas and beans, salted meat, and cheese. The spring with its abundance of fresh fruit and vegetables saved them. It was amongst seafaring men that the disease was commonest, particularly when in the sixteenth century and onwards men began to go on long voyages of discovery often lasting several years, away from land and without fresh food for many months. It was a well-recognized and dreaded hazard of long sea voyages.

Jacques Cartier, the French explorer, wintering on the shores of Newfoundland, records that in the winter of 1535 'not ten of his 110 crew had escaped the disease'. He cured them by following a recipe of the Indians, a decoction made from the tips of the spruce trees.

Again in 1600 four ships sailed from England to establish the East India Company; in three of the ships 105 men died from scurvy on the voyage to Bombay; in the fourth ship they received a daily ration of lemon juice and all arrived at Bombay fit and in good health.

Lord Anson sailed round the world with a squadron of ships starting in 1740; in 1741 more than half the men had died from scurvy and the rest were severely disabled by the disease.

The first experiment on the cause of scurvy is the famous human trial made on H.M.S. *Salisbury* in 1753 by Dr. James Lind, a physician in the Navy. He banished from the British Navy two of the greatest killers of seamen—typhus and scurvy. The first, he realized, was brought on to ships by the infested clothing of the press-gang victims and he issued strict instructions for their disinfestation. The cause of scurvy had already been suggested by the experiences of men like Jacques Cartier and Lord Anson, and so, like Jenner and Hunter, he decided to experiment. Fortunately he had in the Navy the ideal conditions for an experiment using human beings as guinea-pigs. I doubt if they were volunteers. He was in no doubt as to the ravages caused by the disease. In his own words: 'The scurvy alone during the last war proved a more destructive enemy and cut off more valuable lives than the united efforts of the French and Spanish arms.'

In 1753 he published in Edinburgh his famous book, *A Treatise of the Scurvy*, in which he describes in some detail the actual experiment which proved his point. I can do no better than quote the relevant passages from his book:—

On the 20th of May 1747, I took twelve patients in the scurvy, on board the *Salisbury* at sea. Their cases were as similar as I could have them. They all in general had putrid gums, the spots and lassitude, with weakness of their knees. They lay together in one place, being a proper apartment for the sick in the fore-hold; and had one diet common to all. . . . Two of these were ordered each a quart of cyder a-day. Two others took twenty-five gutts of *elixir vitriol* three times a-day, upon an empty stomach; using a gargle strongly acidulated with it for their mouths. Two others took two spoonfuls of vinegar three times a-day, upon an empty stomach; having their gruels and their other food well acidulated with it, as also the gargle for their mouth. Two of the worst patients, with the tendons in the ham rigid . . . were put under a course of sea-water.

Of this they drank half a pint every day, and sometimes more or less, as it operated, by way of gentle physic. Two others had each two oranges and one lemon given them every day. These they ate with greediness, at different times, upon an empty stomach. They continued but six days under this course, having consumed the quantity that could be spared. The two remaining patients, took the bigness of a nutmeg three times a-day, of an electuary recommended by an hospital-surgeon, made of garlic, mustard-seed, *rad. raphan.*, balsam of *Peru* and gum myrrh; using for common drink, barley-water well acidulated with tamarinds. . . .

The consequence was, that the most sudden and visible good effects were perceived from the use of the oranges and lemons; one of those who had taken them, being at the end of six days fit for duty. . . . The other was the best recovered of any in his condition; and being now deemed pretty well, was appointed nurse to the rest of the sick. . . .

Captain James Cook proceeded to demonstrate in a practical way the importance of this finding. During his three years' voyage round the world from 1772 to 1775 he did not have one single case of scurvy. This was unheard of before that time and was due entirely to the fact that he obtained ample supplies of fresh vegetables and fruit wherever he landed.

Lind worked hard to try to get a regular issue of lemon juice for the British Navy, but it was not until forty years after the publication of his book that success was achieved, when in 1795, ironically enough one year after Lind's death, an allowance was made of 1 oz. of lemon juice served daily after two weeks at sea. Senior naval executive officers asserted that this was equal to doubling the fighting force of the Navy, as previously because of scurvy the fleets had to be relieved every ten weeks by fresh crews of equal strength. The immediate consequences were startling; scurvy had disappeared from the British Navy by the beginning of the nineteenth century. During the Seven Years' War (1756–1763) it was quite usual for the fleet to call at Spithead with 2000 cases of scurvy. The admissions to the Royal Naval Hospital at Haslar in 1780 were 1457; from 1806 to 1810 they were but 2.

Sir Edward Hawke was quick to grasp the lesson of Lind's experiments and when he was blockading the French off Brest in 1759 he insisted on a regular supply of fresh vegetables and fruit. At the battle of Quiberon Bay which followed, out of 14,000 men under his command, there were less than 20 sick. If scurvy had been manifest, there might have been a different story to tell! The tragic part of the story is that the crews of the supply ships who were carrying the fresh foodstuffs to the fleet were themselves decimated by the disease. In the Napoleonic wars this discovery had a profound effect upon the health of the sailors and it enabled the British Navy to remain many months at sea blockading enemy ports.

It is highly probable that the history of the British Empire and of Europe would have been very different but for Lind's discovery, and yet the naval history books give little mention of Dr. Lind.

Unfortunately, a tragic mistake was made in the Admiralty about 1860 when a change was made from Mediterranean lemons to West Indian limes and from this time doubts began to be expressed about the value of fresh fruits as a preventive.

In 1875 an expedition set out to discover the North Pole under Sir George Nares. It was well supplied with lime juice, but in a few months scurvy broke out in the party. The Jackson-Harmsworth expedition to Franz Joseph Land in 1894 found that their base party developed scurvy although supplied with lime juice. People had forgotten Lind's work and did not realize that the term 'lime juice' was used indiscriminately for the Mediterranean lemon or the West Indian lime.*

Subsequent analysis has shown that whilst lemon juice is rich in vitamin C, lime juice contains very little. As a result new theories arose, the most popular being that scurvy was due to tainted meat. The National Antarctic Expeditions of 1901 and 1910 were provisioned on this theory, and as a result scurvy was rampant. Captain Scott and his party were suffering from scurvy when disaster overtook them. If they had followed the advice of Dr. Lind put forward 150 years before they would have in all probability survived.

In the First World War scurvy broke out amongst the troops in the Middle East who were still being issued with lime juice. In 1918 tests made on guinea-pigs showed that lime juice possessed only one-quarter the potency of lemon juice as a preventer of scurvy, but what is even more important, lemon juice retains its potency when concentrated and preserved whereas lime juice does not. A striking demonstration of this was the experience of Augustine Courtauld of the British Air-Route expedition to Greenland. He lived for seven months alone, on a diet containing no vitamin C apart from one dessertspoonful daily of concentrated lemon juice. He remained in perfect health and the lemon juice was found subsequently to have retained its potency. The clock then had gone full circle. It had taken 170 years to show once more the protective value of lemon juice, whilst in the meantime scurvy had again caused death and disaster. Today scurvy is a rare disease, but it still occurs in old men whose wives have died. We call it 'widower's scurvy'. The bachelor has learnt by a lifelong experience how to cope with problems of food, but the man suffering sudden bereavement is depressed and apathetic, not interested in food and not knowing how to prepare it, living on a diet of tea, bread, and margarine and jam; he is the candidate for scurvy.

Between the two world wars research went on rapidly and the chemical nature of vitamin C was determined. During the Second World War, however, diet and nutrition had to be carefully planned to ensure an adequacy for all without undue excess or waste. We could not afford to waste those precious vitamins, particularly in England where over 50 per cent of our foodstuffs had to be imported by sea. Every cargo was precious and paid for in human lives. In 1938 the League of Nations had estimated that the daily requirement of vitamin C for an adult was 30 mg.; the National Research Council of America had recommended 70 mg. There was little scientific

---

* The British sailors became known as 'lime-juicer's' and eventually the term 'limey' was applied indiscriminately to all Britishers, particularly by the Americans.

information available; these estimates were barely more than intelligent guesses. There was a great need for research to find out the vitamin C requirements of human beings. This was carried out in Sheffield between 1944 and 1946 on conscientious objectors who had offered themselves as human guinea-pigs. Nineteen men and one woman took part in the trial; to start with all were given large quantities of vitamin C for six weeks; they were then split into three groups, one group continuing on the same intake, the second on a reduced intake of 10 mg. a day, and the third group on a diet containing no vitamin C. During the first seventeen weeks no changes were noted, but in the third group after twenty-one weeks the first signs of scurvy began to appear.

One of the questions which the investigators wished to study was the effect of scurvy on wound healing. Accordingly, experimental wounds were made and their progress watched. After thirty weeks the scars of old wounds became red and livid and new wounds showed a reduced tendency to heal. One man displayed all the symptoms of acute heart failure and would no doubt have died but for the immediate giving of vitamin C. These observations then agreed in a striking manner with the accounts of scurvy given by Dr. Lind and others.

No symptoms were noted in men who had been taking 10 mg. daily for 424 days; clearly 10 mg. a day was sufficient to protect from scurvy. In those who had developed signs of scurvy, cure was gradually effected by a daily dose of 10 mg.

Fortunately, the human guinea-pigs suffered no permanent harm. They knew that their personal safety was at risk when they undertook the trial and by their efforts they increased our knowledge of the amount of vitamin C required to prevent scurvy. Experiments of this nature can only be carried out on human volunteers and all praise is due to them.

So, once more one of the great scourges of history has been conquered; men can explore the oceans and icy wastes and still remain in good health, but the battle has been won only in recent years, and lessons learnt long ago have been forgotten. Scurvy was a typical English disease because the English were sailors and explorers, expanding the confines of the known world and conquering the seas. No other race has suffered so much from its ravages; it is proper therefore that these two controlled experiments should have been carried out by British investigators.

The English people have suffered in the past from deficiency of vitamin C for another very important reason. They are very poor cooks, and of all the food elements most likely to suffer from bad cooking, vitamin C is easily the most important. It is only recently that fresh fruit, orange juice, and tomato juice have become popular in the English diet, but prior to the Second World War the average Englishman obtained most of his vitamin C from potatoes and vegetables. The only way the average housewife knows of cooking vegetables is to boil, boil, and boil, producing on the table a soggy mass of tasteless cabbage or other vegetable devoid of vitamin C. The correct way to cook vegetables is to toss them in a pan for a few minutes with a knob of butter, salt, and pepper. They retain their colour, nutritive value, and what is most important, their flavour. The making of jam is a hopeless waste of good fruit. It destroys the vitamin C and in its place produces a food which because of its high sugar content probably does more harm than good, being an important factor in the production of dental caries in children, together with sweets and chocolates. Today many of our soft drinks are fortified with vitamin C and most sections of the community are getting adequate amounts in spite of the ill treatment of good vegetables. As I have said previously, the widower is the one who is in the greatest danger, and widower's scurvy is about the only frank nutritional disease that we see in England today*. The ultimate source of our vitamin C is the sun because it produces the growth and ripening of fruit and vegetables. The spring and summer months are the times when Mother Nature provides in great abundance for the long winter.

RICKETS

CHILDREN AND THE SUN

Children love to play in the sun; its warmth and light give them added vigour and energy, and what is more delightful to the eye than a smooth, tanned body ?. Sunlight is very necessary for health in a thousand different ways. Unfortunately, there are even today some children who don't really know what it is like to play naked in the sun, and only twenty years ago there were many children whose bodies were deformed and stunted for lack of sunlight, destined to die an early death from respiratory infection, which was particularly prone to attack their debilitated bodies. The particular disease which is caused by lack of sunlight is rickets. Rickets was a product of the Industrial Revolution which started and developed in England in the nineteenth century. It was so common that it was called 'the English disease'. There is very little evidence of it in ancient times for the simple reason that atmospheric pollution was unknown and growing children could receive the full benefit of the life-giving rays of the sun.

The first published description of the disease was by Daniel Whistler in 1645, who wrote that 'Seventy-six years ago the disease was first observed in our country'. He described the symptoms accurately enough, enlargement of the abdomen, swelling of the ends of the long bones, bosses on the skull, bending of the long bones and of the back, flabby tissues, late eruption of teeth, dental decay, and deformities of the chest.

It is pretty certain that rickets occurred in the seventeenth century, but even if it had been known earlier, it can never have been very common. One thing is certain, it increased enormously during the eighteenth and particularly during the nineteenth centuries. Samuel Gee wrote in 1867 that 30·3 per cent of sick children under 2 years of age were rickety. In 1884

---

* I have seen a case of scurvy in an infant whose mother was so hygienically minded that she boiled all the child's food including the orange juice! This is, of course, a most effective way of destroying vitamin C.

there was a country-wide survey of the incidence of rickets; it was shown to coincide with the distribution of the industrial population. This led to the theory that the cause of rickets was poor diet, whilst others said it was lack of sunshine. A wider geographical survey showed that rickets was unknown in parts of India where the diet was very poor, but where there was plenty of sun.* Others, however, postulated different theories: some held that it was caused by syphilis; others propounded infective theories and because it often attacked families they said it was a hereditary disease.

There were some visionaries in those days. Robert Jones, the famous orthopaedic surgeon, was certainly one. In 1888 he gave an address on the 'Hygiene of School Children' in which he concluded: 'We ought soon to eradicate rickets and with it at one stroke the pitiful deformities which follow in its path . . . when it comes we poor physicians and surgeons, many of us at least, may be relegated to the ranks of the unemployed.'

It was Sir Edward Mellanby who, by careful dietetic experiments on puppies, showed that rickets was definitely due to a dietetic error; in other words, a deficiency disease due to the absence of an accessory food factor. This substance was named vitamin D. Puppies fed on diets deficient in this vitamin developed the disease and could be cured by being given the vitamin. There was still much confusion, however, as to the role of sunlight. Rickets had been a terrible disease amongst the children of Vienna during the First World War because of the food shortages; and because of the high cost of cod-liver oil a physician, Kurt Huldschinsky, had tried the effects of ultra-violet light on cases of rickets. He found that in a few months they were completely cured. Immediately there was a great controversy between the two schools of thought on 'diet versus environment'. The problem was finally solved when it was shown that the irradiation of the skin with ultra-violet light produces vitamin D; this was due to its action on a substance called ergosterol present in the skin. Irradiation of this substance in the laboratory will produce vitamin D. Sunlight is very rich in ultra-violet rays, but unfortunately they are easily cut off by smoky atmospheres, by fog, and even by ordinary glass. Children living in our cities therefore are deprived of the beneficial effect of the ultra-violet light, although they can still receive light and heat from the sun.

There are not many natural foods rich in vitamin D. Being a fat-soluble vitamin, it is found in nature in association only with certain fats; the chief source is milk fat, so that full-cream milk, cream, butter, and yolk of egg are good sources; the other chief source is from fish rich in fat, such as herrings, sardines, and salmon. Young children do not normally eat items from the last group and are therefore dependent chiefly on milk products. Before the Second World War, in the 1930's, rickets was still a very common disease, because the consumption of milk by children was still very low and because in our cities they did not acquire vitamin D in their skins. Many poor children

---

* In fact, rickets is common in many parts of India because mothers protect their children from the heat of the sun by keeping them indoors.

never went to the seaside for an annual holiday; this in itself would have been an important preventive measure because vitamin D is stored in the liver, and if sufficient store is laid up during the summer, it can go a long way towards tiding the person over during the winter months. A winter sports holiday is an even better way of filling up the vitamin D stores, but obviously only within the reach of a few. For these reasons, then, rickets was largely a disease of poorer families.

There can be little doubt that the normal source of vitamin D is from the sun, and if one has to rely solely on diet it is very easy to get deficiencies unless special provisions are made. Fortunately there is a very rich source of vitamin D to be found in the liver oils of certain fish, particularly the cod, halibut, and shark. The value of liver was described by Sir Thomas Browne back in 1668 when he was writing about the birds of Norfolk, in the following words: 'Many rooks are killed for their livers in order to cure of the rickets.'

Cod-liver oil had been known for centuries in Scandinavia and used empirically as a cure for rickets, but like many of these discoveries its use had been forgotten. Cod-liver oil was used at St. Bartholomew's in the nineteenth century for various rheumatic complaints, but its use fell into disrepute, and even in 1918 textbooks on medical treatment stated that cod-liver oil was of no value.

During the last war the State stepped in and assumed responsibility for nutrition at a national level. All margarine was fortified with vitamin D, so that today it is as good, if not a better, source of the vitamin than butter. That does not mean to say, of course, that margarine is a better article of diet than butter. Anyone with a palate can immediately tell the difference and he would be a bold man indeed who could guarantee that we had found all the essential ingredients of butter. The more natural our food, the nearer to nature, the better it is for us, not only from a flavour point of view but also from the health aspect. It is regrettable that the lack of ultra-violet light in our smoky cities has led us to use artificial means of supplementing our diets with synthetic vitamins. The milk-in-schools schemes and the provision of special welfare foods such as free cod-liver oil and orange juice played a most important part during wartime rationing in improving the health of mothers and children. There is every evidence that the general level of health of the British nation is now higher than it has ever been. The incidence of dental caries has decreased, rickets is practically unknown, the average height and weight of school children continue to increase, and the infant mortality-rate each year reaches new low records.

WORLD HEALTH AND NUTRITION

In many parts of the world the State plays a great part in ensuring that the people get an adequate diet. In the U.S.A. white bread is fortified with the vitamin B group to replace the important nutrients which are lost in the milling of flour, whilst in Britain during the Second World War a high extraction rate of flour was maintained. Unfortunately, many countries have now gone back to white flour which has had most of its vitamins and minerals removed. Wise people will insist on wholemeal flour for their baking; some people even insist on stone-ground flour from wheat which has been grown without the aid of artificial fertilizers. There is probably a great deal of wisdom in their choice. But there are many people who suffer in the world today because of interference with the basic cereal food of their country. In the East, rice is a staple article of diet; polished rice has had the outer husk removed; as a result the diet of the people is deficient in vitamin B_1. The answer is to supply non-polished rice to the people. A nutritional survey in Burma has made this recommendation recently, although the remedy has been known for over thirty years.

Interference with the age-old customs of the people may cause malnutrition; and well-meaning efforts on the part of would-be reformers can cause trouble.

In Africa and many parts of Asia there are great shortages of animal protein food causing a serious disease of the liver in infants called kwashiorkor. This often depends on the habits of the people who live mainly on a vegetable diet. Strong efforts are being made to make milk popular and to introduce other cheap forms of protein in the diet such as yeast and soya bean. Unfortunately, good quality animal protein is expensive. In 1960 a large-scale outbreak of kwashiorkor occurred in the former Belgian Congo; it was relieved by the emergency issue of skim-milk powder by the U.N.

Anaemia is also common in many parts of the world and is due to poor absorption of iron, proteins, and vitamins. In India, breast-feeding often goes on for two years and as milk is poor in iron the child develops infantile anaemia.

In tropical and subtropical countries, malnutrition is aggravated by the very high incidence of worm infestation of the gut and by such diseases as malaria. This sets up a vicious circle in which the victims are unable to till the land because of weakness from malnutrition and disease, and so food becomes more and more scarce, and the condition becomes worse.

In many parts of the world remote from the sea there are shortages of iodine, producing goitre. This shows itself by enlargement of the thyroid gland in the neck—the well-known 'Derbyshire neck'. It also occurs in some valleys in Switzerland, northern France, northern Italy, the Balkans, northern India, western China, Mongolia, the Andes, and around the Great Lakes and in parts of the Rocky Mountains in North America.

The source of all iodine is the sea, so that people who eat sea food do not get the disease; moreover, rivers and lakes close to the sea are richer in iodine than those remote from the sea; hence the drinking water in these areas is protective. The Japanese do not get goitre because their diet contains seaweed and other marine plants rich in iodine. Goitre can be prevented by the use of iodized salt and this is carried out as a public health measure in Britain and in many states of North America. In many parts of North America fluorides are now added to drinking water to prevent dental caries; this practice is also being carried out in several places in Britain.

Pellagra is an unusual type of nutritional deficiency disease since it occurs in epidemics in localities where there is restricted food intake. It occurs in the southern states of the U.S.A. in the poorer classes following the low winter diet. The areas of the world most affected are Italy, Rumania, Egypt, and the southern states of America, and it has been known for many years in Spain and Portugal. It is due to a deficiency of one of the vitamin B group and can be prevented by enriching corn meal and white flour with the vitamin. Milk is also a useful preventive because it contains a precursor of the vitamin.

Malnutrition is one of the great problems of the world and there is a special nutritional division of the World Health Organization which concerns itself with the problem, whilst the Food and Agricultural Organization (F.A.O.) deals mainly with production and distribution. The problem of feeding the world's growing population is an enormous one, and depends not only on medical knowledge but on adequate financial resources and a thorough knowledge of the habits and customs of the people concerned. The education of people in the proper feeding of infants is of enormous importance (*Figs.* 23–27).

It is tragic to realize, however, that in the Western World many people are ill because of over-eating, whilst in the East millions are underfed. Even with all our knowledge in the West children receive faulty diets; perhaps the greatest error is found in allowing children to eat too many sweets and chocolates at the expense of fresh fruit, vegetables, and milk; apart from any general effect on health such a diet has very definite bad effects on the teeth, producing dental caries.

One thing is certain, there never has been enough food in the world to feed all the people adequately. With the rapid increase in population the gap between production and requirements is tending to become wider. There can be little doubt that as in the earliest days adequate food is the most important, the most urgent, need in the world today.

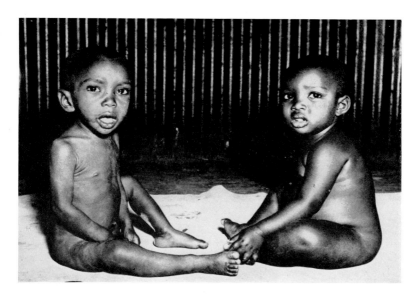

Fig. 23.—A healthy child and a child suffering from malnutrition at a Kenya Maternal and Child Health Centre.

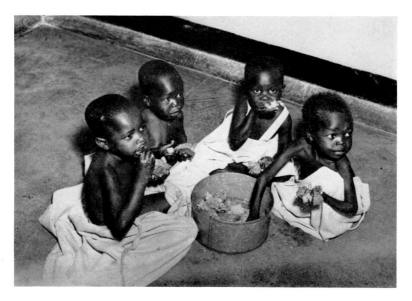

Fig. 24.—Advice on nutrition is part of Kenya's health education programme. Mothers are taught to provide a varied diet for their children to prevent malnutrition.

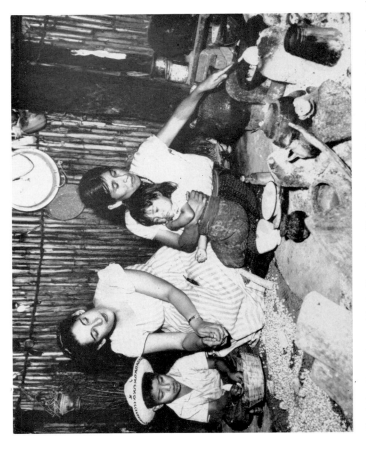

Fig. 25.—Food for the undernourished: Guatemala. The Institute of Nutrition of Central America and Panama (INCAP) is administered by the Pan American Sanitary Bureau. INCAP's activities include laboratory research and health education campaigns to teach people to improve their diet, which too often is based on a single staple. The Institute has succeeded in developing an inexpensive product of high nutritive value, incaparina, which is well liked and widely used in Central America.

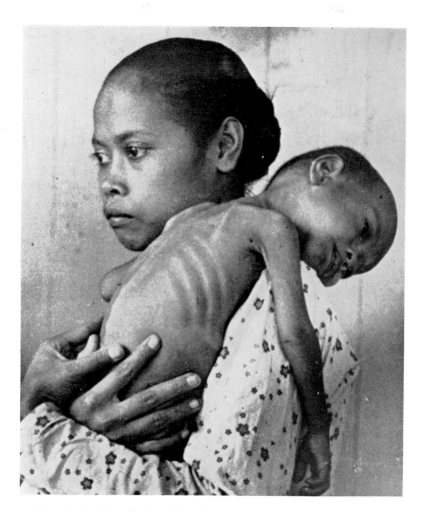

Fig. 26.—A victim of malnutrition in Indonesia. Before his first cry the child has already overcome many dangers and throughout the period of his growth he will continue to struggle until he has found his place in the community. From the age of 1 to 5 years, malnutrition threatens.

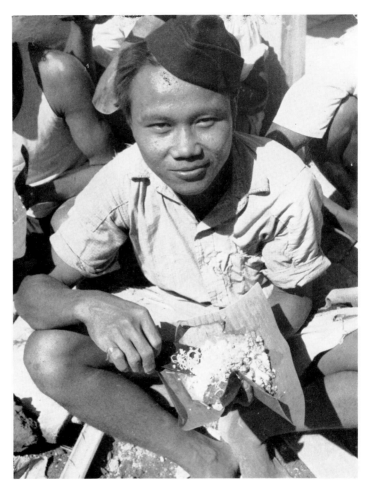

Fig. 27.—This is the lunch of a Javanese worker. His handful of rice, soya-beans, and vegetables costs 1 Rupiol—about 25 per cent of his daily wage. This food is wrapped in a banana leaf.

CHAPTER X

THE WHITE PLAGUE

Where youth grows pale, and spectre-thin, and dies.—JOHN KEATS

THERE are probably some 50,000,000 people at the moment suffering from the disease we call tuberculosis, known to our ancestors as consumption or phthisis; whilst over 3,000,000 die from it every year. It is one of the great scourges which the white man has spread to every corner of the world wherever he has settled. Tuberculosis, like rickets, increased in prevalence as a result of the Industrial Revolution, which started in England in 1760. The same process is now going on in the East and in Africa where urbanization with all its evils is replacing the rural way of life. Overcrowding in factories, in slums, and in schools is a potent factor in the spread of disease. It is a social evil and as such can be prevented by a control of social and economic factors.

Dr. William Budd, of Clifton, as a result of his observations on the prevalence of tuberculosis amongst negroes in Bristol, first suggested that pulmonary phthisis was caused by a specific organism. He wrote: 'The idea that phthisis is disseminated through specific germs cast off by persons already suffering from the disease came into my mind while I was walking on the Observatory Hill at Clifton in the second week of August, 1856. Everywhere where the blacks have come into contact with the whites, phthisis causes a large mortality amongst them.'

It was Robert Koch, however, who discovered the tubercle bacillus in 1870. He was only 39 years old at the time and not very well known in scientific circles, but his discovery shook the medical world and laid the foundation for the control of the disease. He isolated the organism from cases of the disease and cultured it in artificial media. Moreover, he reproduced the disease experimentally by injecting the bacteria into experimental animals. He devised the tuberculin test which enabled him to determine whether people had been infected with the disease. His methods were applied to many other bacterial diseases and led to a great advance in our knowledge of infective diseases in the first two decades of the twentieth century.

The tubercle bacillus can cause destructive lesions in every part of the body, producing in most cases a rise in temperature and loss in weight. The disease may be very rapid in its onset, as in the so-called 'galloping consumption', or very long-acting in its effects. Tuberculosis of the lungs is very infectious because the patient suffers from a severe and frequent cough, often with blood, but many other forms can occur—in the brain (meningitis), skin (lupus), glands of the neck (scrofula), bones, joints, and spine (Pott's disease), and kidneys or intestines.

Evidence of tuberculosis has been found in the skeletons of prehistoric man 6000 years ago and in Egyptian mummies 1000 years B.C., the typical hunchback deformity often depicted in ancient statues being due to tuberculosis of the spine.

The ravages of phthisis were described by the Greeks and Romans as a product of their urban life, but were rarely mentioned in the pastoral life of the Biblical tribes. Later, in medieval times the Kings of France and England were reputed to have the power of curing by touch the swollen glands of the neck called 'the scrofula', and the disease became known as 'the King's evil'.

Tuberculosis became very common in England in the nineteenth century. It has been said that half the people had the disease and the great majority of children suffered from tuberculous glands of the neck. It was unquestionably the greatest killing disease in the Western world at that time, for it was always present. Its greatest mortality occurred amongst young men and women in the prime of life.

The story of John Keats, the poet, is typical of the ravages of the disease. He qualified in medicine at Guy's Hospital Medical School, but soon forsook medicine for the writing of poetry. The Keats family, like so many other famous families of this time, was tuberculous, and Tom, John's younger brother, had suffered from the disease since childhood. The poet shared a room with his sick brother and kept the windows and doors closed, as this was considered the best protection against the disease. This, of course, was the worst thing that could happen. Tom Keats died in December, 1818; by 1820 John also had the symptoms of the dread disease, and ran a high temperature, had a frequent cough, and one day suddenly tasted blood in his mouth; in his own words, 'That blood is my death warrant, I must die'. He was only 24 years of age and had been in ill health for some months before. His resistance, already undermined by inadequate nutrition, was further weakened by repeated bleeding and a starvation diet.

His tragic love affair with Fanny Brawne made matters worse and rendered him morose and introspective. It was under this sort of influence that he began to write some of his finest poetry. In those days it was the fashion to go to the Mediterranean for treatment and in September, 1820, he set out for Italy in a small cargo boat, the *Maria Crowther*, with his friend, Mr. Severn. There was one cabin for all five passengers and one of the occupants was a girl dangerously ill from consumption. The voyage took six weeks and did not improve the health of either. In Italy the doctors kept him on a very low diet, 'a single anchovy and a morsel of bread'. Keats knew that he was dying and his last days were made more miserable by the memory of Fanny Brawne. On 23 Feb., 1821, he died peacefully in his sleep, at the age of 26. He died like so many others, because in the first place he came of a tuberculous stock and because he was heavily exposed to infection. His death was hastened by malnutrition and wrong treatment.

Shelley was also suffering from consumption and in 1818 took his wife and children to Italy. Two children died of typhoid fever; he was spared the fate of Keats and was drowned when his sailing boat capsized.

The growth of Nice as a fashionable resort in the Mediterranean was largely due to the numbers of consumptives who gathered there every winter to forsake the grim mists and fogs of the English winters.

Paganini died there in 1839, riddled with syphilis and tuberculosis, his vocal cords destroyed so that it was difficult to hear him speak. His face was described as 'pallid and corpse like' and he was incredibly thin.

Rachel, the famous French actress, introduced a new intensity into her roles, brought about by her hoarse voice and thin, pallid, face; all this was due to tuberculosis. In 1855 in New York she fainted as the curtain fell, and in her last performance in December, 1855, she knew that she was dying. 'I have done with illusion. I see myself already in the tomb.' She returned to Nice and died in January, 1858, at the early age of 38.

Anthony Trollope had six children and four died from tuberculosis between the ages of 12 and 23 years; much of the best work of Robert Louis Stevenson was done whilst he was severely disabled by the disease in the South Seas where he had gone to recuperate.

It has often been said that consumption fosters literary genius; probably the diminished physical vigour brought about by the disease increases the urge to mental activity.

Many have written of the relief from pain that can be obtained through writing and Balzac believed that up to a point fever could heighten emotion and stimulate the mental processes. He wrote: 'Six weeks with fever is an eternity, hours are like days . . . then the nights are not lost.'

Another effect of tuberculosis was the widespread use of opium for the treatment of the cough and diarrhoea which were so troublesome. Frequent usage rapidly led to addiction. De Quincey, in his *Confessions of an English Opium Eater*, describes how at one time he was taking over 500 grains a day; a normal fatal dose would be 3–4 grains. Under the influence of opium the mind becomes as though detached from the body and produces weird and fanciful thoughts. Coleridge wrote *Kubla Khan* after taking opium. It is probable that every consumptive became an opium addict if he lived long enough; it was one way of finding relief from the physical and mental horrors of the terrible plight in which he found himself.

John Addington Symonds wrote that tuberculosis gave him 'a wonderful Indian summer of experience, the colour of life had become richer, personal emotions more glowing, perception of intellectual understanding more vivid and his power over style more masterly'.

The ideal of feminine beauty in those days was a languorous, pale creature, lying upon her couch, dressed in white filmy drapery. Edgar Allen Poe did much to develop this ideal through his association with consumptive females, his wife and mistress both dying from the disease. He describes one scene with his wife: 'Virginia was dressed in white, delicately morbidly angelic; she was singing and playing the harp in the glow of the lamplight when suddenly she stopped, clutched her throat and a wave of crimson blood ran down her breast.' He regarded the pallor of her skin and her haunting eyes as additional charms.

Many of the artists of the time depicted this type of beauty. Elizabeth Siddal served as a model for some of the pre-Raphaelite painters, such as Rossetti and Millais. She died at the age of 30 from an overdose of laudanum (opium) shortly after marrying Rossetti. The wife of William Morris was also a favourite model of this school and she too suffered from the consumptive disease. This popular conception of feminine beauty became so strong that women abandoned the use of rouge in favour of whitening powder and took to drinking lemon juice and vinegar in order to spoil their appetites.

Alexandre Dumas wrote in his memoirs in 1824: 'It was the fashion to suffer from the lungs; everybody was consumptive, poets especially; it was good form to spit blood after each emotion that was at all sensational and to die before reaching the age of thirty.' The importance of tuberculosis as a killer of young adults pervades the literature and theatre of the time. In *Nicholas Nickleby, David Copperfield*, and *Wuthering Heights* there are classic descriptions of the disease.

The model for Marguerite Gauthier in *La Dame aux Camélias* was Marie Duplessis. She married a young Englishman who died soon after from tuberculosis. She became the mistress of Alexandre Dumas, living a life of gaiety in Paris until her death from tuberculosis at the age of 23 in 1847. Dumas, returning from Spain, learnt of the death of his former mistress and wrote *La Dame aux Camélias* based on her history. It had great triumphs in Paris and New York, and was used as the story for Verdi's opera *La Traviata*.

The original of Mimi in Puccini's *La Bohème* also lived in Paris. She was a flower girl in love with a young architect. Despite his poverty she went to live with him as his mistress in 1847, but already she was very ill and in the following year she died in the Hôpital de la Piété in Paris.

In America, the family of Ralph Waldo Emerson provides a tragic example of familial tuberculosis. The Rev. William Emerson died at the age of 42, in 1811; all his four sons developed the disease. Ralph Waldo was one of those sons. Unfortunately he also married into a tuberculous family; his wife's father and sisters all died young from the disease. Tuberculosis continued to carry off generation after generation of his descendants and a survey published in 1949 by one of these descendants, himself a doctor, shows that the disease had been prevalent in the family for the last ten generations, but the present generation at present appears to be free.

So the story could go on; in every city of Europe and North America there were the same tragic stories of love and death affecting generation after generation.

Before we leave this history of tuberculosis and its effect upon the Romantic era, we must give one final account of a family which has achieved fame because of the disease—the Brontë's of Haworth. The Rev. Patrick Brontë was a true Irishman born of poor parents in County Down on St. Patrick's day, 1777. He left his native heath and finally settled in the wilds of

Yorkshire with his wife in 1820. She died at the age of 38 the next year. His six children were born within seven years; no doubt this contributed to the ill health of his wife. Life at the vicarage at Haworth was extremely austere. The house was damp and cold, and meat was rarely on the menu. The father kept aloof from his children, eating alone, and wearing a high cravat to hide the swollen glands of his neck. The four eldest girls were sent to a semi-charitable institution where the food was even worse than at Haworth. Soon after their arrival an epidemic broke out in the school and Maria and Elizabeth were sent home where they died shortly afterwards from tuberculosis.

During the next four years, Anne, Charlotte, and Emily wrote several books and poems, occasionally leaving home to act as governesses, but always they longed for Haworth. The only boy, Bramwell, was doted on by his sisters, and he, revolting from the austerity of the vicarage, proceeded to find consolation in the village pub. He became a hopeless drunkard and was soon in debt, and seemed quite incapable of holding down any job for long. There was no doubt that in some ways he was a brilliant and likeable personality. However, the ravages of consumption soon produced their ghastly effect. The only thing which could quell his ceaseless cough and give him a few hours' sleep was opium and his end was hastened by his increasing addiction to this drug. He died tragically in September, 1848, after leaving the village pub one night. All this had a profound effect upon his sisters. Emily was now going rapidly downhill and died three months after her brother. Two weeks later the local doctor diagnosed advanced consumption in Anne and she died the following spring in Scarborough where she had gone with Charlotte for her health. Charlotte returned to the lonely vicarage, the last of her generation; she now had a perpetual cough, sore throat, fever, and loss of appetite. In 1854 she married and soon became pregnant. A few months later she died, at the early age of 39.

The Rev. Patrick Brontë lived to the ripe old age of 89 and died of 'chronic bronchitis'.

The tragedies of that lonely household were written by his daughters into several novels and poems, made famous after their deaths. It is quite possible that much of the dramatic poetry and drama written in the nineteenth century would never have been created but for the stimulus of tuberculosis.*

It is clear from these studies that heredity plays a great part in the acquisition of the disease, but after the discovery that tuberculosis was an infectious disease the pendulum swung to the other extreme, and the importance of environment was stressed. It is true, of course, that it is not possible to get the disease without coming into contact with the tubercle bacillus. We can do this in two main ways, either by drinking infected milk from tubercular cows or by inhaling the bacilli when some person with the disease coughs

---

* Besides those already mentioned, other famous persons who have suffered from the disease are Cecil Rhodes (who knows what would have been the history of South Africa but for his illness ?), Watteau, Rousseau, Sterne, Goethe, Schiller, Washington Irving, Elizabeth Barrett Browning, Chopin, and Chekhov.

or spits. The first type, bovine tuberculosis, was fairly common before the last war, but has now almost entirely disappeared owing to the fact that the majority of milk supplies are now rendered safe by pasteurization. (It is as well to remember, however, that until quite recent years something like 40 per cent of the dairy cows in this country were infected with tuberculosis.) As a result, the unsightly scrofulous glands of the neck which were so common have now disappeared, the hunchback from tuberculosis is now never seen, and bone and joint tuberculosis is very rare.

There still remains the disease of the lungs contracted by droplet infection from another person suffering from the disease. In our industrial cities all of us, by the time we have reached adult life, have been in contact with the tubercle bacillus because there are always present in the community open cases of tuberculosis—with the sufferers coughing up live virulent organisms. In 1960 the results of routine mass radiography in England and Wales revealed that there were about 1 in every 625 persons of adult age requiring treatment or close clinic observation. This means that there are over 70,000 such persons at the present time. Wherever we go, then, where there is overcrowding we meet it, and particularly in the winter time, in schools, buses, trains, cinemas, factories, and shops. Even the countryman coming up to town at the week-end comes into contact with the organism. In some, of course, the contact is more frequent and the dosage of organism greater than in others. This is particularly so if we live in a house where there is tuberculosis, i.e., if we are a contact. In these days when tuberculosis is in some people a milder and more chronic disease it is possible for the diagnosis to be missed, and labelled, for instance, 'chronic bronchitis', as in the Rev. Patrick Brontë, and many a child playing on his grandpa's knee has died from tuberculous meningitis as a result. Others at special risk are nurses, doctors, and medical students, particularly those who are looking after cases of tuberculosis. There is a great danger in overcrowded workplaces, particularly in the larger factories where there are many people coming and going. The larger the factory, the greater is the chance of coming into contact with an open case. The safest place is, of course, in the home, particularly if it is in the country, so that young girls who work in factories are more likely to become infected at an earlier age than those who stay at home.

However dangerous industrial conditions may be we must never forget the importance of respiratory infection; the older man is a very great danger to the whole community, because in him the disease tends to run a chronic and insidious course which often remains incorrectly diagnosed. The added risk of infection at work is one of the reasons for the higher incidence in men. There is a higher risk in women when they are employed in industry and are exposed to bad working conditions. In wartime, for example, when many women are working in industry they experience the same high death-rates as men. It would appear that work in unhealthy industrial conditions is one of the important causes of the spread of tuberculosis. Some very interesting investigations have been carried out by Dr. Alice Stewart in the boot and shoe industry in Leicester, since it was known that this is one of the occupations which carry a high risk as far as tuberculosis is concerned. She found that for every person contracting the disease at home there were two who contracted it from fellow-workers, i.e., the occupation is twice as important as the home life. She found also that the larger the working space and the more people in it, the more chance there is of getting tuberculosis. If the person works alone there is very little chance of becoming infected, because there is little chance of coming into contact with an open case. In large factories there is a much greater chance of sooner or later meeting someone who is an open case. In a room of 200 workers the risk of contracting tuberculosis was three times greater than if the person was working alone. There is, of course, also the danger from infection in overcrowded buses, trams, and trains, a danger which affects particularly the worker in cities. An active case occurring in light industry is a greater danger than a case occurring in heavier industry because any person contracting tuberculosis in a light job is more able to carry on with his work than in a heavy job and so he tends to stay on in the industry. The person in whom it occurs in heavy industry immediately leaves the heavy industry because the work is too heavy for him and so there is an automatic sifting of people out of heavy industry into lighter industry. In this respect the boot and shoe industry is particularly dangerous. Dr. Stewart found also that despite the overall fall in total death-rates there was nevertheless a rising incidence of tuberculosis in young entrants into industry because they were no longer immunized in childhood as before. Before the last war most children got their dose of tuberculosis by drinking infected milk. This meant that they had an increased immunity when they went into industry. Today most of our young people leave school without ever having come into contact with the disease; the majority of them are tuberculin-negative and as a result they lack that high degree of immunity which contact with the disease gives. This is a great disadvantage if they are suddenly exposed to a large dose of infection. That is why the whole problem of tuberculosis in industry is centred around the young adult. It is very important to have some scheme for the segregation of persons with tuberculosis in industry. Such schemes have been suggested, but unfortunately many of the manufacturers' associations and trade unions, and even members of the medical profession, are against it. There is no doubt that in theory, at any rate, if we are going to reduce the incidence of the disease we ought to have some scheme for the isolation of the open case in industry. Perhaps in other countries where the trade unions are not quite so powerful it would be easier to bring such a scheme into operation.

I should like to stress the danger of the older worker to the young adult. Dr. Alice Stewart describes the case of a man aged 58 years who died from tuberculosis after being nine years in a factory (incidentally, he had refused mass radiography). At death he had extensive cavities in both lungs. In his workplace of 100 workers there had been 9 cases of tuberculosis in the previous two years, undoubtedly contracted from him.

Let us now consider some more specific hazards. All dusty occupations are potentially dangerous, particularly those associated with silica, such as the mining of anthracite, tin, copper, gold, etc. Other dangerous jobs are to be found in the steel industry, such as fettling and other forms of steel dressing, and also in the making of refractory bricks, abrasive powders, and pottery.

In making a casting, molten steel is poured at a very high temperature into a mould made of silica sand; as the steel sets in a solid mass some of the silica sand adheres to the casting. All traces of the sand have to be removed, either by pneumatic chisels, shot blasting, or wheel abraders. Whatever process is used a large amount of silica dust is produced. The men will not wear the masks which are provided for them and consequently inhale all this dust. When men in heavy occupations, such as coal-mining and steel-making, get silicosis and tuberculosis they do not stay in these occupations because the work is too heavy. They leave and go into some lighter occupation, and hide the fact that they have the disease because employers quite naturally are unwilling to employ such men. Their absenteeism rates are much higher and they tend to drift into less well paid and lighter jobs, still hiding the fact that they have suffered from the disease.

Tuberculosis seems to be a danger in those jobs where there are long and irregular hours of work, as for barmen, stevedores, and costermongers. It is most common in those industries which recruit poor physical types, printers in particular, the boot and shoe industry, and hairdressers. There is also the danger from the misuse of leisure—the young girl just leaving school, having late nights and parties, drinking, spending little money on lunch, with little outdoor life, and burning the candle at both ends. When girls get married and work in the sheltered environment of the home they are much safer. Although we have seen an overall reduction in the mortality from tuberculosis there are still some black spots: localities with particularly high death-rates are Tyneside, Merseyside, Wales, and the west of Scotland. Areas with very low rates are East Anglia and the southern counties. London and the West Riding of Yorkshire have lower rates than the country as a whole, despite the fact that there is much overcrowding and a high density of population.

CONTROL

The control of bovine tuberculosis is relatively a simple matter and can be summed up in the phrase 'the heat treatment of milk', but with the control of human respiratory tuberculosis we are up against a much more difficult problem. First of all there are general methods of control—improvement of working conditions. The Factory Act of 1937 brought about great improvements in places of work despite the overcrowded conditions which followed in wartime. In the years since the end of the last war there have been some very bad housing conditions, almost as bad as they have ever been, caused through bombing, but despite this the fall in tuberculosis mortality has continued. The occupational environment is certainly more important as far as this country is concerned. This does not mean that we should relax our efforts to try to improve housing conditions. Probably housing is more important in the overcrowded conditions we find in Africa and India. Undoubtedly nutrition is of enormous importance in many of the underdeveloped countries of the world, but has become of less importance here where our standards of nutrition are at such a high level. If we concentrate on improving the industrial environment and ensuring better standards of housing and nutrition we shall produce a considerable diminution in the incidence of and mortality from tuberculosis, but we shall never be wholly successful unless we concentrate also on specific measures of control.

Intensive case-finding is very important indeed. Notification in itself is not sufficient because tuberculosis is often very poorly notified. A great many patients die every year who have never been notified. Notification is usually only of advanced cases and is particularly bad in surgical cases. Undoubtedly mass radiography is one of the best methods for early detection of new cases. In 1956 there were 69 mass radiography units in operation in England and Wales, but they are not always used to the best advantage. We should realize that it is more important to concentrate on the most susceptible groups and not waste our efforts on the mass radiography of the whole population. We must concentrate on those industries I have mentioned, and particularly on young people from school who are just entering industry and on medical students, nurses, and teachers. It is no good finding new cases unless one has an adequate organization for dealing with them, i.e., intensive follow-up and home visiting by health visitors. Many doctors and surgeons do not even know that tuberculosis is a notifiable disease and many cases of bone or joint tuberculosis never get notified. But it is just as important to notify the non-infective case in order to trace its origin. Each new case which arises is a challenge to the adequacy of our preventive measures. It means that somewhere there is an open, uncontrolled case of tuberculosis. We should stress all the time the importance of intensive follow-up.

Sir Robert Philip of Edinburgh was the first person to introduce the idea of a tuberculosis dispensary. This is a centre for the control of the disease. It is a receiving house for diagnosis and the supervision of domiciliary contacts, a centre for curative treatment and an information bureau and education centre. I should like to stress the importance of health education in tuberculosis. You can employ men with tuberculosis quite safely if they are intelligent and well briefed on how to look after themselves. Unfortunately, most men in industry are not very intelligent, and there is a great danger in employing the open case in industry. The employment of persons who have had tuberculosis is extremely difficult. There is a Ministry of Health Memo. No. 7/52 advising on the employment of the tuberculous person in industry, but with the best will in the world employers are very loathe to employ them. Their attendance records are very poor and they are a constant menace to other workers. We need more special workshops for the tuberculous person, of the type which has been set up in Birmingham where there is a special Remploy factory for the employment of these people.

Once a person has suffered from the disease there is always the possibility of it flaring up again, and even if it is quiescent the stress and strain of heavy industry may cause a recrudescence of the disease. The healed patients, therefore, should not be employed in heavy jobs or dusty occupations or where there is damp or extremes of temperature, and certainly never where there are young people. They should not be employed where food is involved. This means that there are relatively few jobs available and wherever they are employed they require constant care and supervision. It means that in order to do this we must have some sort of industrial medical service. Such a service is to be found at the Philips works in Eindhoven, Holland, where they look after 32,000 employees and their families. It is much more difficult where there are a lot of small factories, as in this country, where the majority of people work in such factories. However, many of the larger firms have first-class services. If a firm has an industrial medical officer you would think it important that he should be notified of all cases of tuberculosis. Unfortunately, the Ministry of Health has other ideas and has issued instructions that cases of tuberculosis shall not be notified to industrial medical officers because the trade unions made this stipulation when they agreed to the introduction of schemes for mass radiography in factories. I know of several industrial medical officers who are not told about the cases of tuberculosis which arise in their factories. No wonder that the disease continues to spread.

Undoubtedly of great value in controlling the spread are the medical interviewing committees which have been set up by the Ministry of Labour for the placing in suitable jobs of persons suffering from the disease. They consist of representatives of the Ministry of Labour, the Ministry of Education, and doctors and industrial medical officers, and they advise on the sort of jobs that might be suitable for these persons to go into. We must not forget the importance of BCG inoculation for school leavers. After long delay this is only just starting in this country, although in Scandinavia it has been applied with very successful results. The main reason for this was certainly the scare created by the famous Lubeck disaster. Between December, 1924, and April, 1930, 249 newborn babies in Lubeck were inoculated. It was found later that the vaccine had been contaminated with live virulent tubercle bacilli kept at the Lubeck Hospital. Seventy-six babies died from tuberculosis but 173 showed no ill-effects. This is a remarkable example of the natural resistance to massive infection, which is to be found even in the most susceptible groups of the population. Although this was an accident, it was a long time before people became convinced that the vaccine was safe. It is now prepared under the strictest conditions in laboratories devoted exclusively to the work, and despite many millions of inoculations with BCG since that time there has been no similar occurrence and no case of tuberculosis has ever occurred as a result of the inoculation.

We should never forget the great importance of health education of the public as a whole. This must start at an early age, and all schoolchildren should receive education on the fundamentals of health and hygiene. In the factory all new entrants should receive courses of instruction on health and hygiene. The health visitor, the doctor, and the school teacher are key persons in bringing home the facts to the people. Because of tradition and cumbersome methods of control there is no doubt that there are black spots, and we have with us a disease which is preventable but which is still not being prevented. What about other countries of the world ? The impact of the First World War produced serious increases in deaths in those countries engaged in the fighting, particularly Austria, Germany, and Belgium. Again in the Second World War Belgium, France, Germany, Greece, Holland, Finland, Yugoslavia, and Poland all paid their toll in deaths from this scourge following the grave social and economic upheavals of invasion and war.

There is no doubt that the so-called 'white plague' can be eradicated from a country by intensive application of preventive measures, involving the expenditure of much money. In Russia, Sweden, Denmark, and Norway there has been extensive use of BCG vaccination and this, together with all the other preventive measures, has resulted in a great decrease in the disease. There have been several well-controlled experiments carried out on its use, the best of these being a large-scale immunization of North American Indians, 1500 receiving BCG and approximately 1500 acting as controls. It was found in a subsequent follow-up that the inoculated group had a much lower mortality from the disease. This experiment has been criticized on the grounds that whilst it shows the value of BCG in a primitive community with little natural immunity it does not necessarily apply to civilized races. In 1956, however, the Medical Research Council of Great Britain reported on the use of BCG and vole bacillus vaccines in the prevention of tuberculosis in Britain in 56,700 volunteers amongst adolescent boys and girls. The protection given was substantial with both vaccines, the incidence of tuberculosis being 5 to 6 times greater in the unvaccinated group.

An interesting account of the efficacy of BCG is described by J. V. Hyge (1947), in an outbreak of tuberculosis in a school. There were 94 exposed to infection who were tuberculin-negative, i.e., it was their first exposure; of these 59 per cent developed the disease; in 106 who had been vaccinated only 2 children developed the disease; of 105 who were naturally tuberculin-positive, having been exposed before, 4 developed the disease. The disease was spread by a highly infectious teacher and illustrates in a remarkable manner the protective value of BCG.

The value of BCG should not lead us to relax our efforts in follow-up and contact tracing. The early recognition of infective cases still remains the cornerstone of control.

What of tuberculosis in primitive countries ? When this disease was first introduced to communities which had never experienced it before the mortality was enormous. It was the Industrial Revolution in England, for example, which threw many country people into the overcrowded towns and introduced them to massive infection. Friedrich Engels described the typical English working men in those days, 'the pale lank, narrow-chested, hollow-eyed ghosts'. For every Keats or Brontë there were tens of thousands of working-class men dying from tuberculosis. The North American Indians were nearly wiped out by it and their small numbers today are largely due to tuberculosis; however, the present survivors have developed some resistance as a result. The greatest mortality is found today amongst such races as the Eskimoes and negroes, particularly where they have come into contact with civilization, living in unhygienic and overcrowded conditions, eating the poor sophisticated diet of the white man, without any natural resistance whatsoever. (*Figs.* 28, 29.)

The problem of tuberculosis is largely an economic one. In India with 2,000,000–5,000,000 deaths yearly it would require by Western standards 500,000 beds and 15,000 doctors to cope with the treatment of the disease alone. In 1952 there were about 10,000 beds and barely 200 doctors. The policy is now to rely largely on domiciliary treatment with supervision from tuberculosis centres. Fortunately the drug isoniazid is a cheap and effective remedy in most cases. The hospital beds are reserved for those cases which require admittance for some special form of therapy, e.g., surgery.

Tuberculosis can be prevented from spreading by adequate control. In the Papworth Village Settlement, for example, which regards tuberculosis as a family disease, if the disease occurs in one member of the family, say the father, the whole family is brought to the Settlement for several years. Since the inauguration of this scheme there has not been one single case of tuberculosis in any child in these families, despite the fact that the household was a tuberculous one, with its added risks of infection. But such methods are probably too expensive for general application or for poor countries. In these cases, programmes of mass vaccination will probably give the best value for money. The World Health Organization started a BCG vaccination programme in 1951, and from its beginning until the end of 1953, 16,000,000 people had been vaccinated in 26 different countries within the framework of this scheme. Most of these were in India.

Tuberculosis has been almost eradicated from the Scandinavian countries by an insistence on preventive measures such as the large-scale use of BCG vaccination. Let the rest of the world take heed and make sure that this preventable disease is really prevented, so that in the future methods of treatment will no longer be considered, simply because there will be no cases left to treat. Perhaps one day we shall come to the state described by Samuel Butler in his book *Erewhon* (or *Over the Range*), where a murderer was treated as a sick person and the consumptive was regarded and treated as a criminal. There is some justification for this view, for tuberculosis is an evil, a social evil, which can be prevented and which would never occur if we really acted as though prevention were better than cure.

There are some infective diseases of the lungs which are not so amenable to discipline; these are the group of virus pneumonias, of which psittacosis is one example. The disease occurs naturally in parrots, pigeons, budgerigars, and finches, and infection occurs from close association with these birds. Control depends largely on a strict quarantine on the importation of these birds, since treatment by antibiotics is not of much value. In the Faroes the natives get the disease when they catch the fulmar petrels for food in the summer, since this bird suffers from the condition.

Most dangerous, however, of all virus pneumonias is influenza. In 1918 there was a great influenza pandemic which spread throughout the world and caused many millions of deaths in people in the prime of life; the typical heliotrope colour of the face was a well-marked feature. It is estimated that there were 200,000,000 cases and more than 10,000,000 deaths in less than a year; in the U.S.A. alone there were 20,000,000 cases in less than six months. Since that time there have been several serious outbreaks of influenza but not quite on the same scale. Unfortunately, no one knows why it occurred or when a similar epidemic might appear. All attempts at control have been of little value and unfortunately the infection does not respond to any antibiotic yet discovered. Another great epidemic occurred in 1957 of Asian influenza. It started in China and spread across India and Europe to the U.S.A. Fortunately the mortality was very low.

The chief hope for prevention of influenza lies in developing suitable vaccines. Extensive trials have been carried out with various types, and successful results obtained. The W.H.O. Epidemiological Intelligence Service keeps track of the outbreaks and in collaboration with the World Influenza Centre prepares suitable vaccines (*Fig.* 30). A 'break-through' has also occurred in regard to the common cold, several viruses having been isolated and new vaccines prepared.

THE NEW WHITE PLAGUE

There are few diseases which have evoked so much popular attention as that known as infantile paralysis or poliomyelitis; an appeal for money for research will always result in large sums being made rapidly available, but the amount of human suffering it causes is infinitesimal compared with many of the other human afflictions we have been discussing. Because of the great public interest in epidemic paralysis of sudden onset we must devote some pages to a discussion of the problem.

There are no references to paralysis of sudden onset until the late eighteenth century and no account of epidemic paralysis until 1836 when Sir Charles Bell described cases of paralysis on the island of St. Helena, and in the same year 4 cases were described in a small community at Worksop. The disease, however, was not taken seriously until several grave outbreaks had been reported from various countries in Northern Europe. Since 1900 serious epidemics have occurred in Europe and North America and it has now become a great scourge appearing wherever the standards of hygiene are high, but it now appears that poliomyelitis has been common as a relatively mild disease in most parts of the world, breaking out in virulent form when susceptible immigrants visit a country. This has occurred in recent years in the Philippines, Malta, Egypt, India, China, and Korea. Another recent feature of the disease has been the shifting age of incidence. It was formerly called infantile paralysis; today one-third of the victims are adults. Many of those who are attacked die from paralysis of the respiratory muscles, whilst those who survive suffer from atrophy of the muscles of legs or arms with serious disability as a result, a disability which is plain for all to see. This dramatic mode of expression has attracted a great deal of attention and produced much alarm when it was realized that the usual methods for the control of epidemic disease have had no effect upon its spread. Despite a large amount of research we are still ignorant of the precise origin of the infection. During an epidemic the poliomyelitis virus appears in large quantities in the intestinal contents of the person affected and it is found in great abundance in the sewage from areas where the disease is rampant. Flies are often found to be carrying the virus during epidemics. Epidemics occur mainly in the summer months, that is August and September in the northern hemisphere and February and March in the southern hemisphere. With the onset of cold weather there is a sharp decline in the number of cases. In the tropics, however, they may occur at any time of the year. In some epidemics there has been a tendency for them to continue throughout the winter months, particularly in Australia. The cause of this is unknown. For these reasons infection is probably spread by infected food or drink, similar, in fact, to the mode of spread of dysentery and other summer food-borne diseases. It may be possible that dried faecal dust can produce the disease by being swallowed. Unfortunately, there are many difficulties in studying its spread, because of the lack in the past of suitable experimental animals. Anthropoid apes are the best, but they are very expensive; chimpanzees, for example, cost something like £200 each. The most suitable animals to use in any number are small monkeys.

On feeding virulent virus by mouth to such animals paralytic disease can be produced with regularity and the virus recovered in large amounts from the intestinal contents. The virus multiplies in the walls of the intestine and then passes to the nerve-cells of the spinal cord or brain, but not all strains produce paralysis; there are a number which produce infection in the gut and multiply there, but do not necessarily produce paralysis. In human epidemics there are usually many non-paralytic cases which are not diagnosed as such but may only give symptoms similar to the common cold, or in some cases give no apparent symptoms at all. These *in toto* outnumber the paralytic cases sometimes by as much as a thousand to one. In an epidemic a high proportion of the population may be infected but only a small proportion suffer any ill effects. What are the factors which determine whether an infected person will get paralysis or not ? We know some aggravating causes; for example, severe exercise may cause the particular fatigued muscles to become paralysed, or injections in a particular limb may cause paralysis in it. Removal of tonsils or teeth may enable virus to enter the body more easily and attack the nerve-cells. Pregnancy also appears to be a contributory factor.

The virulence of the virus is of the greatest importance, some severe strains causing a high incidence of paralysis, others producing a very low incidence, in some cases none at all, so that a community can be subjected to a wave of infection by poliomyelitis virus and yet be quite unaware of it. Such an event can be of great benefit because it confers a high degree of immunity on the people infected and renders them much more resistant to severe strains which may come along later. It is possible to assess the level of immunity by taking samples of blood and measuring the amount of antibody.

At birth the infant receives some immunity from its mother, particularly if it is breast-fed, but unfortunately this does not last very long and then only as long as the breast-feeding is carried on. The infant then becomes susceptible to infection. In many parts of the world where standards of hygiene are very low there is ample opportunity for infants to pick up infection from infected food and drink, and because of frequent opportunities for passage and growth of the virus it is very common. Most of these strains are of a mild character and so the majority of children of poor families soon become resistant as a result of these infections. In many tropical countries a high percentage of young people have developed antibodies in their blood as a result. We have only just begun to realize that poliomyelitis is a tropical disease, only producing very serious effects when it strays into countries with high standards of hygiene where young children do not come into contact with mild infection and so do not have any immunity. The long period of breast-feeding, up to two years, of many children in primitive countries may also enable them to receive infection under cover of protection from the mother's milk and so develop an immunity without getting paralysis. In these countries the disease smoulders silently, building up resistance. In the Western world breast-feeding is often non-existent or kept up only for a few months. Moreover, the high standards of hygiene and cleanliness protect the child from many infections and so natural immunity is never obtained. A large proportion of children reach school age without any immunity. Such communities are ripe for epidemics which sooner or later appear. Thus the highest incidence of paralysis is found in older children and adults who have had no immunity in infancy. In highly civilized countries also the infant death-rate from all infectious diseases is very low. The outbreaks of epidemic paralysis seen in recent years in such countries as Australia, Scandinavia, the British Isles, New Zealand, Canada, and North America are due to the increasing standards of hygiene in infants over the last forty years. (*Fig.* 31.)

Of course, many isolated communities, such as the Arctic Eskimoes or people living on islands, may remain free from the virus for many years, but once it is introduced the contagion will spread quickly from person to person and often follow trade routes from island to island. This was seen, for example, in 1950 in the Society Islands in the Pacific, and Malta, St. Helena, and Mauritius have all suffered severely.

A tragic example of this rapid mode of spread in a susceptible population occurred in 1948-9 in the Eskimoes of Chesterfield Inlet in Northern Canada. Sixty per cent of the population of all ages was infected with a virulent strain, the resulting paralysis, of course, being a very great handicap in an isolated community which can only support itself by hunting.

It is now possible to predict the effects of a poliomyelitis epidemic on any particular community. It has been found, for example, that in other Eskimo communities in North Alaska and Baffin Island there is a complete absence of antibodies to all the main types of virus, and that if infection were to be introduced it would attack a high percentage of the population of all ages. In Cairo the situation is quite the reverse. By the age of 5 years, 100 per cent of the community have been infected. In Western cities, the position is midway between these two extremes, the percentage of those who have been exposed gradually rises with age from a very low level in infancy to about 80 per cent in middle age. There is some evidence that infection is more likely to be paralytic in older susceptible people than in the very young.

We can now see why the disease has been so prevalent amongst Allied troops serving in China, India, Japan, the Middle East, and the Philippines; the native peoples were immune whereas the Allied troops had no such protection. The disease was also more common amongst officers than amongst men for similar reasons.

The increasing age of attack in more advanced countries is due to successive improvements in hygiene, so delaying more and more the age at which people come into contact with infection. In this respect it closely resembles pulmonary tuberculosis.

OUTBREAKS IN ISLANDS

Poliomyelitis broke out in 1942 in Malta just after the relief from prolonged siege, and again in 1945 and 1950. There was a much higher incidence in troops from the United Kingdom than in Maltese troops working side by side under the same conditions. In the civilians it was a disease mostly of infants.

Mauritius was affected in 1945 with a high attack rate in infants. In St. Helena the first outbreak occurred in 1836, and in 1945 it again suffered a severe epidemic because of the lack of immunity of the population. All ages were attacked. The Nicobar Islands were visited by a similar epidemic in 1947. These deficiencies are probably due to the fact that St. Helena and the Nicobar Islands are isolated and like the Eskimoes the inhabitants have been free from infection for a lifetime, whereas Malta and Mauritius are on the trade routes and infection is brought in at regular intervals, only those who have been born since the last visitation of the disease being attacked. It is possible, by estimating the incidence of antibodies in the blood at various age-groups, to date accurately the various outbreaks of poliomyelitis infection even though the strains may have produced unapparent infection. The Second World War has been an important factor in disseminating poliomyelitis virus throughout many parts of the world where it has never occurred before.

There is no doubt that in some parts of the world there are important racial differences in resistance to the disease. This could be accounted for by a process of natural selection which allows only the fittest to survive. Under many tribal customs a man or woman suffering from paralysis of a limb would have little chance of marrying and allowing such increased susceptibility to be perpetuated. It is interesting to note also that Western

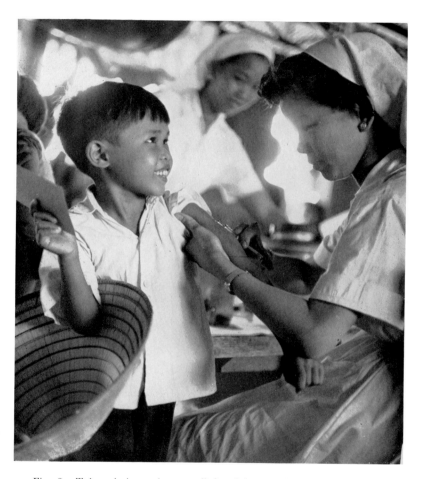

Fig. 28.—Tuberculosis *can* be controlled and its spread prevented. In regions where tuberculosis finds most of its victims there are often no hospitals or sanatoria. To help overcome this lack W.H.O. assists in the establishment of TB centres where national personnel are trained in mass case-findings, domiciliary treatment, and isolation, and in preventive measures such as BCG vaccination, etc. In Viet-Nam, where this unafraid and admiring small boy is receiving a protective BCG vaccination, the government is carrying out an overall BCG vaccination programme in an effort to curb tuberculosis.

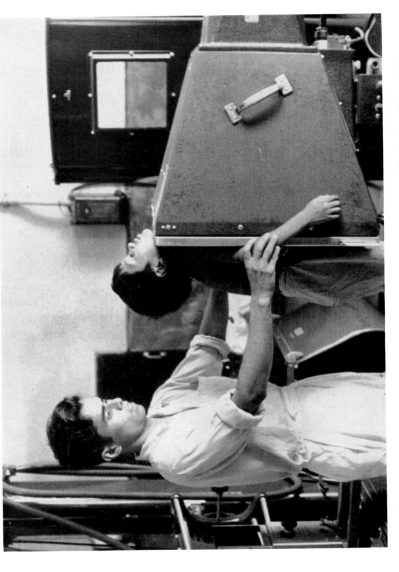

Fig. 29.—A young patient is prepared for an X-ray at the TB Control and Training Institute, Dacca, Pakistan.

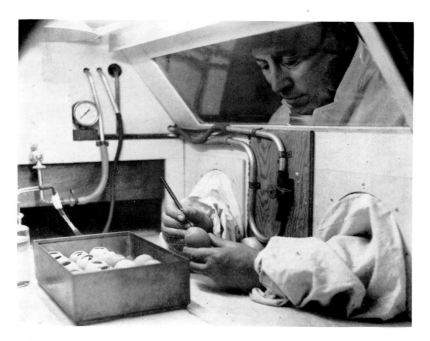

Fig. 30.—Through its world-wide Epidemiological Intelligence Service, W.H.O. keeps track of disease. One of the more elusive is influenza—a potential killer. It is the job of the W.H.O. Influenza Programme to identify quickly the virus responsible for an outbreak and to assist in the development of any necessary new vaccine. Year-round research on influenza is carried out by a network of laboratories in 56 countries in collaboration with the World Influenza Centre, London. Samples of throat-washings, flown to the centre as soon as an outbreak of influenza occurs in any part of the world, are mixed with penicillin and streptomycin and injected into the amniotic cavity of fertile eggs. These eggs are placed in an incubator to allow the virus to grow. After 2–3 days the fluid is removed from the infected eggs in an ultra-violet chamber to prevent bacteriological infection. The fluid extracted is kept for several days in a refrigerator and eventually becomes the vaccine.

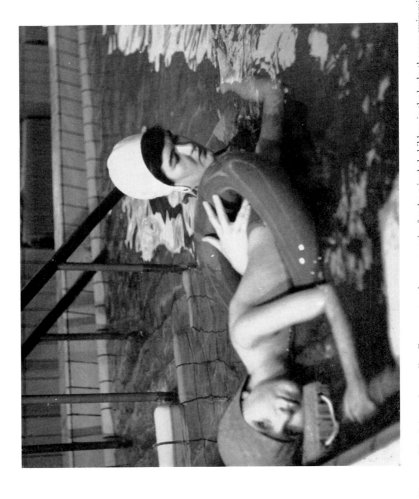

Fig. 31.—The fight against polio. Every gesture becomes easier for the crippled children in the hydrotherapy swimming pool. The hydrotherapist, a young Australian girl, spends four hours a day in the tepid water.

races are more liable to disease of the nervous system than are native races. The Chinese and the Bantu of South Africa rarely suffer from syphilis of the nervous system although syphilis is very common amongst them; the reverse holds good in the Western countries.

Diet appears to have very little effect. Well-nourished Westerners and the malnourished people of places like St. Helena and Malta in 1942 were all liable to epidemics.

At the moment great changes are taking place in Africa and Asia. Millions are being provided with pure water-supplies and safer food. The infant death-rate is falling and there can be little doubt that as in the West the incidence of epidemic paralysis will increase; these countries will have to pay the price for hygienic living and will discover the ravages of the Western epidemic paralysis, unless, of course, some means can be found to control this terrible disease.

Some properties of the virus have important practical implications. It has recently been isolated in crystalline form. This is the first time that any virus has been obtained in such a state. It is one of the smallest and at the same time one of the most resistant to chemical agents. House-dust is not an important source of infection as the virus is killed by drying and also by strong sunlight, and airborne infection is extremely unlikely. The virus is very resistant to freezing but is soon destroyed by temperatures over 70° C. It can probably pass through the pores of water-filtering beds and can certainly resist killing by many of the ordinary antiseptics, particularly in fluids contaminated with sewage. There seems to have been very little realization that water reservoirs can be contaminated by birds; for example, gulls often spend the day on sewage farms and fly to freshwater reservoirs to cleanse themselves, and the properties of the virus are such that under certain conditions and particularly in the summer it might be able to survive filtration and chlorination. One way of treating drinking water to prevent infection is known as the chlorination method; this is *not* an effective means of killing the poliomyelitis virus. Certainly there is every opportunity for the infection of rivers, pools, and bathing beaches. Typhoid bacilli have been recovered from pools of water on the rocks of our seaside resorts and the resistant polio virus could quite possibly be present in the same way.

It is a common practice for raw sewage to be discharged into the sea at many of our coast resorts. Every year there is a migration to our seaside towns and people bathe in rivers, lakes, open-air pools, and in the sea. Water is swallowed regularly, particularly by those who swim and dive, mostly schoolchildren and adults, the very age-groups that are being affected. Is it possible, then, that this summer habit is an important means of acquiring infection ?

Investigation of the source of infection and its mode of spread is very difficult, particularly when there are many unapparent cases and the incidence of notified cases is no measure of the incidence of infection. In some epidemics, however, it is possible to demonstrate case-to-case spread, particularly within households and closed communities such as schools.

It is possible that infection may be kept going in between epidemics by virus reinfecting and growing in immune persons without affecting them. It has been found, for example, that chimpanzees infected experimentally with mild strains can carry the virus for as long as 140 days. It may well be that there are virus carriers just as there are typhoid carriers.

The reason why young children do not get paralysis in areas where the virus is common may be due to the following factors:—

1. Transmission of antibodies from mother to child in the blood-stream. This only lasts a few months.

2. The acquisition of antibodies from mother's milk is a definite possibility. In Cincinnati, for example, it was found that mothers from lower income groups had such substances in their milk. Those in higher occupational groups who lived more 'hygienic' lives did not have such antibodies. The old custom of a 'wet nurse' from a poor family may have been of some practical value after all.

3. In underdeveloped countries where there are frequent chances for the keeping alive of strains of virus, mild strains are constantly being disseminated and producing immunity to the virulent ones. There is ample opportunity for frequent small doses of virus to raise the level of immunity in the same way as the measles virus acts.

4. Probably the nervous system of young infants is less susceptible to damage than that of older persons. It is important for mothers to realize the necessity of rest for children in the early stages of polio and therefore to know something of the first symptoms. The onset occurs suddenly in a previously healthy person. There is fever and almost always vomiting. Pains in the head, neck, back, and legs are very common. Stiffness likewise is a common complaint and sometimes the person may attempt to work it off by exercise. It is essential, therefore, that anyone presenting these symptoms, and particularly during an epidemic, should be put immediately to bed and the doctor called in.

It is clear, then, that the ordinary methods of control of infectious disease are not applicable and the chief hope for the future is in some method of raising the level of immunity by artificial means of people living under 'hygienic' conditions. In recent years several vaccines have been developed. The greatest degree of immunity seems to be given by vaccines made from living strains, but it is very important to ensure that such strains are mild and will not themselves produce paralysis. Unfortunately, there is still some doubt about this, particularly in view of recent mass trials of polio vaccines in which it appeared that the virus had become virulent and cases of poliomyelitis had occurred in one group which had received the vaccine. The same sort of doubts assailed those early workers who were first experimenting with vaccination against tuberculosis. Since May, 1955, the safety standards have been revised and no evidence has cast suspicion on any virus used since then. Other workers have tried using killed vaccines and they would appear to raise the level of antibodies in the blood to the same extent. The final answer can only come from actual field trials in which the incidence of poliomyelitis is compared in groups receiving the vaccine and comparable groups not receiving the vaccine, both being under the same conditions as regards exposure, age, social habits, and so on. Moreover, the number in the trial must run into several millions before effective answers can be given. Extensive trials have been carried out in North America. Thus in one group of nearly 500,000 American children vaccinated with the Salk vaccine the incidence of paralytic disease during the summer of 1955 was 4·0 per 100,000, whereas in an unvaccinated group the incidence was 21 per 100,000.

In Canada, nearly 1,000,000 Canadian children were vaccinated in the spring of 1955 and 1 child per 100,000 of those vaccinated contracted paralysis. Amongst those not vaccinated the corresponding attack rate was 5·4 per 100,000.

By 28 Aug., 1955, 8,500,000 children had been vaccinated in the U.S.A. Vaccination has been carried out in Denmark, where nearly 500,000 people were vaccinated in April, 1955. There have been no cases in this group and vaccination has been extended to Greenland, France, and the Faroe Islands. No ill effects have been reported. Perhaps the unfortunate experience with the Cutter vaccine, when 11 deaths occurred in association with it, will rank with the Lubeck disaster in the early days of vaccination against tuberculosis, when many infants died as a result of contamination of the vaccine. Unfortunately, such experiences delay the use of vaccine for a long time, particularly in conservative countries like Britain, which even now is only using tuberculosis vaccination to a very limited extent.

America and Denmark, which have both suffered very severe epidemics of poliomyelitis, are to be congratulated on their pioneer spirit in going ahead with such heroic efforts to control the disease.

The most recent developments are the use of vaccines grown in tissue culture and inactivated by formalin. This will avoid the criticisms of the anti-vivisectionists. Such strains must contain all three types of poliomyelitis virus and must be non-virulent for chimpanzees. It would appear that one single dose raises the level of immunity quite substantially, but what is more important, it sensitizes the patient to the effect of a second dose, which when given induces very high levels of antibody. This booster dose can be given many months later just before an expected epidemic.

Another important advance is the effective use of mild tissue culture strains non-virulent for chimpanzees and which can be given by mouth. This has been a big advance on the use of injection methods. The main object of vaccination is to find a safe and practical way for doing what Nature does for the majority of the population, but we must do this without incurring the risk of paralysis, for that is the price we have to pay for acquiring immunity naturally.

In 1962 there were 331 cases of acute poliomyelitis in England and Wales, the smallest number for many years; this was no doubt due to the intensive immunization programme begun in 1956. The widespread use of the Sabin oral vaccine not only protects the individual but also establishes a community immunity which should lead to the eradication of the disease.

The public should know about the possible methods of prevention, which should include the following:—

1. Wash the hands frequently, particularly after going to the toilet.

2. Wash all uncooked food and boil all water and milk.

3. Avoid intimate association with others—kissing and shaking hands, communal towels and eating utensils.

4. Rest in bed with any illness, and call in the doctor.

5. Avoid unnecessary travel and crowded places generally.

6. Avoid swimming baths and all bathing places.

7. Immunization for diphtheria, teeth extraction, and removal of tonsils should be avoided during the summer or during epidemics. After all, these procedures can be carried out at any time.

8. Contacts of cases should not handle foodstuffs.

9. The nursing of cases is most important, remembering that the virus is very resistant to chemicals and can easily be present on handkerchiefs, linen, bedclothes, and so on.

This is really the same advice we should give for the control of tuberculosis. Unfortunately in these diseases the reservoir of infection is man, and he is still the most difficult to control. Specific immunization in tuberculosis, influenza, and poliomyelitis offers great hope for the future.

CHAPTER XI

PEOPLE, POISON, AND PARASITES

THIS chapter is concerned with the potential hazards to which people are exposed during their work; whether in the home, in industry, or in agriculture, in the professional classes or in the labouring classes, everyone has some occupational hazard. In prehistoric times the dangers were mostly the physical ones of fighting wild animals, but even in those days men began to till the soil and to dig into the earth for metals. The gold-mines of the Egyptians were notorious for the dangerous conditions in which the conscripted labourers sweated and toiled. In Greek and Egyptian times there was a great prejudice against manual labour, and little notice was taken of occupational disease. It was not until the sixteenth century that anyone bothered to write about such things. Agricola and Paracelsus both wrote about the diseases of miners which were a feature of the Joachimsthal ore mines in Bohemia. These mines supplied Europe with silver for making coins. A standard coin at that time was the Joachimsthaler or thaler; this was called 'daller' by the English and so we get the name 'dollar' today.

The father of occupational medicine was Bernardino Ramazzini. Born in Italy in 1633, he produced his greatest work in 1700 when he was 67 years old. His book was entitled *De morbis artificium Diatriba*, or the *Diseases of Occupations*.

After plague had disappeared from these islands in 1666 the population of England began to rise. Throughout the eighteenth century there was a period of prosperity, with a reduced death-rate and a rising birth-rate. Food was more abundant, wages increased, and gin-drinking, a great evil of the early eighteenth century, declined. The great event which altered the whole face of England, however, was the advent of steam power which enabled factories to be set up independently of sources of water power. The development of expensive machines could only be brought about by large-scale application of capital because the worker himself could not afford to compete. More and more workers came to work in the factories and the industrial cities grew rapidly in size. Several inventions in the weaving trades caused rapid expansions in the production of cotton and wool. The development of canals and railways enabled both raw materials and finished articles to be carried more quickly to their required destination. Life in the slums brought with it ill health and disease from overcrowding, malnutrition, and air pollution, whilst the long hours of work in factory and mine exposed the worker to all sorts of physical hazards, to say nothing of the depression and mental trauma resulting from working in the 'dark Satanic mills'. Arthur Bryant speaks of the 'sinister, sunless city besides the filthy Sheaf whose forges set against the black Derbyshire hills, made the World's finest cutlery'. These changes were aptly likened to a revolution which Friedrich Engels called *Die industrielle Revolution.* (*Fig.* 32.)

Human labour was cheap and easily obtained; the least skilled and the worst paid were the Irish labourers employed on digging the new canals and permanent ways. They brought a new problem to the English towns and villages. There was great resentment against the new machines which it was thought would throw many men out of work.* An organized movement for machine-breaking grew up as a protest, the workmen calling themselves the Luddites. Their activities caused the employers to raise wages. The Chartist movement was another organization for improving the conditions of the 'working man'. One of the gravest abuses was the wholesale exploitation of child labour, particularly of orphans who were often sold for as little as £5 apiece to the mill owners. The appalling conditions under which these boys worked are described with great eloquence in Frances Trollope's novel, *Life and Adventures of Michael Armstrong, the Factory Boy* (1840).

Jeremy Bentham and Robert Owen tried hard to sway public opinion and to introduce legislation to control these abuses. Robert Owen was a great believer in the importance of a good environment for the health of the people. He introduced these ideas into his own mills at New Lanark. Unfortunately the world was not ready for these newfangled ideas and Owen himself lost £40,000. The seventh Earl of Shaftesbury did more than anyone, by his influence and persuasive powers, to bring reforms into effect. It was a long struggle against the industrialists of the time who believed that the State should not interfere in free enterprise. Eventually Acts of Parliament were passed to control working hours and the exploitation of child labour. In 1833 the appointment of factory inspectors became compulsory and the first four men were appointed. At this time we also see the growth of voluntary effort. Mr. James Smith, managing director of some cotton mills in Perthshire, employed a doctor to give advice on the prevention of disease. Leeds, however, was the birthplace of a new kind of preventive medicine, that which concerns itself with a man's occupation. Charles Turner Thackrah was a practising doctor who wrote the first English textbook of industrial medicine. It has a high-sounding and lengthy title which largely explains itself, *The Effects of the Principal Arts, Trades and Professions, and of Civic States and Habits of Living, on Health and Longevity, with Suggestions for the Removal of many of the Agents which Produce Disease and Shorten the Duration of Life*. He was led to write his book from a long experience of illness amongst working-class people in Leeds and because in his own words: 'In many of our occupations, the injurious agent might be immediately removed or diminished—Evils are suffered to exist, even when the means of correction are known and easily applied. Thoughtlessness or apathy is the only obstacle to success.' (*Fig.* 33.)

---

* At the present time we are seeing similar objections to the use of automation.

Unfortunately, Thackrah died from tuberculosis at the age of 37. Sir Thomas Legge wrote of him in 1920 as follows: 'Had he lived, his clinical knowledge and experience would have given prominence in legislation to the need for medical supervision in the factory and workshop.' It is to be noted that this need is only just being realized today and certainly only affects a small proportion of workers. In 1844 power was given to appoint certifying factory surgeons in order to examine young persons. Regulations were brought in for enforcing improved conditions in certain dangerous trades. Some particularly bad examples were the hazards of silicosis in cutlers, called 'grinder's rot', and in potters, the so-called 'potter's asthma'. Women and girls were employed almost exclusively in the lucifer match trade which resulted in a painful disease of the jaw-bone known as 'phossy jaw'.

Conditions were very bad in mines where women and children were used for carrying and hauling the coal to the surface. In the Yorkshire pits women were harnessed almost naked to coal trucks and worked like horses, for cheaper rates than men. The reports of the Children's Employment Commission shocked England; it showed that in some pits children of 6 and 7 years were commonly employed, because they were small enough to work the low, narrow galleries. They were largely used for hauling trucks. In some workings the passages were only 18 in. high, and could not be worked without very young, and cheap, child labour; even these children had to crawl on all fours. Children were also employed for cleaning out the long narrow chimneys—the climbing boys of Dickens and Charles Kingsley. The evil was finally abolished in 1875 by the efforts of Lord Shaftesbury; in the words of the Hammonds, 'his perseverance and his humanity stand out in sharp contrast to the apathy of the politicians and the cynicism of the magistrates'. This great reformer was all the more remarkable since, born into a life of ease and plenty, he preferred to carry out his work and live his life dedicated to the poor; in his own words, 'my business lies with the gutter'. In those days we lived on the sufferings of others.

Today new towns are being created on different and far-seeing plans. There are the dormitory towns to take the surplus population of the world's largest city, already over-populated, whilst the Steel Age has caused new towns to grow in the middle of the countryside, as at Scunthorpe and Corby.

New inventions are revolutionizing industry on different lines. The future industrial era will see a great growth in the use of atomic energy as a source of power; perhaps in our time we shall see the coal-mine disappear, at least let us hope so. The increasing use of electrical energy and automation in factories will radically alter working conditions; more and more men will become machine minders. (*Fig.* 34.) All this will demand an ever-growing army of technologists and technicians and there will be little place for the labourer. We have certainly controlled many of the more obvious physical hazards to be found in industry, but new advances bring new problems to tackle, some of them not always so obvious. Mental ill health is a problem which is becoming intensified as work becomes less satisfying emotionally.

The dangerous effects of radioactivity cannot be seen but they are present in ever-increasing measure. Radioactive substances and X-rays are now used in a wide variety of industries, e.g., in the steel industry for taking photographs of steel castings; and in the textile and printing industry for the elimination of static electricity; gamma- and beta-ray gauges are used for checking and measuring the thickness of steel strip, linoleum, paper, and plastic rolls. The watch-dial industry is one of the most dangerous known, as it uses thorium for painting the luminous dials. Radium is the most deadly poison known; 1/100,000 of a grain is sufficient to cause death years after its ingestion. We need no reminder of the dangers of the H-bomb. Even agriculture is not exempt, with the increasing use of toxic chemicals for spraying crops and their uses as insecticides and weed-killers. Every day new processes are being introduced into all kinds of work which are potentially dangerous and it is very necessary that we should be aware of these dangers.

The worker may be unaware that he is being exposed to a hazard or is handling dangerous materials. This may be due to ignorance on the part of his employer or to his own stupidity; it is seldom due to deliberate concealment on the part of the firm. There are today many proprietary articles used in industrial processes. Paints, lacquers, varnishes, glues, cleaning agents, and solvents are often sold as made-up articles and only the actual makers know their constituents. The workers who use them in other factory processes may be exposed to risks of which neither they nor their superiors are aware. Furthermore, new substances whose action on the human body is often unknown call for a constant look-out for new types of occupational poisoning. Doctors themselves have many occupational risks. Probably the greatest today is writer's cramp! But they have in addition a definite risk of getting coronary heart disease, peptic ulcer, cirrhosis of the liver, and drug addiction. In the past the pathologist was prone to sepsis, and various laboratory workers have died from diseases they were investigating, as Noguchi, Adrian, and Stokes all died from yellow fever, and Rickets died from typhus fever and Yersin from plague. The following medical men lost their lives as a result of working with X-rays: H. E. Albers-Schönberg, L. G. Allen, E. F. Ascheim, F. H. Baetjer, B. E. Baker, J. Bauer, R. Blackall, I. Bruce, E. W. Caldwell, C. M. Dally, J. M. Davidson, W. J. Dodd, C. G. Dyke, L. M. Early, W. C. Egelhoff, H. Fowler, W. W. Fray, W. C. Fuchs, S. C. Glidden, H. Green, F. J. Hall-Edwards, E. H. Harnack, W. Hillier, G. Holden, G. Holzknecht, C. Infroit, M. K. Kassabian, W. Krauss, C. L. Leonard, A. Leray, C. R. C. Lyster, R. H. Machlett, F. Mann, S. Melville, J. T. Morehouse, L. B. Morrison, R. Morton, S. Nordentoft, F. H. Orton, G. F. Parker, G. A. Pirie, J. T. Pitkin, G. E. Richards, J. R. Riddell, F. le R. Satterlee, I. Sims, J. W. L. Spence, H. J. Suggars, F. H. Swett, B. F. Thomas, E. Tiraboschi, R. V. Wagner, T. L. Wagner, L. A. Weigel, C. A. Wilcox, J. C. Williams, E. E. Wilson, and J. Young.

Even domestic work is not exempt from risk, with the danger of dermatitis from household chemicals, whilst housemaid's knee was more common when servants were plentiful. In India the flimsy inflammable sari is an important cause of domestic burns, many of them fatal.

Some industrial poisons have a delayed action in the body and do not show their presence for many years after the worker has left that particular job. For example, increasing breathlessness in an elderly man may indicate the presence of dust disease of the lungs, a legacy from his coal-mining days of long ago. Jaundice may develop in a former munition worker months after he has ceased handling T.N.T., and the long-term effects of radioactivity and lead poisoning may not become manifest until many years after all exposure has ceased. Cancer of the skin may take as long as forty years to appear after exposure to tar has ceased. Another point is the wide variation in the ways in which individual people react to poisons.

It is true, of course, that specific industrial diseases are relatively rare in this country, but in a great many occupations there are conditions of work which aggravate ordinary common conditions. Such things as temperature, humidity, draughts, bad lighting and ventilation, excessive noise, and long working hours can all affect the worker and increase fatigue. There are many occupational diseases due to physical agents, such as heat cramps in stokers, boiler-makers' deafness, miners' nystagmus (a defect of the eyes due to bad illumination at the coal-face), the decompression sickness or the bends found in deep-sea divers and tunnellers, and glass-blowers' and chain-makers' cataract. Cramp of the hand has been described in the following occupations: writers, telegraphists, cotton twisters, tailors, drapers, seamstresses, sail-makers, knitters, hairdressers, ironers, metal workers, hammermen, turners, engravers, goldbeaters, cabinet makers, sawyers, locksmiths, tinsmiths, nailmakers, masons, painters, enamellers, compositors, watchmakers, shoemakers, saddlers, sailors, fencers, diamond cutters, money counters, letter sorters, cigarette rollers, cigar makers, pianists, organists, violinists, violoncellists, harpists, flautists, drummers, orchestra conductors, typists, comptometer operators, waiters, florists, artificial-flower makers, folders of newspapers, and milkers of cows. Rarely the lower limbs are affected as in dancers, sewing-machine workers, knife sharpeners, and trades-men's tricyclists. Identical spasms of the muscles of the head and neck are still rarer; cramp of the lips occurs in trumpet players and other musicians.

Studies of the effects of occupation on health must cover a much wider field than those found solely in industry; even in rural areas a man's occupation has a marked effect on his health. Let us turn for a moment to a consideration of some of these in more detail.

WOOL-SORTERS' DISEASE

Anthrax, or wool-sorters' disease, is an occupational disease which spread to man from horses, cattle, camels, sheep, goats, buffaloes, and pigs. It is a common disease in many parts of the world where no precautions are taken to prevent it, as in Russia, Siberia, China, Japan, the Middle East, India, Tibet, Egypt, South Africa, and Peru. It is rare in Britain, the U.S.A.,

Australia, and New Zealand, because strict measures have been taken for its control. There is a constant fight to keep infection from entering these countries. The disease is found in persons whose job involves handling animal products, such as hides, skins, and fleeces. The bacilli form very resistant spores which can remain alive for years; thus if an animal has died from anthrax, its blood will be teeming with the organism and this can easily contaminate skins and hides which are the source of disease-producing dust. It may be inhaled, swallowed, or enter the skin. The disease was extremely fatal before the use of antibiotics in treatment.

The human disease affecting the lungs was first described in Bradford and the French still call it *maladie de Bradford*. It was also common at Kidderminster, from the importation of animal products from the East. Shaving brushes were also liable to be infected.

In Britain there is now a disinfecting plant at Liverpool, using the Duckering process for rendering harmless the most dangerous kinds of wool and hair. All wool and hair from Egypt has to come through this port, but there are legal loopholes in the Anthrax Prevention Act and certain imported articles are exempt. As a result, although anthrax is still very rare in Britain, cases do occur from time to time. In 1953 there were 29 cases with 1 death; 9 were in contact with wool, and 11 with hides and skins; several cases occurred in dock-workers handling Indian bone-meal, showing how the anthrax spore can withstand all sorts of rough treatment. In 1954 there were 18 cases with 1 death; 9 were in contact with wool and 5 with hides and skins; others were dealing with such animal products as glue and gelatin, and in tanneries. Nearly all these cases were associated with the importation of animal products from foreign ports. There is a clear need for tightening up control and making it compulsory for all imported materials to go through the Duckering process.

Anthrax is obviously a global problem and as such has received serious consideration from the World Health Organization. Measures recommended for its control are as follows:—

1. All dusty operations in leather and wool industries which handle suspected anthrax-contaminated material should have adequate exhaust facilities and should be isolated from other operations.

2. Floors, walls, and vehicles should lend themselves to ready cleaning by wet sweeping or suction methods.

3. All dust, dirt, and sweeping should be burned.

4. Protective clothing should be worn by employees in all occupations where exposure to anthrax is likely.

5. Employees should be thoroughly instructed as to the cause, nature, and control of anthrax. All cuts, scratches, abrasions, and pimples should be reported immediately, and adequate medical attention given.

6. All animal by-products likely to be contaminated by anthrax such as wool, hair, hides, skins, bone, and bone-meal should be treated so as to render them non-infective. The method and process already in existence in the United Kingdom and the United States are recommended.

HOOKWORM

One of the most common of the infestations of the intestine in the world today is hookworm. Stott has estimated that one-sixth of the world's population is infected, nearly 500,000,000 people. It is associated with malnutrition and poverty and is found in those who have to work for a living in wet fields. The worm produces chronic anaemia and malaise and contributes considerably to the malnutrition, thus rendering the victim less capable of agricultural work. The life cycle is most extraordinary and is as follows. The adult worm lives in the intestine of man, attached to the wall and sucking blood from its victim. The eggs are passed in the excreta and hatch out in a few hours under suitable conditions of warmth and moisture, into small larvae. These can survive for several weeks and infect man by entering through the skin. From here they migrate in the veins to the lungs where they are coughed up and swallowed to reach the intestine where they grow to adult worms and so complete the cycle. During the stage when they are in the lungs they produce coughing and sputum. The female worm may lay as many as 20,000 eggs a day.

This disease is common in tropical Africa and Asia and was brought to the New World by negro slaves. It is now common in the southern states of North America, in Central America, and parts of South America, where it is called the American or New World hookworm. The temperate zone hookworm is common around the shores of the Mediterranean and Asia Minor. Farther north it is found mostly in mines. It was common, for example, in the construction of the St. Gotthard tunnel in 1879. When the tunnel was completed the labourers, returning to their homes, spread the infection to England, France, Belgium, Holland, Hungary, Sicily, and Spain. In 1898, as a result of effective preventive measures, no cases occurred in building the Simplon tunnel. It occurred in the French coal-mines, but fortunately the coal-mines of Britain remained free.

The disease was once common in the Cornish tin-mines. The site of entry of the larvae produces intense itching of the skin. This dermatitis was known as the 'miner's bunches'. The arms were affected because they were kept bare and came into contact with the rungs of the ladders. In the Dolcoath mine, the parasite is still referred to as the Dolcoath worm. In the old days there was no sanitation and the mines became infested with eggs from the faeces of the men; the larvae remained alive because of the damp conditions and the warmth due to the great depth of the mines. One carrier can easily infect a whole community.

In tropical and subtropical countries, as in mines, infection is due to those human habits which deposit faeces in moist shady places. Another causative factor is the use of human excreta as a fertilizer for crops. This is a common practice in China in the cultivation of the mulberry tree for the silkworm. The women who pick the leaves walk barefooted and suffer the most. They first of all get 'ground itch', also known as coolie itch, water itch, and water pox; this is followed by cough due to the migrating larvae, then later by anaemia. The sweet-potato gardeners in Szechwan and Fukien provinces also get a very high rate of infestation.

Indiscriminate defaecation amongst the trees also provides a source of infection in the coffee groves of Puerto Rico, the orange groves of Palestine, and the tea plantations of India.

The negro is much less susceptible to hookworm than any other race, no doubt because of centuries of association with the disease; it may also be due to the thicker skin of the negro which makes it more difficult for the larvae to enter.

As can well be understood, hookworm is a special danger to troops. They get infected easily by bathing in infected pools.

It may seem at first a simple matter to eradicate the disease, but it is not easy to change overnight the habits of millions of people who are living below the poverty line. The use of privies and the wearing of shoes are important preventive measures. The Rockefeller Sanitary Commission has waged an intensive war against hookworm disease with conspicuous success. Family education has been an important factor in reducing the incidence in the southern states of America. This should remind us of Florence Nightingale's maxim, that the nurse can do more real good in the home than in the hospital, by teaching the principles of healthy ways of living. The Georgia Health Department has made extensive surveys in the schools, and home contacts were made, giving advice and treatment. Assistance was offered in the construction of an effective privy.

Mass treatment of populations with tetrachlorethylene is another useful method of attack.

Although hookworm is the most important intestinal worm, there are many others, such as round worms, whip worms, and thread worms. None of them produces so much economic loss, however, as the hookworm—that is why the World Health Organization is devoting much of its energy to its control.

FLUKES

Flukes are flat worms which have intermediate stages in freshwater snails. They are an important class of parasites which produce disease in the animal world, but there are a number which have serious effects in man. They can be divided into liver, intestinal, lung, and blood flukes. They are common in many parts of the world and the constant movement of troops in these areas is a grave threat in wartime, not only to the men themselves, but also because of the danger of importing flukes into the countries from which the men came. Thus large numbers of American soldiers were infested with oriental fluke in the Philippines during World War II. Infection is by ingesting the eggs in food, but in the case of the blood fluke the larvae enter the skin from water in the same way that hookworm larvae enter from moist soil, so that wading in canals and lakes is a common mode of infection.

Liver flukes are prevalent in the Far East where raw fish is taken in the diet. They are particularly important in Cambodia, Laos, Vietnam, Korea,

Southern China, and Japan. A similar type of parasite occurs in Eastern Siberia. Many of the fish raised in artificial ponds are infected. They are shipped from Southern China to Canton and used raw in various dishes.

Intestinal flukes are common in China, in Northern Chekiang province, where more than 1,500,000 people are affected. Their presence is due to the cultivation in shallow ponds of water nuts for eating purposes. These ponds harbour a snail which acts as an intermediate host; the eggs of the parasite enter the water in enormous numbers when the crop is fertilized with 'night soil'. Infection occurs when the contaminated nuts are peeled with the teeth.

Lung flukes occur in the Far East, particularly in Southern Korea, Formosa, Central China, Japan, and the Philippines. A closely allied species has a wide distribution in Northern America. Infection is spread by eating improperly cooked freshwater crabs or cray fish which harbour the intermediate stages of the parasite. The larvae then hatch in the intestine and migrate to the lungs. Dogs, cats, and pigs can all act as reservoirs of infection.

Blood flukes cause the disease known as schistosomiasis or bilharzia. British soldiers in Egypt used to call it 'Bill Harris'. The disease in man is one of the most widespread of all parasitic diseases, and it seems to be spreading. A large proportion of the people living in the valley of the Nile are affected and it occurs in many parts of Africa and the Middle East, including Arabia, Israel, Iraq, and Iran; it is spreading in Turkey. Stott has estimated that there are 40,000,000 cases of this disease in the Middle East. The adult worm lives and migrates in the blood-vessels, so that it can affect many parts of the body; with the Middle East type the bladder and lungs are frequently affected.

Another type is found in Africa from where it was carried to the New World by negro slaves. It is now a great problem in Brazil where it is on the increase; a recent estimate puts the number of cases there at 6,000,000. It is also found in Central America and Puerto Rico.

The oriental type is found in China, the Philippines, and Japan. The estimate for this type of disease is 46,000,000 cases. This is a very serious disease in humans, having effects on the intestines and liver. Dogs, cats, cattle, pigs, and rats contribute to the spread.

In Egypt the system of perennial irrigation is responsible and the extensive system of canals has enormously increased the habitation available for snails. The water of canals and ditches is constantly being infected by the Mohammedan need for water when defaecating.

In China and Japan the wet cultivation of rice is largely responsible, together with the use of human manure as fertilizer.

The World Health Organization is attacking this problem with considerable vigour because the inadequacy of control measures makes it a worldwide problem. Many of these fluke diseases are most common in the trouble spots of the world, the Far East and the Middle East, and any flare-up of war here will contribute to their spread. New schemes of agriculture and irrigation can seriously upset the balance of nature, and, of course, the most potent agent of all in this respect is war.

A number of non-human flukes can penetrate the skin when a person is bathing, and cause swimmers' itch; one of these belongs to the duck; it has a widespread distribution in the lakes of North America. It is clear that bathing in infected waters has its hazards and before leaving this group of interesting diseases we should mention a form of infective jaundice which occurs in Great Britain. It is known as Weil's disease, after the man who first described it. The organism can enter through the skin like the hookworm larva, and it is found in the excreta of rats. If is found, therefore, whenever people come into contact with places infested with rats. Thus it is an occupational disease of sewer men in Glasgow and London, coal-miners in southern Scotland, fish-gutters in Aberdeen, rat-catchers in East Anglia, tripe-scrapers in Glasgow, and sugar-cutters in Queensland. In all these cases the organism enters through the skin when the victim comes into contact with mud or slime contaminated with rat excreta. A number of people have been infected by bathing in dirty rivers, ponds, or streams. In Holland it is now quite a serious problem because of the heavy rat infestation of the canals.

In recent years it has been shown that dogs can harbour a similar type of organism and spread infective jaundice to human beings.

INDUSTRIAL MEDICINE

Some of the greatest achievements of preventive medicine have been carried out in the field of industrial medicine. They have certainly not been due solely to the efforts of medical men; indeed, the efforts of the legislator have probably been far more effective than the discoveries of the scientist.

In industry, co-operation is of the greatest importance. Perhaps the most important person of all in this is the managing director, together with the top flight of management, for without them little can be achieved. This idea of prevention should infiltrate from them throughout all branches down to the humblest apprentice. In the past the trade unions themselves have been a great obstacle for advance, often viewing new measures to their benefit with great suspicion. Only when given this co-operation can the engineer, chemist, or doctor play his full part in prevention.

LEAD POISONING

Lead poisoning has been known from Roman times and a review of its history will illustrate the importance of prevention in industrial medicine.

Lead was used by the Romans for making pipes and tanks for their water-supplies. It was mined mostly in Spain and Britain. Hippocrates described the symptoms of lead poisoning and they were later confirmed by other Greek physicians; constipation, colic, anaemia, and paralysis were those most frequently noted. The most dangerous jobs in nineteenth-century England were pottery glazing, the manufacture of lead compounds, and the smelting of lead ores. A great advance in prevention was made when in 1883 strict regulations were laid down with regard to ventilation, protective clothing, and hygienic conditions generally. The employment of women and children in certain lead processes was prohibited.

Intensive studies of industrial hygiene conditions were carried out at the beginning of the twentieth century by such pioneers as Sir Thomas Oliver and Sir Thomas Legge. As a result of their work the incidence of lead poisoning was markedly reduced. Thus in 1900 over 1000 cases were notified, but in 1950 only 57.

Let us turn for a moment to the writings of a great novelist for a description of a typical lead works. In *The Uncommercial Traveller* (1867), Charles Dickens describes a visit he made to a white-lead works near Limehouse Church, London. Two intelligent managers of the works, brothers and partners with their father in the concern, showed him everything quite freely.

The purport of such works is the conversion of pig-lead into white-lead. This conversion is brought about by the slow and gradual effecting of certain successive chemical changes in the lead itself. The processes are picturesque and interesting, the most so being the burying of the lead, at a certain stage of preparation, in pots, each pot containing a certain quantity of acid besides, and all the pots being buried in vast numbers, in layers, under tan, for some ten weeks.

Hopping up ladders, and across planks, and on elevated perches, until I was uncertain whether to liken myself to a bird or a bricklayer, I became conscious of standing on nothing particular, looking down into one of a series of large cocklofts, with the outer day peeping in through the chinks in the tiled roof above. A number of women were ascending to, and descending from, this cockloft, each carrying on the upward journey a pot of prepared lead and acid, for deposition under the smoking tan. When one layer of pots was completely filled, it was carefully covered in with planks, and those were carefully covered with tan again, and then another layer of pots was begun above; sufficient means of ventilation being preserved through wooden tubes. Going down into the cockloft then filling, I found the heat of the tan to be surprisingly great, and also the odour of the lead and acid to be not absolutely exquisite, though I believe not noxious at that stage. In other cocklofts, where the pots were being exhumed, the heat of the steaming tan was much greater, and the smell was penetrating and peculiar. There were cocklofts in all stages: full and empty, half filled and half emptied; strong, active women were clambering about them busily; and the whole thing had rather the air of the upper part of the house of some immensely rich old Turk, whose faithful seraglio were hiding his money because the sultan or the pasha was coming.

As is the case with most pulps or pigments, so in the instance of this white-lead, processes of stirring, separating, washing, grinding, rolling, and pressing succeed. Some of these are unquestionably inimical to health, the danger arising from inhalation of particles of lead, or from contact between the lead and the touch, or both. Against these dangers, I found good respirators provided (simply made of flannel and muslin, so as to be inexpensively renewed, and in some instances washed with scented soap), and gauntlet gloves, and loose gowns. Everywhere, there was as much fresh air as windows, well placed and opened, could possibly admit. And it was explained that the precaution of frequently changing the women employed in the worst parts of the work (a precaution originating in their own experience or apprehension of its ill effects) was found salutary. They had a mysterious and singular appearance, with the mouth and nose covered, and the loose gown on, and yet bore out the simile of the old Turk and the seraglio all the better for the disguise.

At last this vexed white-lead, having been buried and resuscitated, and heated and cooled and stirred, and separated and washed and ground, and rolled and pressed, is subjected to the action of intense fiery heat. A row of women, dressed as above described, stood, let us say, in a large stone bakehouse, passing on the baking-dishes as they were given out by the cooks, from hand to hand, into the ovens. The oven, or stove, cold as yet, looked as high as an ordinary house, and was full of men and women on temporary footholds, briskly passing up and stowing away the dishes. The door of another oven, or stove, about to be cooled and emptied, was opened from above, for the uncommercial countenance to peer down into. The uncommercial countenance withdrew itself, with expedition and a sense of suffocation, from the dull-glowing heat and the overpowering smell. On the whole, perhaps the going into these stoves to work, when they are freshly opened, may be the whole part of the occupation.

But I made it out to be indubitable that the owners of these leadmills honestly and sedulously try to reduce the dangers of the occupation to the lowest point.

A washing-place is provided for the women (I thought there might have been more towels), and a room in which they hang their clothes, and take their meals, and where they have a good fire-range and fire, and a female attendant to help them, and to watch that they do not neglect the cleansing of their hands before touching their food. An experienced medical attendant is provided for them, and any premonitory symptoms of lead-poisoning are carefully treated. Their teapots and such things were set out on tables ready for their afternoon meal, when I saw their room; and it had a homely look. It is found that they bear the work much better than men; some few of them have been at it for years, and the great majority of those I observed were strong and active. On the other hand, it should be remembered that most of them are very capricious and irregular in their attendance.

American inventiveness would seem to indicate that before very long white-lead may be made entirely by machinery. The sooner, the better. In the meantime, I parted from my two frank conductors over the mills, by telling them that they had nothing there to be concealed, and nothing to be blamed for. As to the rest, the philosophy of the matter of lead-poisoning and workpeople seems to me to have been pretty fairly summed up by the Irishwoman whom I quoted in my former paper: 'Some of them gets lead-pisoned soon, and some of them gets lead-pisoned later, and some, but not many, niver; and 'tis all according to the constitooshun, sur; and some constitooshuns is strong and some is weak.'

Retracing my footsteps over my beat, I went off duty.

Alice Hamilton, in her book *Exploring the Dangerous Trades*, describes the hazards of vitreous enamelling in Pittsburgh:—

I remember a foreman saying to me, as we watched the enamelers at work, 'They don't last long at it. Four years at the most, I should say, then they quit and go home to the Old Country.' 'To die?' I asked. 'Well, I suppose that is about the size of it', he answered. It was not the lead, as I discovered then, that did the greatest harm, but the silica dust. Many of the doctors I talked to told me that there was where my attention should be turned, to the pulmonary consumption; lead poisoning was a minor evil. But lead dust was my job, not silica.

The lead dust was bad. In the enameling rooms of the plants, this would be the picture. In front of the great furnaces stood the enameler and his helper. The door swung open and, with the aid of a mechanism which required strength to operate, a red-hot bathtub was lifted out. The enameler then dredged as quickly as possible powdered enamel over the hot surface, where it melted and flowed to form an even coating. His helper stood beside him working the turntable on which the tub stood so as to present all its inner surface to the enameler. The dredge was big and so heavy that part of its weight had to be taken by a chain from the roof. The men during this procedure were in a thick cloud of enamel dust, and were breathing rapidly and deeply because of the exertion and the extreme heat. I found that I could not stand the heat any nearer than twelve feet but the workmen had to come much closer. They protected their faces and eyes by various devices, a light tin pan with eye-holes

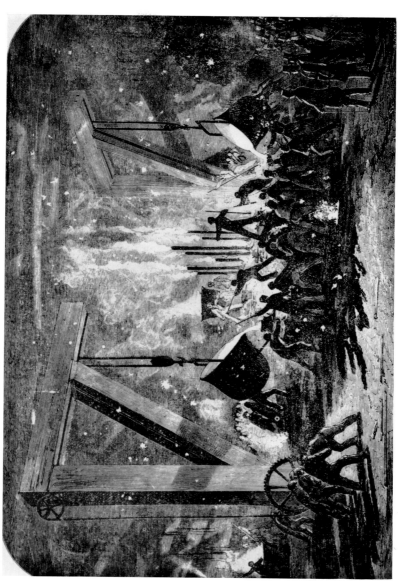

Fig. 32.—'Dante's inferno'. Working conditions in the nineteenth century. The casting of a giant cylinder in 1854. From the *Illustrated London News*, 1854, p. 440.

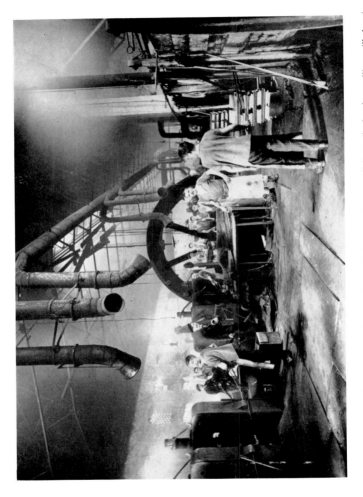

Fig. 33.—The old. Early attempts to improve hot and dusty working conditions. A view in a rolling mill showing the Sturtevant 'Cold Air Douche' system introducing a stream of cool air directly upon the workers.

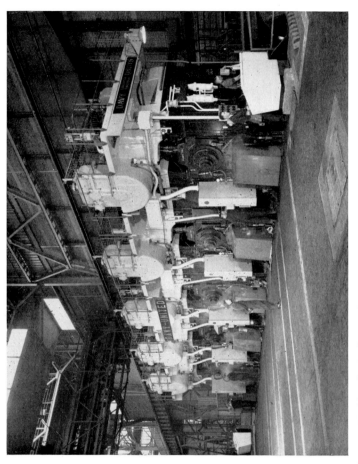

Fig. 34.—The new. Health and safety in a modern rolling mill. Modern high-speed strip rolling at the Velindre works of the Steel Company of Wales Ltd. This mill rolls tin plate gauge steel strips up to 38 in. wide at a finishing speed of 5000 ft./min. in outputs of the order of 10,000 tons a week. There is complete extraction of rolling oil fumes and little or no danger from the operation of the mill. Automatic control of mills of this type is increasing, and it is now common practice to incorporate mechanical handling equipment at all stages of the process. This reduces the physical effort required on the part of the operator to a minimum and provides a very high safety factor. The motors driving this mill total over 18,000 h.p. and are housed in a separate motor room.

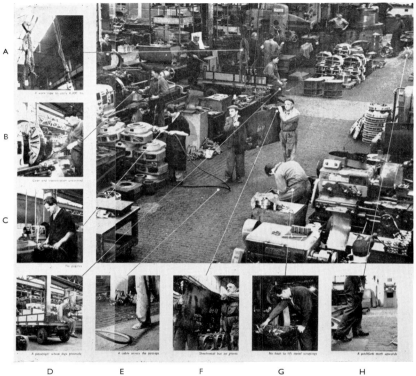

Fig. 35.—The factory's best product is its safety. Each year in Europe between one-ninth and one-quarter of all workers have a disabling accident. In the United States, out of a total of 91,000 accidental deaths from all causes, almost 14,000 are due to industrial accidents. In the Siemens-Schuckert factory in Vienna, the works safety engineer and workers staged a series of accidents that should not happen : A, A worn rope to carry 4000 lb. B, Gear and transmission uncovered. C, No goggles. D, A passenger whose legs protrude. E, A cable across the passage. F, Sheetmetal but no gloves. G, No hook to lift metal scrapings. H, A pitchfork teeth upwards.

and a hoop to go around the head, or a piece of wood with eye-holes and a stick nailed at a right angle so that it could be held between the teeth.

Apart from those employed in producing lead compounds, people engaged in a wide variety of occupations were exposed to the hazard of lead, including police officers, who used white lead for taking finger-prints, vitreous enamellers, colour manufacturers, accumulator pasters, fitters, coopers, rubber compounders, foundry workers, painters, file cutters, paper hangers, type setters, welders, ship breakers, bullion refiners, and embroidery stencillers: no doubt there were others. Today most of the cases occur in ship breaking, where the oxyacetylene burners cut through the plates of the ship, vaporizing the lead paint, and in lead accumulator makers. A new hazard arose when ethyl petrol was used; cleaning out the tanks was particularly dangerous.

In prevention, the most important points are personal hygiene, education of the worker, and periodic medical examination. Most of the cases which occur are due to neglect in not wearing masks or in lack of cleanliness.

In recent years several cases of lead poisoning have occurred domestically in children who pick the lead paint off fences and other things and eat it, or suck lead soldiers. In some households poisoning has occurred where old lead accumulators have been used as fuel. Similar descriptions could be given of poisoning by a whole range of chemicals, new and old.

The outstanding contribution in preventive medicine in industry was provided by Sir Thomas Legge, who enunciated four all-important principles:—

1. Unless and until the employer has done everything—and everything means a good deal—the workman can do next to nothing to protect himself, although he is naturally willing enough to do his share.

2. If you can bring an influence to bear external to the workman (i.e., one over which he can exercise no control) you will be successful; and if you cannot or do not, you will never be wholly successful.

3. Practically all industrial lead poisoning is due to the inhalation of dust and fumes; and if you stop their inhalation you will stop the poisoning.

4. All workmen should be told something of the danger of the material with which they come into contact and not be left to find it out for themselves—sometimes at the cost of their lives.

It is clear, however, that there are still many hazards in industry which have not been prevented because these maxims have not been fully carried out. Let us turn to a consideration of some of these.

ACCIDENTS

The most important cause of absenteeism in industry is injury. It has been estimated that there are 15,000,000 minor injuries and one-third of a million serious injuries per year in this country. This is clearly a most important drain on our manpower resources. At the moment we are fighting for economic existence and increased productivity. The prevention of accidents and the prevention of undue loss of time from accidents are, therefore, of the utmost importance. The prevention of accidents is the responsibility of the Safety and Welfare Committees of the various organizations which investigate the cause of all accidents. In the majority of cases accidents are due to the personal factor. It has been found, for example, that there is a particular person who is accident-prone, and that the majority of accidents are experienced by a small percentage of people, and it is still difficult to get men to wear protective devices regularly, such as masks, goggles, safety boots, and proper gloves and aprons. (*Fig. 35.*) The prompt and efficient treatment of minor injuries is all-important in preventing sepsis and loss of working time. The majority of such accidents are treated by the Works Casualty Services which are either staffed by first-aiders or nurses, with or without the supervision of doctors.

INDUSTRIAL DERMATITIS

It is estimated that half a million working days are lost annually by employees suffering from industrial dermatitis. The engineering industry produces annually a large number of cases. Unfortunately the incidence appears to be increasing and there is no doubt that many cases are due to sensitization by various therapeutic agents used in treatment, e.g., penicillin, procaine, etc.

OCCUPATIONAL CANCER

True occupational cancer is rare. It is, of course, of very great interest, as it is one of the few types of cancer in which we have a knowledge of the causation and which can be prevented, but which unfortunately is not always prevented. In fact, prolonged treatment of skin disease with perforations of arsenic has produced cancer in the past.

We know that cancer of the lung is an occupational risk also in gas workers, workers with arsenic, chromates, asbestos, and radioactive substances. Cancer of the lung has been known as an occupational disease for several centuries since Paracelsus in 1531 described the 'mala metallorum', a disease of the lungs which affected men in the prime of life in the Schneeberg ore mines in southern Germany. In Bohemia are the uranium mines of Joachimsthal, where Madame Curie first discovered radium; lung cancer is also an occupational risk here. In both these mines it is probably due to radioactivity. These mines now form an important source of uranium for Russia.

Skin cancer also occurs with those who work in contact with soot and oil, e.g., cancer of the scrotum in chimney sweeps, mule-spinners' cancer and epithelioma of the forearm in those who work with cutting oils in the engineering industry. Cruikshank, in a recent survey, showed that 80 per cent of the workers in a particular engineering works suffered from a pre-cancerous condition, i.e., oil folliculitis. It also occurs in those who work with arsenic, e.g., makers of sheep-dip. Occupations which have a high incidence of cancer of the skin are those of lathe operator, gunsmith, oiling coolie, chimney sweep, tar, pitch, anthracene, and creosote worker, briquette maker, shale oil worker, cotton mule spinner, and sheep dip worker.

Cancer of the nose occurs in those who work with nickelcarbonyl and cancer of the bladder in the aniline dye industry.

DUST IS DANGEROUS

One of the greatest of all occupational hazards is dust.

The historian may discover references to lung diseases in workmen engaged in dusty occupations, but it is only in comparatively recent years that we have really learnt how and why the inhalation of dust can cause diseases of the lung. There are references in the writings of Hippocrates (460 B.C.) and Ramazzini (1700). References in the text of Bensons Patents of 1776 and 1732 give us information on the effects of grinding flints: 'Any person other so healthful or strong working in that business cannot probably survive above two years, occasioned by the dust sucked into his body by the air he breathes, which, being of a ponderous nature, fixes there so closely that it is now very difficult to find persons which will engage in the business to the great obstruction and detriment of the said trade.'

Flint-knapping was probably the earliest occupational dust disease known; it occurred when flints were broken for the production of flint arrow-heads and axes. This produced dust, which, on inhalation, produced lung disease. It is interesting to note that the process is still carried on at Brandon, in Norfolk, where the local inn is called the 'Knappers' Arms', and the flints are still obtained from the same quarries that were used by our Stone Age ancestors. Flints were formerly exported in large numbers to Africa and at one time supplied most of the needs of the British Army. Today, however, the flints are exported for use by a certain body of American sportsmen who still use the flint-lock gun; they consider that the modern hammerless gun is too unsporting.

Thackrah, of Leeds (1832), drew attention to the short life of operatives subjected to dust. The disease then was incurable, as it is now, and therefore our only method of control is prevention.

In *The Vital Statistics of Sheffield* (1843) G. Calvert Holland, who was physician to the Sheffield General Infirmary, wrote as follows:—

The analysis of the trade of fork grinding will present a vivid but painful picture of the condition of an extensive class of artisans in this town. It is perhaps more destructive to human life than any pursuit in the united empire. Wet grinding is generally confined to saws, scythes, and edge-tools; the dry to an extensive class of small articles, such as razors, scissors, pen and pocket knives, forks and needles. Fork grinding is always performed on a dry stone, and in this consists the peculiarly destructive character of the branch. In the room in which it is carried on there are generally from eight to ten individuals at work and the dust which is created, composed of the fine particles of stone and metal, rises in clouds and pervades the atmosphere to which they are confined.

The dust which is thus every moment inhaled, gradually undermines the vigour of the constitutions, and produces permanent disease of the lungs, accompanied by difficulty of breathing, cough, and a wasting of the animal frame, often at the early age of twenty-five. Such is the destructive tendency of the occupation, that grinders in other departments frequently refuse to work in the same room, and many sick clubs have an especial rule against the admission of dry grinders generally, as they would draw largely on the funds from frequent and long-continued sickness. In 1,000 deaths of persons above 20 years of age, the proportion between 20 and 29 years, in England and Wales, is annually 160, in Sheffield, 184; but among the fork-grinders, the proportion is the appalling number 475; so that between these two periods, three in this trade die to one in the kingdom generally.

Between the ages of 30 and 39, a still greater disparity presents itself. In the kingdom, 136 only in the 1,000 die annually between these two periods. In Sheffield, 164; but in the fork-grinding branch, 410; so that between 20 and 40 years of age, in this trade, 885 perish out of the 1,000; while in the kingdom at large, only 296. Another step in the analysis, and we perceive that between 40 and 49, in the kingdom, 126 die; in this town, 155; and in this branch, 115, which completes the 1,000. They are all killed off. For in carrying forward the inquiry we observe that between 50 and 59, in the kingdom, 127 die; and in Sheffield, 155; but among the fork-grinders, there is not a single individual left. After this period of life, there are remaining in the kingdom, of the 1,000, 441; and in the town, 339; but none in this branch of manufacture.

Grinders' asthma in its advanced stages admits neither of cure nor of any material alleviation. In the early stages the only efficient remedy is the withdrawal from the influence of the exciting cause; but how is this to be effected by men who depend from day to day upon their labour, and whose industry from early life has been confined to one particular branch? Here then, is the melancholy truth that nearly one-third of this class of artisans, in addition to the poverty and wretchedness common to the whole is in a state of actual disease—and disease which no art can cure. Fiction can add no colour or touches to a picture like this. Truth transcends the gaudy embellishments of imagination. The distempered fancy has here no room to exercise her powers.

Further evidence of the wretched state of the fork-grinders—and the remark applies with great truth to grinders generally—is the low state of education among them. Of the 197 men and boys, 109 can read only, and 69 can write. Thus, in a Christian country—a country that expends vast wealth in attempting to educate and enlighten the dark heathen—one half of an important body of human beings, near this source of benevolence and comprehensive charity, actually cannot read, and about two-thirds cannot write! The inability to work, and yet the necessity to labour, creates a degree of wretchedness and suffering easier to imagine than describe. But the wretchedness is not confined to the individual. A wife and increasing family are involved in the accumulated evils. Poverty, yoked with disease, embitters and shortens life in a thousand forms, but all forms of misery. We do not hesitate to assert that this is a picture of wretchedness, which has no parallel in the annals of any country, or in the records of any trade.

It was the need for action to alleviate such conditions and to protect the workers which resulted in the passing of the Factory Acts.

Originally it was thought that all dusts were harmful to the body. Later, however, with the discovery of the effect of silica on the lungs, dusts were classified as harmful or inert, depending upon their silica content. We realize today, however, that although silica still remains probably the most important cause of lung disease resulting from exposure to dust, there are very many modifying factors, and from the hygienist's point of view we want to know whether a particular dust exposure may be harmful to the health of a worker. In assessing exposure, information is required on the following factors:—

1. Chemical composition of the dust.
2. Size of the dust particles.
3. The concentration of the dust in the breathing zone of the worker.
4. The severity of exposure and total length of exposure.
5. The severity of the work.
6. General health of the worker in relation to other factors, e.g., nutrition, housing.
7. The efficiency of preventive measures.

The chemical composition of the dust is particularly important, and we can classify it into mineral dust and animal dust and vegetable dust.

MINERAL DUST

It is the mineral dusts which are responsible for the most severe type of disease, and free silica is the harmful agent. There has been considerable controversy as to the manner in which silica produces its harmful effects on the lung. It has been quite definitely disproved that it is due to the sharpness of the particles, and it is undoubtedly due to a specific chemical action on the lungs.

It is important to realize also that it is the very small particles which are dangerous. Most of the larger particles settle out of the air before it is breathed, or are trapped in the secretions of the nose and throat and either eliminated in the black spit of the miners or are swallowed. The very small and dangerous particles are invisible, and they are the ones which reach the lung and produce their harmful action. That is why in the wet-drilling of hard rock there may be very little visible dust produced, but there may be a very high percentage of dangerous dust because the larger particles are trapped in the wet process, while many of the finer particles escape.

The concentration of the dust is also of importance. It is important to realize that there is a wide variation in individual susceptibility of two men working at the same job and in the same exposure over a period of years; one may develop severe dust disease of the lung, while the other remains quite unaffected.

The severity of the work is also of importance. If a man is engaged on hard manual labour he has to breathe in and out much larger volumes of air than normally and this will increase the amount of dust which is inhaled. A hot atmosphere will also have the same effect. That is why many of the worse examples of dust disease are to be found in the very hot and deep mines, e.g., the Cornish tin mines and the South African gold mines.

The general health of the individual person is also important. Other things being equal, the healthy, well-nourished person is likely to resist disease more than the thin, undernourished one. There is also undoubtedly a hereditary influence which may explain differences in individual susceptibility.

Dust disease of the lung is now referred to as pneumoconiosis. The definition of this under the National Insurance (Industrial Injuries) Act, 1946, is as follows: 'Pneumoconiosis means fibrosis of the lung due to silica dust, asbestos dust or other dust.' Throughout our industrial history dust diseases of the lung have created serious problems and today they constitute as never before a major social problem. There are comprehensive statistics available from the records of the Ministry of National Insurance, and of the industries which contribute the greatest number of persons suffering from this disease, easily the most important is the coal-mining industry. Between 1939 and 1947 over 19,000 persons were certified as being disabled by reason of the disease. Undoubtedly the coalfields of South Wales are the most important from this point of view; the rest of the country is relatively free.

The anthracite mines of the west part of the coalfield seem to be the most dangerous. There is at present a Medical Research Council Unit at Cardiff investigating various aspects of the disease, but we still do not know why anthracite causes such a severe type of disablement. It appears that ordinary coal-dust is, if anything, protective, and the coal-miners of Yorkshire and Nottinghamshire have very little incidence of lung disease. It is true that they have produced the well-known black spit of miners, but, as indicated previously, this is evidence that the respiratory passages are functioning in a healthy manner in eliminating the large coal-dust particles. It is probable that the increasing mechanization of the coal-mining industry has been responsible for an increasing incidence of the disease because with mechanical cutters there is a much greater amount of dust produced.

Preventive measures have, of course, been instituted in the form of wet drilling and the infusion of water behind the coal-face, but this does not necessarily eliminate all the harmful particles, as we have seen, and it may make the atmosphere look relatively clear, when, in fact, it contains particles of a size which are harmful to human beings when inhaled.

The other dangerous industries include the manufacture of pottery, sandstone and stone masonry and stone drillers, sand blasting and steel dressing, the making of refractories, and asbestos, metal grinding, metalliferous mining, slate mining, and haematite mining. Taken altogether, however, these industries only account for 9 per cent of the cases to be found in the coal-mining industry. One reason is, of course, that there are very many more people exposed to risks in the coal-mines than there are in these other industries. In Sheffield there has been a great decrease in silicosis in the metal grinding industry owing to the replacement of sandstone grindstones by carborundum stones.

The loss to the community from the effects of dust disease is enormous even if we only take it on the basis of compensation payments involved. It is estimated that for each case certified an average of £1000 is paid out. In the coal-mining industry alone this involves an annual liability of £2,000,000. More important is the fact that the most highly skilled workers are lost to the industry and the problems of finding alternative employment are particularly serious.

So far we have discussed the most important of all dust diseases, i.e., the pneumoconiosis of coal-miners, and we have seen that the causation is not yet fully understood. It will be of interest to describe some of the other diseases which, though less important from a numerical point of view, are nevertheless of considerable interest.

In the steel and refractory industries, silica sand is used for making the moulds into which the molten steel is poured. When the casting has cooled there is a layer of sand fused to the outside of the casting. This has to be removed by various means. In sand blasting, sand is propelled under force against the outer surface of the casting in order to remove the fused material.

For large articles the blaster works in a specially constructed room and is protected by a helmet which is provided with air under pressure. With smaller articles the worker passes his arms through guarded holes on to the article in a closed cabinet. Sand has now been replaced by metal shot and in some cases by the hydroblast. Nevertheless, there is a considerable amount of dust left in the atmosphere for some time after the process has ceased. This used to be an extremely dangerous process with a short period of employment and the rapid progress of the disease. Now, however, the preventive measures have almost eliminated the danger. In other cases the casting is treated with a drill or abrasive wheel in order to finish the article. This is an extremely dangerous process and a large amount of dust is evolved, and there is very little protection available to the worker, though down-draught ventilation has been installed to try to diminish the amount of dust. Workers have also been provided with masks, but the men simply will not use them as they are a nuisance and a hindrance to efficient work, and, in fact, any preventive measure which depends on the personal element is usually of little avail.

Furnace dismantling and furnace bricklaying is also a hazardous occupation as the men are working in furnaces whilst they are still hot and large volumes of siliceous dust are produced.

Sandstone grinding in the Sheffield area was a most important cause of silicosis. In 1926 about 1600 natural grindstones were in use in the Sheffield district. This number was reduced to about 200 in 1933, and there are only one or two wet sandstones still in use today.

The manufacture of abrasive soap is particularly dangerous. In this process, a highly siliceous rock containing 98 per cent of silica is mixed with powdered soap, soda, and other substances. This is one of the few industries in which females contract dust disease of the lung.

The quarrying and working of siliceous rocks is, of course, another very important source of silicosis. It occurs in those employed in the quarrying, mining, and dressing of sandstone, and in masons in builders' and sculptors' yards; stone masons are particularly affected. Cases in which the greatest degrees of silicosis have been described occur in those working in red sandstone and in men employed in tunnelling for sewers or railway tunnels where sandstone is involved.

The refractories industry is another important source of the disease as gannister is a special form of sandstone found in the mould measures. It contains 92–98 per cent of silica.

Granite is not quite as dangerous as sandstone as it rarely contains more than 30 per cent of free silica. Nevertheless, masons, rock getters, drillers, and crusher men in the granite industry can all get severe dust disease of the lung.

Welsh slate quarried in North Wales contains about 60 per cent of free silica and is also a source of disease. About 10,000 men are employed in this industry, which has a high risk.

Other forms of mining which are dangerous in this respect are gold mining in South Africa, tin mining in Cornwall, and haematite iron-ore mining in Cumberland, because in the mining of these metals there are associated loads of granite or sandstone which have to be worked by the rock drillers in order to get the metal ore. In other words, it is not the metal—gold, iron, or tin—which is responsible, but the free silica in the other rocks associated with the metal.

In the pottery industry the manufacture of earthenware and china is particularly dangerous and the ingredients contain free silica. As long as the process is a moist one it is relatively harmless, but during the baking and subsequent finishing of the pottery much dust is evolved. In countries in which flint is not used in the manufacture of pottery respiratory disease appears to be much less prevalent in the workers.

So far we have discussed the dangers of lung disease from the inhalation of dust containing free silica, and undoubtedly this is by far the greatest risk. There are, however, other substances apart from free silica which are capable of causing serious disease of the lung when inhaled. Asbestos is one such substance. Today it is used for a wide variety of purposes—in the manufacture of fire-fighting suits, safety curtains, and boiler mattresses, in the composition of lagging material, in steel pipes, the panelling of rooms, tiles, the lining of chemical pans, the coating of bulkheads of ships and marine piers, and in the brake linings and clutch rings of motor vehicles of all descriptions. Since it is recognized as a dangerous agent there has been widespread legislation within the industry which has been generally effective in controlling the disease. Since 1931 all entrants to the industry have been medically examined, initially and annually, by a panel of experts. Dust exhaustion has received special attention in one factory; spinning rooms are totally enclosed with perspex, with an ingenious device which admits free access to the bobbins. Most of the cases now certified have industrial histories beginning prior to 1931.

The disease of asbestosis is particularly interesting as an excess mortality for cancer of the lung has been found associated with it, and several workers have drawn attention to the fact that cancer of the lung also occurs fairly frequently in association with asbestosis.

In recent years other mineral substances which have been implicated as a cause of dust disease of the lung are aluminium, beryllium, kaolin, and graphite. The inhalation of iron oxide in welders, however, appears to be relatively harmless. Calcium, tin, and barium can also produce X-ray changes which do not cause much disability. It must be realized also that harmful effects can occur from the inhalation of metallic dust and fumes in a wide variety of industries. This would lead to poisoning from a particular substance involved, and in the days when lead poisoning was more common than it is today the inhalation of dust containing lead was a quick way of absorbing the poison. All these hazards, however, are extremely rare today.

VEGETABLE DUST

So far, then, we have considered the mineral dusts. We next come to consider vegetable dust. It is only in recent years that the importance of vegetable dust as a cause of respiratory disease has been realized. This is apparently due to the fact that the condition of chronic bronchitis which sometimes results from their prolonged inhalation is not accompanied by any characteristic X-ray picture, as is found in pneumoconiosis. The chronic effects of these vegetable dusts are, therefore, less easily recognized; their mode of action is obscure, and it is not known whether it is the vegetable substance itself or some contaminating toxic material. Vegetable material always contains bacteria and fungi, some of which are known to be harmful. Many of these moulds and fungi may have an irritant action on the lung and cause asthma. We know that the absorption of foreign substances can cause asthma and hay fever in this way. Such a phenomenon is spoken of in medical circles as an 'allergic phenomenon'.

One of the most important vegetable dusts is to be found in the cotton industry, and the term 'byssinosis' has been applied to a respiratory affection occurring in the workers exposed to this dust. At first, complaints are noticed only on Monday mornings, hence the term 'Monday morning fever'. Those affected develop a feeling of irritation in the throat and chest and a sharp dry cough, which gradually subsides during the course of the week, and symptoms return again each Monday morning. After a number of years the conditions gradually become worse. Removal to other work might result in some improvement, but a return results in further recurrence of symptoms. A similar acute fever often occurs when new entrants enter a works. This is known as mill fever, comas fever in the hemp mills, and hackling fever and flax fever in the flax mills. Grain fever and malt fever associated with grain and brewing are probably also similar conditions.

Weavers' cough is another condition which occurs in those associated with the handling of mildewed yarn. It is probably due to the inhalation of moulds and fungi; a similar condition occurs in farm workers who have been handling mouldy hay. Workers who handle bagasse or dried sugar-cane also get a similar condition.

Chronic bronchitis has been reported in workers exposed to all kinds of vegetation, such as cotton, grain, flour, flax, hemp, tobacco, and tea. It differs little from the chronic bronchitis which occurs quite commonly in the older age-groups of the general population. It is probable that the most severe of all these conditions is the chronic respiratory disease due to continued inhalation of cotton dust. This can result in severe disability. Acute asthma following exposure to dust has been noted in a great variety of occupations.

ANIMAL DUST

There are very few reports of harmful effects from animal dust. Anthrax or wool-sorters' disease was caused by the breathing of infected wool, but is now extremely rare. It is also possible to get acute asthma from the inhalation of dust from feathers and animal skins.

One of the greatest dangers from dusts of all kinds is the risk of explosion, particularly from such things as flour, starch, sugar, dried milk, and coal. One thing we should not lose sight of is that, while considerable effort is usually made to extract dust and fumes from industrial processes in an all-out effort to protect the worker, rarely is much effort made to render the extracted material harmless to the community as a whole. Whilst the burning of fuel coal is the most important cause of air pollution, the quota is added to by all sorts of dusts and fumes from a wide variety of industries.

There is a great need for dust suppression officers in all dusty jobs; they must be fully trained and have the authority to insist on proper control measures being taken. A great onus rests on the manufacturers of mining and other machinery; only rarely is the human element considered when such machinery is designed; in the future we must design machines for the benefit of the men who work them; the engineer is not necessarily the best fitted for this task—he expects men to conform to the machine and is often oblivious of the dangers he may have created.

RADIOACTIVE DUST

One of the greatest dangers from the explosion of atomic bombs is the 'fall-out' of radioactive dust many miles away from the site of the explosion. Fall-out depends upon the type of weapon tested and on how close to ground or water it is set off; in other words, it is controllable to a certain extent. In fact, the Americans claim to have developed a hydrogen bomb which is 'safe', meaning that there is only a small amount of radioactive fall-out. There are three kinds of fall-out:—

1. Local fall-out, which is geographically restricted.
2. Trophospheric fall-out, which stays in the lower atmosphere and then descends to earth in the latitude of the test site.
3. Stratospheric fall-out, which circles the earth for several years before returning to earth.

The last two types are the most important because they distribute radioactive particles over a large area of the surface of the earth. The most dangerous of these particles is strontium 90 because it can be absorbed and accumulated in bone, and in sufficient dosage can cause cancer and leukaemia. Genetic effects, on the other hand, are produced by the short-lived particles which have lost much of their potency by the time they descend.

It has been estimated that the increase in genetic mutation from fall-out amounts to 0·2 per cent spread over the world's population; this would appear to be of minor significance. This increase is smaller than that which comes from the medical use of X-rays or from moving to higher altitudes where cosmic radiation is more intense. (*See* World Health Organization (1957), *Effect of Radiation on Human Heredity.*)

The latest evidence shows that man-made radiation from strontium amounts to about 1/200th of the dose which is usually considered well within safe limits. There is an added danger in calcium-deficient soils where poisons may absorb more than five times these amounts. We still do not really know, however, what are the minimal exposure limits over a lifetime and possibly only time alone can tell us.

HEALTH AND RADIOACTIVITY

The effects of heat and light rays from the sun were already recognized when in 1895 a new kind of radioactivity was discovered, namely, X-rays, which had the power to penetrate solid objects. It was soon realized that they also had profound effects on living tissue. This was followed by the discovery that certain substances, such as uranium and radium, found in the earth's crust were capable of emitting similar rays. Later came the identification of cosmic rays which reached the earth from outer space; these are filtered by the earth's atmosphere so that the dose at sea-level is less than that at the top of a mountain or in a high-flying aircraft.

A great deal of information about the effects of radiation on man has come from experience with occupational hazards.

The first to be affected were the early medical workers who used X-rays for taking radiographs and for treating inoperable cancer; many lost their lives as a result (*see* p. 152). Some developed skin damage which led to skin cancer or damage to the bone-marrow. Luminous dial painters absorbed thorium or mesothorium and developed bone cancer. Men working in the Joachimsthal and Schneeberg mines developed lung cancer from the inhalation of the radioactive gas, radon. There is no doubt that exposure to radioactivity can cause leukaemia—the survivors of Hiroshima and Nagasaki bear witness to this fact. Exposure to X-rays also produces a greater risk of developing this disease. Irradiation during pregnancy can produce abortion or stillbirth, and if the child is born alive, mental retardation can occur. Unfortunately the harmful effects of radioactivity are not limited to those directly exposed to its effects; future generations may suffer in consequence. It is as yet too early to say what the effects of increasing radioactivity will be on future generations.

The Medical Research Council published in 1956 and 1960 two reports entitled *The Hazards to Man of Nuclear and Allied Radiations*. Estimates were given of the existing and foreseeable levels of exposure to radiation; the unit of measurement used was the roentgen, expressed as 'r' for short. From all natural sources the dose over a 30-year period is about 3 r; in addition the medical use of X-rays contributes another 22 per cent, occupational sources about 1·6 per cent, and the luminous dials of watches and clocks, television sets, and shoe-fitting X-ray apparatus about 1 per cent. From atomic bomb explosions up to 1956, Britain can expect to receive over the next fifty years from 0·02 to 0·04 per cent of the radiation which will be received from natural sources. There is a great deal of fuss about the possible dangers of this, but what about the much more dangerous use of X-rays for medical diagnosis, which are contributing 22 per cent of the natural source, a hazard which is from 500 to 1000 times greater than that from radioactive fall-out?

The harmful effect of radiation depends upon the type and dosage received, the duration of the exposure, and the part of the body exposed. In the atomic bomb explosions those who received an immediate dosage of 500 r became ill shortly afterwards and at least 50 per cent died; if the dosage were of the order of 50 r illness would be rare and very few would suffer any after-effects. In the miners who developed lung cancer the total dosage received over seventeen years' average exposure was at least 1000 r. The bone-marrow seems particularly sensitive, and dosage of as low as 1 r per week can cause change in susceptible people.

The figure recommended by international bodies as the maximum permissible level is 0·3 r per week, while the total dosage should not be more than 200 r, spread over a lifetime.

The following is a summary of the recommendations made in the above report:—

1. *Limitation of the Use of all Sources of Radiation.*—Adequate justification should be required for the employment of any source of ionizing radiation on however small a scale.

2. *Fall-out from Test Explosions of Nuclear Weapons.*—

a. The present and foreseeable hazards from external radiation due to fall-out from the test explosions of nuclear weapons, fired at the present rate and in the present proportion of the different kinds, are negligible.

b. Account must be taken, however, of the internal radiation from the radioactive strontium which is beginning to accumulate in bone. At its present level no detectable increase in the incidence of ill-effects is to be expected. Nevertheless, recognizing all the inadequacy of our present knowledge, we cannot ignore the possibility that, if the rate of firing increases and particularly if greater numbers of thermonuclear weapons are used, we could within the lifetime of some now living be approaching levels at which ill-effects might be produced in a smaller number of the population.

3. *Recommendations regarding Specific Uses of Radiation.*—

a. All sources of radiation, both medical and industrial, should be under close inspection in order to ensure that the high standards of protection now attainable against the absorption of ionizing radiations, and against radioactive materials, are generally observed. Those using radiations should be instructed in the precautions to be taken, and no unnecessary or unauthorized persons should be allowed to engage in such occupations. A personal record, not only of doses of radiation received during occupation, but also of exposures from all other sources, such as medical diagnostic radiology, should be kept for all persons whose occupation exposes them to additional sources of radiation.

b. Present practice in medical diagnostic radiology should be reviewed, with the object of clarifying the indications for the different special types of examination now being carried out and defining more closely, both in relation to the patient and to the operators, the conditions which should be observed in their performance.

c. The uses of radiotherapy in non-malignant conditions should be critically examined.

d. The small amounts of irradiation from miscellaneous sources, such as X-ray machines used for shoe-fitting, luminous watches and clocks, and television apparatus, should be reduced as far as possible.

4. *Collection of Vital Statistics.*—As an essential basis for future studies of the genetic effects of radiation, further data are required on the genetic structure of human populations; so there is an urgent need for the collection of more detailed information when births, marriages, and deaths are registered.

The setting up of atomic energy establishments has brought into being a new concept of occupational health in which the most elaborate precautions are taken by the health physics team. As many as 70 inspectors would be required for the inspection and supervision of the health of 1500 workers. Workers must wear a sensitive photographic film at all times; this is called the personnel monitoring meter, and its purpose is to detect the amount of radiation received. Mobile Geiger counters are used to check the contamination of floors and walls, whilst static instruments will sound an alarm when the radiation rises above a certain level. Special barriers of lead and concrete are always needed and remote control is essential, sometimes by the use of television. Protective clothing and special soaps and barrier creams are also provided. Ventilation is necessary to prevent excessive airborne contamination. The disposal of liquid and solid wastes is a great problem; they may be burned or dumped in the deep parts of the sea. These waste products can be harmful for many years to come. Despite all these precautions some persons may still receive harmful radiation, and so finally the health team must use as its final check routine tests of the workers' blood, sputum, urine, faeces, and expired air. Needless to say, continuous and extensive health propaganda is essential.

PSYCHONEUROSES

The family doctor is, of course, well aware of the high incidence of psychoneuroses in general practice. He is certainly in a position to understand tensions within the family which may predispose to these, but he also needs to understand something of the emotional difficulties which occur at a man's place of work. We are in the process of a second industrial and social revolution. From being a nation of craftsmen we are becoming a nation of machine minders. Industry no longer gives the sense of satisfaction which the village craftsman finds, and other incentives are necessary. There is, of course, the financial incentive, but the sense of participation in a great and important enterprise can be even more important. When a man is frustrated and unhappy and has no sense of satisfaction in his work he gets a high accident rate and a high incidence of psychoneurosis. That is why the understanding of human relationships in industry is of the very greatest importance. An instructive illustration of this was the very low accident and sickness rate of those employed on the construction of the Mulberry Harbour in Normandy during the last war, despite the fact that the job was a very hazardous one. A great deal can be done in the selective placement of individual workers. This is particularly important in the very young, in the elderly, and in the disabled. Much is being done in the selection, for example, of medical students and personnel for the fighting services. Selection is also important in preventing industrial dermatitis; for example, those with a past history of

173

eczema or allergy ought not to be employed in contact with irritants. Blondes do not tolerate degreasing agents and are more sensitive to dust; brunettes and very hairy persons develop oil acne easily. Those with dry skins should not work in water or alkalis. The testing of colour vision and visual acuity is very important in the transport services.

EMPLOYMENT OF THE ELDERLY

It has been said that employment is the only means known to delay the effects of ageing. In the light industries there is plenty of scope for placing older men and women in suitable jobs. I know of one old lady who has been with a Sheffield firm for sixty-seven years; she refuses to sit down at her work and she is doing a useful job. Another old man of 84 still continues his work as a commercial traveller and goes to dances three times a week. His chief worry seems to be the fact that he is being chased by a gay young thing of 55 with a view to matrimony. Others I have talked to say that sooner than retire they would prefer to continue working without pay. In the cutlery and silversmith trades there are craftsmen of over 80 who will be virtually irreplaceable when they retire. The position in the heavy industries and particularly in unskilled work, however, is more difficult. One firm in Birmingham has already set up a special workshop for its older workers and at least one Sheffield steel firm is considering the setting up of a light industrial factory to cater for its aged and disabled workers. I am not so sure, however, that this always provides the right answer. Many older persons to whom I have spoken do not wish to be treated differently from their fellow workers. They are particularly sensitive about the disparaging remarks of the younger men. This is a most important factor in making them retire. It is probably better to try to employ them wherever possible within the same factory. We have already seen that they cannot compete with a younger worker on a time and stress basis. What jobs then can the elderly unskilled do, particularly those who were employed in heavy industries? I suggest the following as suitable occupations: warehousemen, storekeepers, lift men, boiler men, cleaners, gate keepers, sweepers, servants, and waiters. Many of the heavy industries employ their elderly workers in these particular jobs.

Industrial medicine has an important part to play in achieving these results and I would name particularly two major functions. The first is diagnostic: the management requires information on the type of work which the individual person can do and requires to know when the change of occupation is to be desired. The second function is a therapeutic one: the periodic health examination should help men to overcome their physical and mental disabilities by sound advice and counselling. (*Fig.* 36.)

All this is particularly important in view of the widespread individual differences between people. Some of these principles have already been applied in the United States of America. The Dodge, Chrysler, and Ford Works all have schemes for the employment of their elderly workers. The Standard Oil Company at New Jersey has what is called a pre-retirement counselling programme, where employees are interviewed five years before

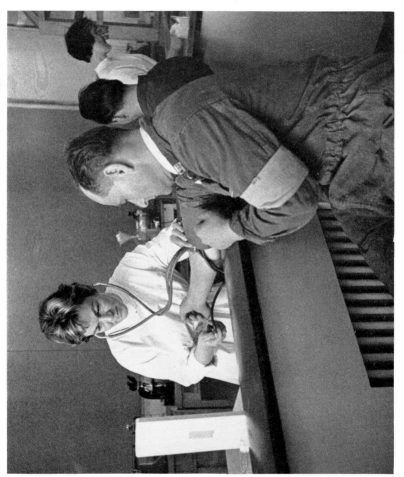

Fig. 36.—Factory health in Germany. Six medical teams (8 doctors, 31 nurses, of which 6 are male, 2 masseurs, 1 masseuse, and 12 laboratory workers) look after the factory's health 16 hours out of 24.

retirement is due to enable them to continue in a suitable occupation, should they so desire. One of the most important functions of industry in this respect is educational. This should be directed towards workers of all ages. The disparaging remarks of younger workers are a frequent cause of retirement. It is only by a suitable programme of education that the younger workers can be made to understand the problems of their older associates and to realize that they in turn will meet with the same problems. Moreover, preparation for old age is a lifelong undertaking and not something to be considered when retirement age is reached. The factory stands to the adult as the school does to the child in this respect. The difficulty is, of course, during periods of unemployment; with increasing productivity and mechanization all men should have more leisure and the old should tail off gradually.

Let us turn now to a consideration of the industrial medical services. Every person who works needs at some time the following type of health services:—

1. Environmental and preventive health services to minimize routine industrial health hazards. This includes health education.

2. Personal health services which provide for first aid and emergency treatment and rehabilitation.

3. Routine examinations for particular jobs. Many firms now demand pre-employment examinations of all workers; it is a good opportunity to get to know the men and to talk to them about the health aspects of their job. An important aspect is the training of supervisors of the work of nurses and first aiders. In this respect the industrial medical officer is rather like the R.M.O. in the army or the school doctor in childhood.

Anybody who has been in industry is aware of the large amount of time which is lost by workers having to attend hospital and often being laid off work unnecessarily, and workers will not leave work if it involves loss of several hours' working time. Prompt treatment on the spot prevents sepsis.

Dr. Donald Stewart has shown that since the introduction of an industrial medical service to a particular works the number of lost-time accidents complicated by sepsis fell from 3 per 100 workers before the service to 0·2 per 100 after the service. I hope, therefore, that I have made the point that an industrial medical service can be of great value to the community.

In America and Europe great efforts have been made to make the occupational environment a healthy one; there is still considerable scope for improvement, particularly in many of the smaller and older firms. At the moment, the Ministry of Labour is considering what steps can be taken to improve existing medical services in industry. As far as the underdeveloped countries are concerned, there is enormous scope for improving community health by attention to the working environment. The setting up of new large-scale industries enables planning for health to start right from the beginning; so that the industrialization of Asia and Africa should proceed in a healthy manner, based on the accumulated knowledge and experience of the West. Let us not forget, however, that new diseases are arising in the Western world which require rather different methods of approach. We turn now to a consideration of some of these.

CHAPTER XII

DEATH IN THE CITY AND THE DIRECTORS' DILEMMA

CHRONIC BRONCHITIS

MANY elderly people, particularly in the north of England, suffer from a wheezy cough each winter which becomes progressively worse with the years. They cough in an effort to try to bring up the tough, tenacious, mucus in the lining of their air-passages which is so troublesome to them. Many of these people also get short of breath very easily. At first this occurs only when they are walking up hill and it is not an uncommon sight to see these sufferers wearily plodding homewards up the hills of Lancashire and Yorkshire after their day's work. Soon they are quite unable to tackle the smallest incline and can only walk either downhill or slowly on the level. The noise of their wheezy chests can be heard several yards away and the blueness of their lips denotes the heavy load which the heart and lungs are having to cope with. Soon the sufferer is unable to leave the house at all, except on fine sunny days and then only for a short stroll around the houses and only on the level. Now even at rest coughing brings on an attack of breathlessness. Many of these people are an easy prey to respiratory infection and death from pneumonia, whilst others succumb to a failure of the right side of the heart.

Although there are many other serious conditions of the heart and lungs, in the absence of these the condition is usually called 'chronic bronchitis'. Not only does it kill in large numbers but it seriously interferes with the ability to earn a living, especially in hilly districts. These people are fairly happy when they are at their place of work, but it is the journey to and from work which causes the trouble. Sometimes they can overcome the difficulty if there is suitable public transport. There is one patient I know who lives on a steep hill, has a tram route at the top of the hill and a bus route at the bottom. He walks downhill to the bus in the morning and in the evening he returns by tram, walking downhill to his home. In the south-east of England the disease is far less common, and because most places are flat it causes far less interference with getting to and from work.

There were over 31,000 deaths reported from bronchitis in England and Wales in 1961 and the death-rate has remained unchanged despite the introduction of the antibiotics, and is particularly high in men as opposed to women. Bronchitis flourishes in the damp and dirty atmosphere of industrial

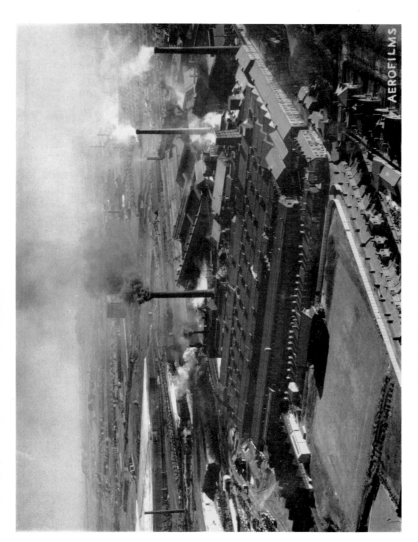

Fig. 38.—Smoking factories, north-east England.

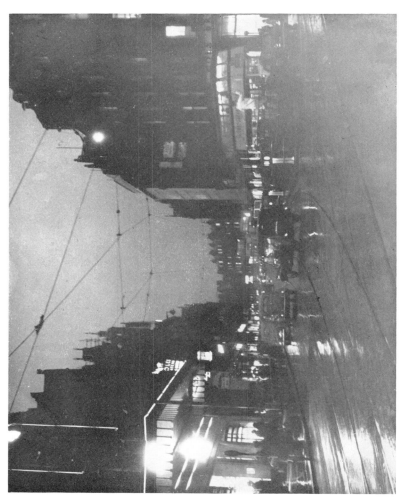

Fig. 39.—Smog. Sheffield—mid-afternoon! (*Sheffield Telegraph*)

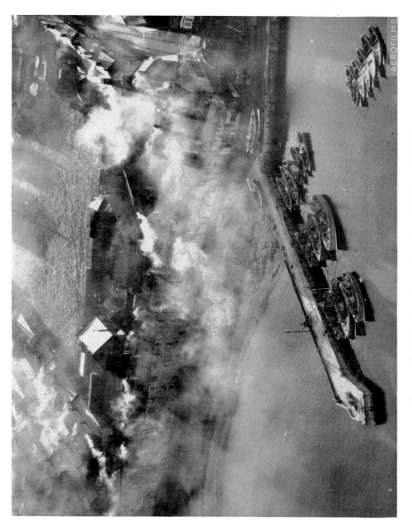

Fig. 40.—Pollution from houses in north-east Northumberland.

England. Thus the death-rate for males in 1948 in England and Wales was 17·8 for every 10,000 of the population. (*Fig.* 37.) In Norway the corresponding figure was 0·2 and in Sweden 0·4. In other words, the death-rate was nearly 100 times greater in England and Wales than in Norway. It is

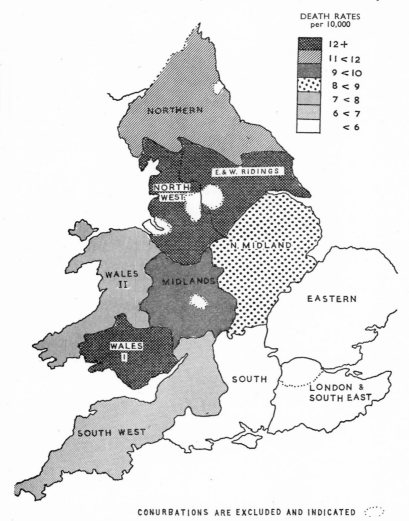

Fig. 37.—Map of chronic bronchitis, showing the density and death-rates per 10,000 for England and Wales in 1948.

interesting to note that a line drawn from the mouth of the River Severn to the Wash divides England and Wales into two contrasting areas. The southern half has low death-rates for infants, tuberculosis, and chronic bronchitis; at all ages of life, in the very young, during adult life, and in old age, the story is the same—there is a healthy part of the country in the south and east and there is an unhealthy part in the north, north-east, west, and Midlands; south-east Lancashire is particularly bad. In a steel city like Sheffield bronchitis accounts for 13 per cent of winter illness in industrial workers and a much greater amount in older people. It is the old-age pensioner who suffers the most, and in a survey undertaken in Sheffield we found that 44 per cent of men and 38 per cent of women were affected by the disease. The incidence was more marked in the industrial steel area at the east end of the city; here 50 per cent of old-age pensioners of both sexes were affected. These figures indicate the vast amount of ill health and disability produced by living under the shadow of our large steel works; the majority had lived there all their lives. (*Fig.* 38.)

Irrespective of geographical areas the death-rate in industrial areas is more than twice that in rural areas. Thus Greater London has twice the rate of the surrounding districts. Atmospheric pollution, dusty working conditions, and frequent infection from overcrowding are all important causes, and there is no doubt that heavy smoking is an aggravating factor. Doll and Bradford Hill, in an analysis of deaths from chronic bronchitis in doctors, found that the death-rate in non-smokers from this disease was 0·12 per 1000 and 0·72 per 1000 in heavy smokers.

From time to time in various parts of the world there have been repeated sudden dramatic episodes in which many people have died from acute respiratory disease owing to the blanketing of the area in a smoke fog (smog). The first recorded episode of this nature occurred in the Meuse Valley in Belgium in 1930 when 60 people died after a few hours' illness. In 1948 a similar occurrence took place in Donora, a steel town in Ohio, U.S.A. One-third of the total population was affected, nearly 6000 in number, although the number of deaths was not as high. The following is an account by Dr. Townsend of the episode:—

It was that familiarity with smog in Donora which prevented the people of the town from suspecting anything unusual when a smog blanketed the town on a Wednesday of the last week in October of 1948. It was the smog season. But this one stayed longer than usual and became worse than usual. And the longer the blanket kept the air bottled up, the heavier became the concentration of contaminants in that stable air. The first death occurred about 2 a.m. on Saturday morning. By late Saturday night 17 deaths had occurred and hundreds were very sick. On Sunday afternoon the rain came, and shortly thereafter the smog went away; but this time the town was thoroughly scared and they had no scientific knowledge to tell them whether or not the smog was gone for good.

The town council of Donora had no idea how to fight this new and unidentifiable menace. They called for officials of the State Health Department and asked for emergency aid for the sick, but there was little else that could be done. And while the smog had disappeared, hundreds were still sick and there was no way of knowing when the smog might return.

The worst episode so far recorded in Britain was in the London fog of December, 1952, when in 4 days there were nearly 4000 deaths, mostly in elderly persons suffering from chest or heart disease; there were also several deaths in healthy cattle at the Smithfield Show which was being held during this time. One thousand deaths a day from atmospheric pollution; this was as dramatic as the worst days of the plague or cholera.* There can be little doubt also that atmospheric pollution is an important, though not the main, cause of cancer of the lung (*see* p. 186).

What evidence there is on the formation of this dense, dirty fog points to the fact that sulphur dioxide absorbed into sooty particles is to blame, so that the burning of coal is the chief cause of what we now call smog. Smog occurs when there is a heavy fog associated with smoke. Under normal atmospheric conditions smoke is quickly dispersed into the upper atmosphere, but under certain atmospheric conditions the smoke cannot get away. Fog occurs when there is a sudden cooling of the air and little or no wind. The water vapour in the atmosphere condenses around particles of soot and grit and so fog occurs more frequently in heavily populated areas. It is to be noted that domestic smoke, as much as industrial smoke, is responsible for this. The absence of wind usually means that the fog is not easily dispersed, or sometimes a light wind may bank the fog up against mountain ranges; thus the prevailing westerly winds affect Lancashire most of all, and when the winds are easterly conditions are aggravated in the West Riding of Yorkshire. Even under these conditions, however, smoke will often disperse fairly quickly, but sometimes if the temperatures near the ground are lower than those in the upper atmosphere the smoke cannot get away and accumulates close to the ground. Conditions like this may arise when a layer of warm moist air flows into a depression or against a hillside where the ground is very cold. Conditions such as these caused the accumulation of harmful gases in Donora and the Meuse Valley. The sulphur dioxide content of heavily polluted areas, such as Billingham or Bessemer Road, Sheffield, is often as much as fifty times greater than in the country, and it is much higher during dense fog.

AIR POLLUTION

I was able to observe and note for myself the harmful effects of smoky cities every winter when I had to make the journey from Sheffield to Leeds by car. I remember a typical journey in late November when I left the centre of Sheffield at 3 p.m. (*Fig.* 39.) The city was engulfed in fog, the shop and street lamps were already lit, their light penetrating the yellow haze for only a few yards. It was still the middle of the afternoon, but everything was as black as night, the traffic proceeding at a slow pace because of the poor visibility, and the general atmosphere was one of deep depression; the fog seemed to be weighing down on everything; the irritant effects of the atmosphere could be felt in the back of the throat, and taking a deep breath produced

---

* The experience of 1952 caused Dr. W. P. D. Logan, of the General Register Office, to make further inquiries; he showed that similar incidents occurred in the years 1873, 1880, 1882, 1891, and 1892; thereafter until 1948, although fogs remained, none produced a high mortality. The latest recorded episode was in December, 1962. We do not know why there was such freedom from serious effect between the years 1892 and 1948.

a violent bout of coughing. As we crawled along in the slow stream of traffic we could hear the raucous coughing of pedestrians groping their way along the pavements. Many of the worst sufferers would no doubt be at home on such an afternoon. As we reached the outskirts of the city the ground began to rise and soon the speed of the traffic in front began to increase, a sure sign that we were running out of the fog. As we left the city behind us the light became brighter and brighter and suddenly at the top of the hill we emerged into bright sunshine. It was a beautiful, still, sunny day, with a clear blue sky, and even in midwinter the birds could not refrain from singing. Behind us in the valley lay the gloom of Sheffield and we could see the dense yellow haze blanketing out the view. Here and there on higher ground a tall chimney poked its nose through the haze and belched forth its quota of pollution, but for the most part the chimneys were hidden in the shroud of smog. We gaily stepped on the accelerator and pushed on to Barnsley. Here again, the same story repeated itself, the increasing haze as we approached the outskirts of the town, the decreasing pace of the traffic, and the coughs of the passers-by. We were soon once more enveloped in haze. Once again on leaving Barnsley we left the murk behind us. Wakefield was exactly the same, and if anything Leeds was even worse than Sheffield. When we think of the psychological effects on human beings living their lives under such conditions it is hard to believe that we do, in fact, know how to remove such conditions.

There have been complaints about the use of coal for the last six centuries. In the reigns of Edward VI and Elizabeth I there were proclamations prohibiting the use of coal whilst Parliament was in session. In 1661 John Evelyn wrote his famous pamphlet called *Fumifugium, or the inconvenience of the Aer and Smoake of London Dissipated, together with some remedies.* '. . . That men whose very Being is Aer, should not breathe it freely when they may; but (as that Tyrant used his Vassals) condemn themselves to that misery and fumo praefocari, is strange stupidity; yet thus we see them walk and converse in London, pursued and haunted by that infernal smoake. . . . Her inhabitants breathe nothing but an impure and thick Mist, accompanied by a fuliginous and filthy vapour, which renders them obnoxious to a thousand inconveniences, corrupting the Lungs, and disordering the entire habit of their Bodies, so that Catarrs, Phthisicks, Coughs, and Consumption rage more in that one City than in the whole Earth besides.'

We should not believe, however, that all smoke is bad, otherwise where would be some of the delectable English delicacies of the table, such as the various smoked fish, the herring, haddock, trout, eel, salmon, buckling, cod's roe, and even the lordly turkey, to say nothing of bacon, ham, and venison ?

The use of coal increased rapidly after 1800; the yearly output was then about 10,000,000 tons; by 1900, in the course of a century, the output had risen to 220,000,000 tons, and the inland consumption is now about 200,000,000 tons a year. During the Second World War users were encouraged by every means possible to produce as much smoke as possible in order to camouflage the cities. Now that the war is over they are finding it very difficult to forget the habit and the usual excuses are made of shortage of adequate equipment and finance. The existing legislation is quite inadequate to deal with the problem, and remedies promised for the future will be slow in materializing. It is particularly difficult to deal with the problem of domestic smoke; one answer is the provision of smokeless zones, as in Manchester and other cities, where only smokeless fuels may be burnt in firegrates approved for the purpose. (*Fig.* 40.) But is this the correct answer? Although they do not produce smoke, smokeless fuels still produce the gas, sulphur dioxide.

Meanwhile, in America, where they work faster than here, the problem of atmospheric pollution has been tackled with customary vigour. Pittsburgh is like Sheffield, a steel city. Once it was referred to as 'Hell with the lid off'; today it is a city with a clean atmosphere. In St. Louis and Los Angeles there are practically no open fires. Special regulations are enforced with heavy penalties for non-compliance. Heating appliances must be notified and approved and only special fuels are allowed. The worst offenders in the industrial field are gas works, electrical power stations, steel rolling mills, smelting works, and iron foundries. They should be built away from residential areas and the latter should be declared smokeless zones. The widespread destruction in Germany has enabled this sort of planning to take place in their newly built cities. Unfortunately, we are still left with our legacies of ancient mills, factories, and hospitals, which should have been replaced long ago.

Apart from the effect on health the economic cost to the country is enormous; at least 3,000,000 tons of coal are lost annually in the ordinary domestic grate, to say nothing of the cost of chimney sweeping. The burning of coal in an open grate is a most wasteful use of energy, the majority of the heat and the waste gases going up the chimney. In addition, there is the cost of cleaning houses, renewing paint, and the laundering of clothes and linen. It has been estimated that smoke costs us £100,000,000 per annum.

There are two other effects of pollution. Experiments carried out in Leeds showed that lettuces and other vegetables grown in the centre of the city were much smaller than controls grown outside.

Another serious effect is the corrosion of many of our public monuments and buildings by sulphuric acid.

Today over 7,000,000 tons of pollutants are produced annually, distributed over a very small area of this country where people are most densely crowded. In some of our worst cities, like Leeds, Manchester, and Sheffield, the yearly deposits of soot are of the order of 400 tons per square mile in the centre of the city. The real answer seems to be in the use of electricity for all heat and power, produced if necessary in power stations situated away from the centres of population, operated either by coal, by water power, or by atomic power. The sooner we can abolish coal the better, not only from the point of view of the population as a whole but also because of the person who has to mine it. Man was never meant to labour in the bowels of the earth, subject to every sort of hazard from falls of rock, explosions, and inadequate lighting, to clouds of irritant dust. The inhalation of coal dust kills the miner slowly but surely (particularly in the anthracite mines of South Wales), just as the burning of coal kills many old people in our cities today. The advance of science has brought within our grasp the weapon of atomic power, which should see within the next few decades the abolition of the diseases of coal-miners (there are over 1,000,000 of them in this country) and a marked reduction in the incidence of chronic bronchitis. Let us remember, however, that in addition to the burning of coal there is much pollution from diesel and petrol engines, and tobacco smokers not only pollute the air they themselves breathe, but also the air of cinemas, buses, trams, and other such public places.

There are three main types of pollutant from the burning of coal. First of all, smoke; this consists of soot and tarry matter. It is not difficult to remove these from domestic and industrial smoke, and the Clean Air Act should go a long way to deal with this, but it will probably take at least seven years before anything really effective can be achieved. It is, of course, no good placing smokeless housing zones in the middle of cities if they are surrounded by industrial plants which are still allowed to produce smoke. The enforcement of the Clean Air Act will naturally be expensive. It will mean that the extra amounts of smokeless fuels required will enable their price to be put up by several pounds per ton. Electricity will also go up by something like 12 per cent. It has been estimated that the removal of smoke from the chimneys of electricity undertakings alone will put another £200,000,000 per annum on the cost of electricity.

What is needed in the home is a really efficient space heater which has a thermal efficiency of something like 60 per cent when burning smokeless fuels.

If, however, smokeless zones can be created the dirt, fogs, and waste will be removed, making our cities cleaner and brighter. Probably the harmful effects of smoke on the lungs are mainly due to soot and tarry matter.

The second main pollutant from the burning of coal is grit. It is fairly easy to remove the large particles but difficult to remove the smaller ones, and very expensive. Probably, however, grit is not so important.

The third main pollutant is the gas, sulphur dioxide, which oxidizes in the air to produce acid substances. It is very difficult and expensive to remove. The content of this in the air is increasing for various reasons. Poorer quality coal, for example, which is now being used in greater quantities contains more sulphur, and the sulphur content of fuel oils is increasing. Although sulphur dioxide can produce ill-effects under certain conditions, probably its main effects are due to its association with soot and tarry matter. The smokeless cities of America still produce plenty of sulphur dioxide. Unfortunately, in our present state of knowledge we do not know sufficient about the ill-effects of the various pollutants on human beings. In some occupations in which there is exposure to high concentrations of sulphur dioxide alone, the workers appear to be quite free from lung complaints.

The practical solution would appear to be to ensure by every means in our power that smoke is removed from our cities and to allow no loopholes. The elimination of fine grit and sulphur dioxide would be a practical impossibility because of the cost.

It is, of course, not going to be easy to get public support for all this, and no piece of legislation can be completely successful unless it has an informed and co-operative public behind it. Education of the public is here of enormous importance, but I am afraid we shall not get very far with the older ones; we must start with the young; and what we have to do, first of all, is to get everyone to realize that the old idea of an open fire is completely impossible in the future. Our ideas in the home will have to undergo radical changes. Why, for example, should the miner get more coal than he wants at reduced rates, when the rest of the country is short, the price going up, and the quality falling? He is one of the worst offenders in atmospheric pollution because he can afford to keep his coal fire banked up all night. Will he be very happy when he is forced to buy expensive smokeless fuels and fit a different type of heating appliance?

Most of the industrialists I have spoken to are very open-minded in this matter. They realize that clean air will cost them money and no doubt the price of steel and all other things will go up accordingly.

In the meantime, what can the individual person do? Certainly those with chronic bronchitis should stay indoors during a fog and in very bad smogs. Those who have to go out can wear a mask which should remove the smoke. Experiments are being carried out on the possible neutralization of the sulphur dioxide content using a bottle filled with ammonia and fitted with a wick; this ensures evaporation of ammonia gas into the air in sufficient quantities to neutralize the sulphur dioxide without being offensive. It is too early yet to say whether this is effective. Perhaps the best advice to chronic bronchitics is to go and live in a better climate. This may not be so difficult as at first appears. There are many clean engineering works in the south of England, for example, around Bournemouth, where the skilled worker can get a job. For the man who owns his own business this is not an easy matter; he may have to decide whether it is better to continue making money in Lancashire or retire prematurely to live on a smaller income in Bournemouth. We may call this the first of the directors' dilemmas.

The final answer to the problem of clean air must come from the development of atomic power and the elimination of the coal mine.

In conclusion, we should not forget that the pollution of cities can travel hundreds of miles. The heather of the Pennines is, of course, impregnated with soot and the sheep are all black; even the moths have produced black varieties indigenous to the area. The Welsh mountains also get deposits of solid matter from the Black Country, and the Lake District even has its quota from the dark Satanic mills of Lancashire. Even country districts have their sources of pollution; at Fort William in Scotland cattle have died from fluorides emitted from the aluminium works there, and in the Hope Valley of Derbyshire the white cement dust spreads its mantle on the green fields. This latter, however, is probably more harmful to the eye than to the lungs. It has even been suggested that if the cement works were sited in the middle of Sheffield it would be a good thing because the alkaline dust of the cement works would neutralize the acid gas from the steel plants.

SMOKING AND CANCER

We should perhaps be thankful that chronic bronchitis is not on the increase, but unfortunately there is one respiratory disease which is increasing rapidly and that is cancer of the lung. I shall never forget one personal experience with lung cancer. My bank manager was a young man, 38 years old to be exact; he had everything a man could wish for—a pleasant home, charming wife and family, and good prospects for further promotion. He was a heavy smoker. One day the mass radiography service came to X-ray the employees in his bank; there was young Miss X, a little chesty, best to have a check-up on her lungs, and the young lad who had just left school— he looked pale and thin. The manager himself was well proportioned, with a ruddy countenance from his week-end golf, and had an air of self-assurance which gave confidence to the customers. It certainly was not necessary for him to be X-rayed; well, just to show willing he went through with the others. When the results came through there was only one abnormal X-ray; it did not belong to Miss X or to the pale lad who had just left school; it belonged to my friend, the manager. There was a round mass in his chest which looked suspiciously like a new growth. At first he was quite facetious when it was suggested that he should have an operation; he was in perfect health, not a single abnormal sign or symptom. In the end he was persuaded to undergo an operation; he had an inoperable cancer of the lung. In a few weeks he developed a cough with blood-stained sputum and in six months he was dead. This story illustrates one of the most tragic features of this type of cancer; it attacks many men in the prime of life, unlike most other cancers, which are essentially diseases of old age.

The deaths per annum from this disease are now considerably more than those from tuberculosis and greater than those from any other form of cancer.

In 1900 the annual death-rate attributed to lung cancer was 8 per 1,000,000 persons in England and Wales. By 1954 it had risen to 370 per 1,000,000. There were 22,000 deaths in 1960, compared with 3105 from pulmonary tuberculosis. There is every reason to suppose that this trend will continue. Many doctors have said that this is due to better diagnosis and to a greater 'awareness' of the disease amongst general practitioners; whilst part of the recorded increase is no doubt due to these factors, there can be no question at all that there has been a real increase for the following reasons. The disease is still increasing despite the many years which have elapsed since attention was first drawn to it. It is now so common that had the increase been merely one of getting the right diagnosis it would mean that fifty years ago 95 per cent of the cases were wrongly diagnosed as something else.

Routine post-mortem examinations at hospitals show an increasing proportion of deaths due to this disease. The increase is greater in men than in women and the disparity is increasing; this increase has been the same

184

in general practitioners in whom the disease would be more likely to be diagnosed accurately.

At an international convention on lung cancer held in Belgium in 1952 it was generally agreed that a large part of the recorded increase represented a real increase in the number of people suffering from cancer of the lung. This increase has taken place in many civilized countries.

This disease has every right to be called an English disease because the highest rates are recorded here. Taking the 1949 statistics, England and Wales and Scotland had rates of 288 and 256 deaths per 1,000,000; then came Finland with 171, followed by Switzerland, Holland, France, U.S.A., West Germany, South Africa, Canada, Denmark, Australia, and Eire in that order. The disease is almost unknown in India and in South African natives. It is, of course, very difficult to get accurate figures from many of the under-developed countries with insufficient medical services and lack of vital statistics. In Iceland the disease was very rare before the Second World War, but has now begun to occur in some numbers.

The mortality generally is greater in towns than in the country, Greater London, for example, having twice the rate of rural areas. These are the facts of the case; now for the causes. Factors which have been considered are tobacco smoking, atmospheric pollution, and exposure to the fumes from internal combustion engines, but pollution has been present for years, and in order to explain the sudden rapid increase there must have been some potent environmental factor which has recently become more prevalent.

We know, of course, that chronic irritation is the cause of a number of types of cancer of the skin and that there are a number of special occupations which have a high incidence of lung cancer. Thus the workers in certain mines of Central Europe have been known for years to suffer from an excess mortality from cancer of the lung, we think probably from exposure to radio-active substances in the mines. Paracelsus, in 1567, described the ' mala metallorum', a malady of the lungs which killed the Schneeberg miners of the ore mountains between Saxony and Bohemia. It is also prevalent in the Joachimsthal uranium mines, made famous by Madame Curie when she discovered radium there.

Cancer of the lung has also occurred with greater frequency among workers in chromates, asbestos, in the manufacture of arsenical sheep-dip, and in gas workers.

However, there are very few persons dying annually from the disease who are employed in any of these industries and we must seek the cause of the general increase elsewhere. Those who are exposed to the fumes of internal combustion engines, such as garage hands, bus drivers, and roadmen, do not show any excessive mortality from the disease. One of the most obvious suggestions is that it might be due to smoking and in particular to cigarette smoking. All the facts fit in with this theory. It is not always realized that cigarette smoking only came to be at all popular after 1900, when it became fashionable, particularly in this country and more so in males. Later the habit was taken up by females, but not to the same extent. Naturally we should expect a certain lag period, perhaps ten to twenty years, before the increase in cigarette smoking produced any effect, and in fact that is exactly what has occurred. The rise in the cancer death-rate began in about 1920 soon after the end of the First World War. Cigarette smoking increased in many of the other civilized countries, but it has never been common in India, for example, and in Iceland it was practically unknown before the Second World War when the arrival of American and British soldiers introduced the Icelander to cigarettes; cases of lung cancer began to appear soon after the war, all in heavy cigarette smokers, and the rate is rising. In some vocations, such as coal-mining and the police force, the rates are low. This is in keeping with the fact that in neither of these occupations is smoking allowed on duty. Now all this does not amount to proof, and a more detailed investigation was required. Several independent investigations in different parts of the world have shown that cigarette smoking is an important factor, although not the only one, in producing cancer of the lung. The first study of the relationship between cancer of the lung and smoking was carried out in 1939 by Müller in Germany. He found that in patients with lung cancer, 65 per cent were heavy smokers, and in those without lung cancer the percentage was 35 per cent; the percentage of non-smokers also was much lower in the cancer group. Similar results were obtained in America and by independent workers in this country. For example, Professor Bradford Hill and Dr. Richard Doll have carried out some research into the epidemiology of this disease and its relationship to smoking in sufferers from lung cancer. Another investigation has recently been carried out in North Wales by Dr. Percy Stocks in which he expresses in more definite terms the death-rates from cancer of the lung in town and country and in relation to smoking habits. His results are so important that they are worth discussing in some detail. He investigated 10,000 cancer deaths in North Wales, Cheshire, and Liverpool, and was able to compare the death-rates from lung cancer in relation to smoking habits and to residence in urban or rural areas.

The following table illustrates his findings:—

Death-rates from Lung Cancer per 100,000 *Men, aged* 45–74 *Years*

	Cheshire	Liverpool
Non-smokers	0	131
Pipe smokers	25	143
Cigarette smokers: Light	153	297
Medium	213	287
Heavy	303	394

Light smokers were those smoking less than 100 cigarettes per week; medium, those smoking between 100 and 249 cigarettes a week; and heavy, more than 250 cigarettes a week.

It shows in a remarkable way the effect of residence in an industrial city, the death-rates being higher in every category of smoking habits in the city compared with the country. The effect of smoking is also indicated by the increasing mortality in cigarette smokers, increasing as the number of cigarettes increases. We should note that cases occur occasionally even in non-smokers who have lived in the country. There can be many explanations of this: buses, trams, public halls, and cinemas are heavily polluted by tobacco smoke, whilst the air is polluted by diesel and petrol fumes from the roads and by smoke pollution which can be carried by prevailing winds many miles from industrial areas; all these constitute a menace to the non-smoker who lives in the country.

The moral of this story is to live in the country, and if you must smoke, use a pipe. There are clearly two important factors—atmospheric pollution and smoking. Unfortunately there are still many ostrich-like human beings in this world who bury their heads in the sand and refuse to see what they do not want to see.

Many cigarette smokers will not believe the story, and it is for this reason that I have given the evidence in some detail. There are still a few doctors, unfortunately, who tell the public that cigarette smoking is harmless; they are worse than the ostrich, not only are they blind, but ignorant of the facts in addition.

Further confirmation of these results has been afforded by a follow-up study by Bradford Hill and Doll of the cause of death in doctors in relation to their smoking habits. A questionnaire was sent to all doctors in the United Kingdom in 1951, and there are about 40,000 medical men and women now classified according to their smoking habits. The cause of death of every doctor on this register is being noted and, in this way, accurate information can be obtained on the relationship between smoking and lung cancer. So far, the results have confirmed in a striking fashion the results obtained by other workers. In a report published in the *British Medical Journal* on 10 Nov., 1956, Bradford Hill and Doll reported 84 deaths from lung cancer, and there was a steady increase in the death-rate from lung cancer with increasing amounts smoked; the death-rate per 1000 for non-smokers was 0·07, for light smokers 0·47, for moderate smokers 0·86 (15–24 cigarettes daily), and for heavy smokers 1·66 (25 and more cigarettes a day). In other words, in heavy smokers the death-rate was 20 times greater than in non-smokers. Another interesting feature of these results showed that deaths in non-smokers were concentrated in the older age-groups, whereas many of those in heavy smokers occurred in middle age. It would appear that atmospheric pollution takes longer to kill than cigarette smoke.

The evidence showed also beyond doubt that giving up smoking reduced the liability of a smoker to develop lung cancer. Pipe smoking appeared to be about one-third as dangerous as cigarette smoking at all levels, and there was insufficient evidence relating to the smoking of cigars. Another point, the total mortality from all causes was much higher in heavy smokers (18·84 per 1000) than in non-smokers (13·25 per 1000); this is important, because some people have suggested that if a person does not die from lung cancer he will die from something else. No doubt he will eventually, but it is clear that heavy cigarette smoking is an important cause of premature death after middle age. In this revealing inquiry the methods used were such as to constantly underestimate the effect of cigarette smoking. A similar study in America on 187,783 men reported by Hammond and Horn in 1958 has confirmed these findings in a striking fashion; they concluded that all smoking shortens life, cigarette smoking being by far the worst offender, and the risk goes up with the amount smoked. It will be several decades before these human guinea-pigs are all finally laid to rest and the answer will be cut and dried, by which time it will not concern either you or I very much. But the results may at least persuade future generations to smoke either a pipe or cigars as did our grandfathers before us.

Further experiments have isolated a chemical substance from the air and from cigarette smoke which is a well-known cancer producer in experimental animals. This substance is benzpyrene, produced by the combustion of coal and diesel fuel. Not only has the consumption of coal increased but also the use of fuel oils for road transport vehicles. Diesel-engined road vehicles did not come into use in this country until 1930 and now the yearly fuel consumption is over 1,000,000 tons; in addition an increasing number of petrol engines continue to pollute the air with a variety of toxic substances discharged at ground level. Let us not forget either that the density of road traffic in our cities is one of the highest in the world; the fact that it is and also that it moves more slowly than anywhere else only aggravates the situation. The quantities in air and cigarette smoke can be calculated. The amount in the 'air', if we can call it such, of our industrial cities is many times greater than in the air of rural areas; thus in Liverpool it is eleven times greater than in North Wales. The amount of benzpyrene taken into the body per year in town and country in the various grades of smokers can thus be calculated. These bear a direct relationship to the lung cancer death-rates.

There is now evidence that both cigarette smoke and the products of atmospheric pollution can produce lung cancer in experimental animals, but, as many 'ostriches' have pointed out, these results are not necessarily applicable to man; they do not need to be, we have all the evidence we want from man himself without quoting animal experiments.

From mid-1952 to mid-1954 there were 539 deaths from cancer of the lung in men in Liverpool; if the death-rates had been for non-cigarette smokers living in rural areas the number would have been 63; in other words, 476 deaths occurred which could probably have been prevented. Similar calculations applied to the population of England and Wales show that something like 10,000 lung cancer deaths are due to causes which could be removed.

The estimation of benzpyrene is a very complicated and tedious business and cannot be carried out as a regular routine throughout the country, but the insoluble deposit is measured as a routine in many stations in tons per square mile per month. It is in this fraction that the carcinogenic substances are to be found.

In the middle of the last century, just about a hundred years ago, Dr. John Snow showed the way in which cholera was spread, although it was not until the end of the century that the precise causative agent was isolated. As a result the last major cholera epidemic occurred in 1866 and cholera was brought under control. In those days the disease was brought from the East by ships. Today we are in a similar position regarding lung cancer. There has been a recent rapid increase due to the introduction of a new habit—the smoking and inhalation of cigarette smoke. Although we do not know the precise causative agent we have a shrewd idea what it is. Nevertheless, that should not prevent us from applying the measures which will bring the disease under control. Those measures are the concern of every man, woman, and child in this country. It is no longer a medical matter, but should be a Government policy to warn everyone by every means in its power of the danger of smoking cigarettes. So far there is no evidence of such a policy.

One final word. Comments have been made on the fact that the consumption of cigarettes is much higher in America than in this country but the lung cancer death-rate is higher here; to anyone who has been to America and seen the ashtrays full of half-smoked cigarettes the answer is clear. Ever since the outbreak of World War I, we in Britain have had to smoke our cigarettes down to the last half-inch; some of us have even used pins in times of shortage. It is this last inch which causes the trouble; a cigarette acts as a filter for the cancer-producing tars and the dangerous material is collected in that last inch. The average American takes a few puffs and when the cigarette begins to burn and taste unpleasant he stubs it out and so throws away the cancer-producing tars in the unsmoked portion.

A recent survey of cigarette filters in America has shown that the most efficient is that type which actually uses a whole cigarette as the filtering medium; it removes 50 per cent of the tarry matter and soon becomes black and sodden and has to be thrown away. If you must smoke cigarettes, then use a filter tip or a filter with a cigarette holder, and only smoke half the cigarette. We do not know yet what is the most effective way of removing the carcinogen (cancer-producing substance), but research is proceeding apace, much of it financed by the tobacco companies, and eventually we shall probably be able to produce a harmless cigarette. Until that time I think it is best to stick to a pipe. Of course, as in all things appertaining to health, prevention is better than cure, and it is better never to have started. A good way of achieving this is to be given a pipeful of old string at the age of 12. I used to use 20 cigarettes a day despite the fact that I smoked blotting-paper as a youth, and I gave up smoking cigarettes completely two years ago. I only hope I gave it up in time.

DRUG ADDICTION

Smoking.—Pearl (1938) showed that smokers of 10 or more cigarettes a day, aged 30–45 years, have death-rates from all causes more than double those of non-smokers. The evidence incriminating cigarette smoking as a cause of lung cancer has already been reviewed, but in addition heavy cigarette smokers suffer an increased mortality from chronic bronchitis, coronary heart disease, and peptic ulcer. There is evidence that the high death-rates from pulmonary tuberculosis in older men are due to a break-down of old lesions as a result of smoking. Since there appears to be a real case against tobacco on health grounds it is appropriate to consider it in more detail.

The use of tobacco was made known in Europe when Columbus returned after landing on San Salvador on 31 Oct., 1492. It was first brought into this country by Ralph Lane and popularized by Sir Walter Raleigh. In 1603 James I published a pamphlet pointing out the bad effects of tobacco smoking. In Russia the Tsar Michael punished his soldiers with the rack and knout for smoking, whilst several Popes forbade its use in churches. The Puritans condemned it, but John Evelyn records in his diary that the soldiers at Cromwell's funeral took tobacco. Smoking was used as a preventive against the plague, and in 1665 the boys at Eton School were made to smoke pipes to ward off the evil. In those days tobacco was taken either in a pipe or in the form of snuff. Cigars became popular in Regency days, but it was not until 1861 that the first cigarettes were made in this country by John Theodori, a Greek who lived in Leicester Square. He imported the idea from Spain. (The cigarette was a South American invention of the 1750's.) It was not until the turn of the century, however, that they became at all popular. In 1900 the annual consumption of tobacco in the form of cigarettes was less than $\frac{1}{4}$ lb. per head; today it is about 4 lb. The use of cigarettes has by now become universal throughout the world. America has actually taken steps to combat the use of tobacco. The twentieth amendment to the Constitution of the U.S.A. prohibits the manufacture, sale, and consumption of cigars, cigarettes, pipe tobacco, cut plug, and snuff, with powers to appoint enforcement officers. I should hasten to add that it has never been ratified! In 1848 smoking in the streets of Berlin was prohibited, whilst today the sale of cigarettes to minors is prohibited in many countries.

Tobacco smoke contains pyridine bases and ammonia which are intensely irritant and produce the smoker's cough. It also contains poisonous substances such as carbon monoxide, arsenic, nicotine, and 3 : 4 benzpyrene found in the tarry oils. This latter substance is the probable cause of lung cancer. The immediate ill-effects of excessive smoking are due mainly to nicotine since the other substances are present in such small amounts, although the amount of arsenic is greater than that allowed in foods. This probably comes from the chemicals which are used in spraying the tobacco crops.

The ill-effects of nicotine are first of all increased secretion of the glands of the alimentary tract, giving increased salivation and gastric secretion, loss of appetite, nausea, and dyspepsia and vomiting when taken to excess. Some people are much more sensitive to these effects than others. It has also a laxative action, particularly in those unaccustomed to it. Later there is diminished secretion, causing a dry furred mouth and tongue often accompanied by halitosis. The pulse-rate is increased with a small rise in blood-pressure. This may be partly responsible for increased breathlessness on exertion, a phenomenon well known to athletes and mountain climbers at the beginning of the season! It certainly reduces the vital capacity of the lungs and is 'bad for the wind'. Osler showed that an angina-like pain could occur after heavy smoking, together with more serious effects on the heart such as palpitation and various disorders of rhythm. Arteriosclerosis can easily be produced in animals by injecting nicotine and there is considerable evidence that it causes constriction of arteries. This may be the reason for an added risk from coronary heart disease in heavy smokers.

Nicotine acts as a mild sedative to the brain. This is the reason for its widespread use in producing a feeling of well-being. Excessive smoking may produce anxiety, insomnia, headaches, neuralgia, giddiness, and tremor.

Blindness due to excessive intake of cheap wet tobacco was due to the large amount of nicotine ingested, but it is very rare today. Finally, we should not forget the stained fingers and foul breath.

As with all drugs, people become rapidly tolerant to the intake of nicotine. This tolerance may disappear, however, with age or during severe illness, particularly febrile illness. It is well known that many people lose their desire for tobacco during an influenza attack, for example. The pleasant effects of smoking can be produced by injecting nicotine. Finally, nursing mothers should remember that nicotine is excreted in their milk if they smoke heavily.

The habit of smoking, then, is a drug addiction to nicotine, although not quite in the same category as the heroin or cocaine addict who is usually powerless to stop his habit without outside help. An addict takes his particular drug in order to free himself from the cares and worries of the world. He is fearful of the consequences of withdrawal and of the craving which follows.

The consumption of cigarettes per head is greater in Britain than anywhere else. We, as a nation of drug addicts, contribute £800 million to the National Exchequer for this privilege. Clearly the Government has a vested interest in smoking; in fact, this tax pays more than the whole cost of the National Health Service. In 1962 the Royal College of Physicians issued a report on the subject of smoking and lung cancer. They recommended that the Government should increase further the tax on cigarettes and decrease the tax on cigars and pipe tobacco.

Tobacco smokers pollute the air of public places so that not only they, but non-smokers, too, have to breathe the pollution. The financial side of the problem needs consideration, too. I know of one family of a father and mother and six children in which the father smokes 50 cigarettes a day and the mother 20. He earns £8 per week, out of which £4 3s. is spent on cigarettes. That is more than half his wages and yet they seem powerless to stop smoking. The children are inadequately clothed and fed as a result. There must be many families today in a similar position. No wonder so many people are asking for more wages! In China the habit of opium smoking is a similar problem; it injures the health and physical powers, especially in the poorer classes, so that some families have to go without clothes so that the parents can satisfy this habit. Opium is still called the great curse of China. Future generations may say that cigarette smoking was the great social evil of the Western World.

Why do people smoke? In the first place the youth considers it manly to smoke and cissy not to; it is considered grown up and sophisticated because father or mother do it. Freud considered that the pleasure of having something in the mouth may form part of an urge which is similar to the pleasure the infant gets from sucking at the breast. Certainly many men suck empty pipes and non-smoking women suck sweets and chocolates, and Americans chew gum. It is also said that one of the causes of overeating is the need for something in the mouth in those who are emotionally maladjusted. Certainly in smoking there is also the sedative action of the nicotine and the addiction which follows. This urge to smoke is reinforced by the powerful advertisements issued by the tobacco companies and by social factors, such as the handing round of cigarettes and the ritual of smoking after meals. Smoking may be a good thing after breakfast, bringing into play an urge to defaecate. The worst habit is smoking during meals, introduced from America and now considered fashionable in some circles. In these cases smoking replaces food for those people who have no taste for good wine or food.

The cocktail habit is another product of America where a quick fillip is needed to pep up the overworked business man; he needs a cigarette at the same time to soothe his nerves. It is noteworthy that chain smoking and the cocktail habit are opposed to the appreciation of good food and wine; that is why there are so few gourmets in America.

It may be that as a result of reading this chapter there are people who wish to stop smoking. It can be done.

How to Stop Smoking

There is only one way and that is to cut it out completely. The craving for the drug effect of tobacco reaches its peak 1–2 days after stopping, and then declines. The psychological craving, however, may take longer. The first week is undoubtedly the worst and if the smoker can weather this he can tell himself that it will become progressively easier. Absolute conviction that smoking is harmful is the first necessity. I hope that my remarks in this chapter have succeeded in convincing the reader. Secondly, he should withstand all invitations to smoke. As one who has given up smoking several times, I know that this is the most difficult part. It is very difficult to refuse a cigarette which is offered; perhaps it has something to do subconsciously with the idea of getting something for nothing. You must be prepared to withstand the leg-pulling of your friends; perhaps one good way is to be ready with a counter blast about their furred tongues, stained fingers, and foul breath. One thing, you should throw away all smoking appliances, pipes, matches, lighter, and cigarettes. The whole thing then is psychological; you can reinforce this strongly by thinking about the ill-effects last thing at night until you go to sleep. Suggestion under hypnosis can also help.

As far as tablets are concerned there appear to be no particular drugs which have any definite action in curing smoking, but of course any tablet which is thought to have this action will be of value in reinforcing the will to stop. For that reason I would not necessarily condemn them. Unfortunately they are often far too expensive for the substances they contain. One well-known tablet, for example, contains ferrous sulphate and alum, giving an unpleasant taste in the mouth when the person smokes. Another reputed remedy is a few brushes on the tongue with a silver nitrate stick; the tongue is then rolled round the palate; if a cigarette is taken it produces an unpleasant taste. There is a danger of silver poisoning from this, so it is hardly to be recommended except perhaps for the first two days of stopping. For the first week or so, sweets or chewing-gum may help to relieve the craving. There is no doubt that the weight will go up at first, but this can be adjusted later and it is best not to worry about it initially. It may cause also increased irritability and nail-biting; treatment of this by a doctor could help to minimize the ill-effects.

If the urge is overwhelming the smoker can try a small whiff or cheroot as being less harmful, but I regard this as an undesirable compromise because it continues to keep up the vicious circle which we are trying to break. One régime which has been advocated in the columns of the *Lancet* is as follows: 'Having decided to stop smoking fix a definite date five days ahead when all forms of smoking will cease. In the meantime carry out deep breathing exercises, taking in a large breath, preferably through the nose, then pause for five seconds, and exhale forcibly. This should be repeated as often as desired; while the exercises are being carried out the person should concentrate on the date fixed for stopping.'

Another tip to try is to write down all the undesirable features of the smoking habit and to read them over twice just before going to sleep.

The whole onus, then, is on the individual person's will-power and I am convinced that the great majority of heavy smokers can give it up if they follow these instructions, but they must *want* to.

Of course, the best thing is to never start, and there is a great onus placed on teachers and parents to tell children the truth about cigarette smoking. Unfortunately, too many old wives' tales are about which fool no one. There can be little doubt that social pressures are the most difficult to overcome; for example, following a broadcast on the subject, I received an anonymous letter with the word 'Windy' printed inside.

There are also strong vested interests working against the person who wants to stop smoking; for example, the tobacco companies, and the Government, which would be faced with the very difficult problem of finding £800,000,000 from other sources.

ALCOHOL

With tobacco smoking goes the drinking of alcohol. Today it is the cocktail habit and the cigarette; in the old days it was the beer and baccy, the latter being smoked in a pipe. Whereas tobacco smoking is of recent origin, the drinking of fermented liquors goes back for many thousands of years. The Romans cultivated the grape for the health-giving wine it produced, which, drunk in moderation, had no harmful effects; similarly with beer, which in parts of Africa has nutritional significance providing substantial quantities of vitamin B as in Kaffir beer. Interference with this habit by well-meaning but ignorant 'white' administrators has on occasions resulted in vitamin B deficiency. In Ancient Egypt, bread and beer were the poor man's food as they were in nineteenth-century England. Drunkenness occurs when men drink spirits distilled from fermented liquors. In the eighteenth century drunkenness reached its height in Britain with the drinking of gin. The evils this brought are depicted by Hogarth in his celebrated picture 'Gin Lane'. The drinking of hard liquors, particularly cocktails, on an empty stomach is bad for health.

Wine drinking, however, is in a different category. It was recommended in Biblical times when wine, corn, and olive oil were the staple articles of diet, and in Grecian times the frugal diet of Sparta included wine. Hippocrates and Galen both wrote about its virtues. There is a general opinion that it is conducive to longevity. Pearl (1928) compared the longevity of moderate drinkers and total abstainers, however, and could find no difference. Wine is useful as a sedative, as a medicine, or as a food, and as an aid to digestion and appetite, particularly in the elderly and sick. Wine drunk with a meal greatly enhances the flavour of the various dishes, and the delectable aromas and flavours which good wines possess are a great delight in themselves.

Narcotic Drugs

The taking of habit-forming drugs is common in many parts of the world, particularly in the East and in various Indian peoples. It is now becoming increasingly common in the underworld of America and its use by teenagers has caused widespread alarm in the U.S.A. China is cursed with opium, which is usually smoked in pipes; in the West marijuana is taken in the form of cigarettes known as 'reefers', whereas cocaine is usually taken in the form of snuff, and the morphine addict takes his drug by injection. Often the needles and syringes are dirty and transmit other diseases such as syphilis and malaria. Heroin is probably the most dangerous form of addiction known. It is taken in the form of small pills, known as 'red pills'. In 1955 the British Government decided to prohibit its use even in medicine, but later reversed its decision.

In the nineteenth century opium was a common drug for the relief of coughing and so was given in cases of tuberculosis and to keep fretful children quiet. Apparently opium was taken in large quantities by the poor people of this country during the last century. It was sold in the form of pills or penny sticks. At Spalding, for example, 7 druggists sold 27 st. 3½ lb. of opium in a year; this gives an average of 127 grains per head per annum. It was also used to quieten babies whilst the mother went to work, and it was, of course, a very good palliative for cough and diarrhoea, the former common in the winter and the latter prevalent in the summer. The Commission on Employment of 1867 gave evidence of the widespread use of 'Godfrey's Cordial' in Lincolnshire, each shop preparing its own mixture containing opium. Dr. Hunter stated that narcotic agents were also put in the beer, and described the opium-eating babies as 'wizened like little monkeys'. (*See* Gillett and Hughes, 1955.)

Many of the writers and poets of this period were consumptive and produced much of their work under the influence of opium. De Quincey, who first took it for toothache, writes in his *Confessions of an English Opium Eater* that at one time he was taking the equivalent of over 500 grains of opium a day;* the normal dose is ½–1 grain.

Hashish and marihuana are smoked in cigarettes to give erotic dreams and to act as aphrodisiacs; their use is bound up with the white slave traffic. Hashish is prepared from Indian hemp and its use has increased since the Second World War; a single cigarette costs 50–100 francs in Paris and even more in New York. Very often an unsuspecting girl has started on the path to drug addiction when she has lightheartedly accepted a 'reefer' from her 'admirer', sometimes unknowingly. There is no viler criminal on earth than the pedlar in narcotic drugs, who makes enormous profits at the expense of human lives. Thus in China a kilogram of opium sells for the equivalent of £2, but as the material changes hands it gradually fetches exorbitant prices; in Egypt it costs the equivalent of £250 a lb.; as a result, the most amazing deceptions are practised to smuggle these dangerous drugs across the frontiers. These enormous profits make the drug traffic so difficult to stamp out. For these reasons a special section of the World Health Organization is concentrating on the control of the habit-forming drugs.

Drug addiction is an occupational hazard of those who handle dangerous drugs in their work, particularly doctors, nurses, and chemists. William Stewart Halsted, one of the greatest surgeons of the Johns Hopkins School of Medicine, was a cocaine addict.

There are several tribes of Indians, for example the Incas and Aztecs, who habitually use plants containing narcotic drugs, such as mescal. They give strong visual hallucinations, which have been likened to seeing a Walt Disney silly symphony; no wonder the Indians like to repeat the performance!

Another form of drug addiction, which can produce cancer, is the chewing of the betel leaf or nut; it produces betel chewers' cancer of the inside of the mouth from chronic irritation.

How common drug addiction is, it is difficult to say, but in the United Nations Bulletin on Narcotics of January, 1951, it was stated that 'it may be concluded that a considerable fraction of the world's population (the figure of 200 millions has been mentioned) indulges in the consumption of hemp as an inebriant; there were 3,000,000 drug addicts in India, and in all Mohammedan countries the taking of drugs is used in place of alcohol,

---

* The raw opium in those days was not standardized in any way, and it is probable that part of this 500 grains was made up of impure substances in the opium.

which is forbidden, whilst in China it was estimated that there were probably 40,000,000 opium addicts. Figures collected by the Bureau of Narcotics in the U.S.A. since 1953 show that there are 60,000 addicts in the States, centred chiefly in New York.

The three great smokes of the world are tobacco, opium, and Indian hemp. Perhaps we should be thankful that tobacco is probably the least harmful of the three, at any rate if smoked in a pipe. In fact, in the Congo the smoking of tobacco has been encouraged as a substitute for hemp, with beneficial results.

Before leaving the question of addiction, we should not forget that tea and coffee taken in excess can become a form of addiction just as much as an excess of alcohol or tobacco; which is the worse is a matter of opinion. The custom of tea drinking first originated in China, where the plant is common; it has probably been of great benefit to that country because the water has to be boiled in order to make the necessary infusion; this prevents many of the intestinal diseases which are so prevalent there.

The effects of tea and coffee are due to a stimulant, caffeine. In parts of Turkey, Egypt, China, and India strong infusions of coffee are drunk as dark, syrupy liquors containing enormous amounts of this drug. This produces increased excitability, sometimes mania, delusions, and adverse effects on the heart and circulation. The habit becomes a necessity, and the victims spend considerable sums of money to get the potent sources of their 'beverage'. If the person cannot give up the habit and suffers ill-effects as a result, then what can be a pleasant habit becomes a compulsive necessity. I know of one or two tea drinkers in this country who might classify for this latter category. One can hardly, however, call it common. In eating, drinking, or smoking, let us remember that moderation is the important thing.

We have today become a nation of medicine takers, and large quantities of sedatives, purgatives, and vitamins are taken. The drug bill under the National Health Service has reached enormous proportions despite measures taken to try to reduce it (for example, charging 2s. for each article on each prescription). Older people with their aches and pains are constantly demanding palliatives and placebos; unfortunately, some doctors take the easy way and prescribe many useless remedies for their patients. This state of affairs has been spoken of as 'medicated survival'. The yearly bill for vitamin preparations prescribed by doctors is at a conservative estimate something like £2,000,000, to say nothing of the large quantities bought privately. We are not perhaps quite as bad in this respect as America, where enormous sums are spent in advertising proprietary medicines. Another drug which is being used in increasing amounts is amphetamine or dexedrine; although in law it can only be obtained on a doctor's prescription, many chemists supply it quite freely without one. It is much in demand as a stimulant in those who need pepping-up for a party and many of the London barmen will supply it to counteract a hangover. It is a well-known stimulant for students taking examinations, for long-distance drivers, and for dance-band leaders, as it keeps the person awake. It is also much used in weight-reduction to reduce the appetite. Unfortunately, it may be necessary to take pheno-barbitone to get to sleep and there is an enormous sale of this drug, too, it being a very favourite prescription for 'nerves'. It is not uncommon for those who have to entertain the public, and even for business executives, to take their benzedrine in the morning, alcohol at lunch time and in the evening, nicotine all the time, and phenobarbitone at night. In Japan this problem is particularly acute amongst young people between the ages of 15 and 20 years. The Japanese Pharmaceutical Association assumes that there are 1,500,000 misusers of what are called the 'wake-amine' drugs, and there is considerable increase in the numbers admitted to psychiatric hospitals as a result of mental impairment from addiction to the drug. There have been several cases reported in this country of prison inmates eating the contents of benzedrine inhalers for their stimulant effect.

The latest group of drugs which can cause addiction are the tranquillizers. The excessive use of these drugs in anxiety states is a threat to Western society; they can seduce patients into a state of bogus health and weaken adaptive capacity.

There is also a great use of purgatives, particularly in women. It is probably true to say that most of the constipation in elderly females is due to the habitual use of purgatives.

All these habits are a product of the Western way of life with its mental and emotional stresses and strains and its high tempo.

THE DIRECTORS' DILEMMA

In the highly industrialized areas of Western Europe and North America the widespread application of preventive methods has done much to elimi-nate the infectious diseases, and as a result we have been left with a legacy of those chronic diseases which occur most frequently after middle age. Increasing attention is now being directed to the ultimate cause and possible prevention of these conditions. We already know that a number of types of cancer are preventable, particularly those of an occupational nature. The study of the variation in the incidence of disease in relation to various factors, such as age, sex, time, occupation, geographical location, and personal habits, is an important means of discovering causative factors. It is the whole basis of the epidemiological method. This method has been applied in brilliant fashion to answer the conundrums concerning the cause of cancer of the lung. There are other forms of cancer for which similar clues are available; thus cancer of the womb is rare in virgins and Jewish women, and circum-cision of the male goes a long way to prevent this cancer in the female. Thus a time-honoured custom which is practised by many races throughout the world is of great importance in preventive medicine. Cancer of the stomach shows important social and geographical variations which are probably due to local variation in methods of cooking. Investigation is now taking place into this aspect. Other forms of cancer which have shown recent increases are leukaemia (a form of cancer of the blood), brain cancer, and cancer of the prostate. Recent work has indicated that part of the increase in leukaemia may be due to the increased use of X-rays during pregnancy which affects the child. Leukaemia has become more prevalent (for similar reasons) in the cities of Japan devastated by the atom bomb. It may be that part of these increases are due to better standards of diagnosis in recent years, but it is clear that the epidemiological method offers great scope for the study of preventable causes. Unfortunately it is time-consuming and very expensive to undertake, requiring teams of workers to carry it out.

We still have to consider the great group of diseases due to degenerative changes in heart and blood-vessels; these are easily the most important cause of death today. It is true, of course, that many are the end-results of ageing and for their prevention we must look for some means of delaying the ageing process.

The expectation of life has increased enormously, and now when we are born the normal expectation is 68 years in the case of men and 73 years in the case of women. This has been brought about mainly by removal of those causes of death which kill in the early or middle stages of life. There has been little effect upon the expectation of life after we have reached, say, 60; to put it in another way, although many more men now survive to old age, we have not increased the maximum allotted span, which is still around the old Biblical estimate of three score years and ten.

Needless to say, there is now a great deal of research into the biological aspects of ageing and how to prevent it. There are some encouraging signs that we have at any rate found out some important causes. In the first place, if we turn to animal experiments, the only known way of prolonging life is to feed our animals on a spare diet. This work has been carried out on rats and shows quite definitely that rats on high-calorie diets have shorter lives than those fed on low-calorie diets, care being taken to ensure that both contain the necessary dietary essentials. This is in keeping with our knowledge of human beings. The Metropolitan Life Insurance Company of New York has shown that people over middle age who are overweight have a decreased expectation of life and increased mortality from a number of conditions such as diabetes, high blood-pressure, heart disease, and nephritis.

It is well known that varicose veins and arthritis cause more trouble in people who are overweight. Weight-reduction is a very important part of the treatment of many of these conditions which are commoner in older middle age. One particular disease which has been increasing enormously in Western Europe and North America is coronary heart disease, whilst the condition is rare in Asiatics and Africans. In the United Kingdom alone nearly 92,000 deaths from this disease, the greatest killer of them all, were registered in 1960. In this country the disease is found more commonly amongst the well-to-do; doctors and company directors are particularly prone.

In those Western countries with low dietary standards, such as Italy and Sardinia, there is a low incidence of coronary heart disease. In the Mediterranean countries olive oil has been used for thousands of years without manifest ill effect, and most of the population live active lives. Interesting evidence comes from Norway which, when it was occupied by the Germans, had a considerable fall in deaths from coronary heart disease; at the same time there was a fall in the intake of fat. This is a clear indication of the importance of dietary habits. Further experimental work on the blood of persons living in the U.S.A., Great Britain, Italy, Spain, Sweden, South Africa, and Central America shows that the intake of animal fat in the diet plays an important part in producing those conditions necessary for the development of the disease.

This work has been confirmed in animal experiments on dogs and rabbits. Although this is certainly not the only factor there is evidence that coronary artery disease occurs more frequently in those who have an excess of animal fat in the diet. Certainly another predisposing factor is the question of physical activity. In London the conductors of double-decker buses have less coronary artery disease than the bus drivers, whilst postmen suffer far less than do their colleagues who sit without exercise in the post offices. Labourers, coal-hewers, and policemen have a very low death-rate from the disease. There is evidence too that the excessive smoking of cigarettes is associated with a higher death-rate from this disease. This may be due to an indirect effect in that heavy smokers cannot take severe exercise. The miner and policeman are, of course, forbidden to smoke on duty. It may be that physical exercise can protect to some extent against dietary habits.

Temperance in eating and drinking was accepted in early Chinese medical writings as a cause of longevity. Cicero lived on wholesome food and wine, and in his book *De Senectute* advocated a spare diet as the only means of achieving longevity.

The Western way of life has brought with it certain diseases such as cancer of the lung and coronary heart disease. They are due to habits which have developed as a result of this way of life—the smoking of cigarettes (we are now too lazy to smoke pipes and cannot afford cigars), riding in motor cars, sitting in office chairs, and eating far more than our sedentary habits require of us.

It seems perhaps that the ancients knew something about healthy living after all. The answer to us moderns should be clear; after the age of 40 we should have a low-calorie diet, maintain a reasonable weight, and ensure that we get sufficient exercise. Once more the preservation of health depends upon the strict attention to personal habits of living. Food should not be fried because it absorbs a lot of fat; grilling, boiling, or roasting are much better. Certain foods, such as nuts and herrings, are quite rich in fat and are best avoided in middle age, although, of course, herrings are a very rich and nutritious food for the young—and how delicious they can be if fresh! Nearly all sea food has a low-fat content, but it must be fresh to be any good. The native cottage cheeses of this country are a very good form of diet for the middle aged, rich in protein and low in fat. Some of the less well known are excellent, such as Caerphilly, Dorset, Double Gloucester, Lancashire, Leicestershire, or Wensleydale, apart from the more familiar Cheddar, Cheshire, and Stilton. Remember, then, that fat control is important after middle age—spare your calories and live longer. The younger generation will only be too glad of your share of butter, cream, and eggs.*

Unfortunately, the social habits of our times make it very difficult to reduce weight. The business-man's lunch and a large dinner at night cause excess weight in many. Many men get a large percentage of their calorie intake from alcohol and even though they eat very little they are still surprised when they put on weight. Beer is particularly fattening. It is all right, of course, if the person takes plenty of exercise but the company director never has the time. That is why coronary thrombosis takes such a toll today of our higher executives; it can well be called the company directors' disease. Everything conspires against him and he must be strong willed indeed if he is to remain healthy. He should certainly try to get some vigorous exercise daily; squash rackets is an ideal way for the younger man, golf is very suitable for the older, but not many men can afford the time to play it regularly and the English winter is against it. If he gives up smoking he immediately puts on weight. Truly the disease is a director's dilemma. He should also take note that the hazard from being a stone overweight is greater than that from smoking 25 cigarettes a day.

The following verse by Sir Alan Herbert is an amusing commentary on our times:—

'The Bottle—and the Bite'

They say, with whispers or with winks,
'Poor Smith! The trouble is—HE DRINKS'.
But doctors worry more for Brown
Whose gluttony has got him down.
They know, as some of us do not,
The plate's as deadly as the pot.
The sober diner may depart
From Fatty Something of the Heart,
While he whose wickedness is wine
May totter on to 99.
But no one whispers on the streets
'Poor Brown! The trouble is—HE EATS'.

(*With acknowledgements to the 'Sunday Graphic'*)

We know that there are lies, damned lies, and statistics, but the following figures may give wine-bibbers some consolation and an excuse for their glass of wine (if they need one!). The mortality-rates from arteriosclerotic heart disease (annual death-rate per 100,000 of the population in 1958) in high wine-drinking countries were as follows: France 106, Italy 120, Switzerland 173, Germany 194; compare these figures with those for low wine-drinking countries—U.S.A. 660, Canada 550, New Zealand 492, Finland 483, England and Wales 372.

---

* A most useful aid to those who wish to control their weight is *The Vest Pocket Calorie Counter* published by Garden City Books, New York. It can be obtained (price 4s. 6d.) from H. K. Lewis & Co. Ltd., 136 Gower Street, London, W.C.1.

CHAPTER XIII

GENESIS

ONE of the great problems for the future is the control of inherited disease. In the case of certain diseases, we can give advice on the chances of abnormal offspring being born when there is evidence that some inherited abnormality is present in a particular family. There are many commoner diseases in which inheritance plays an important part, but the precise mode of transmission is complicated. We know, for example, that in tuberculosis, diabetes, epilepsy, mental deficiency, and in many forms of mental illness, nature as well as nurture is of importance. The interplay between genetic and environmental factors is very complicated and varies with differing circumstances. The more we do, however, to remove and control adverse physical factors the more important become genetic factors. Take tuberculosis of the lung, for example: we cannot contract this disease without coming into contact with the tubercle bacillus, but in actual fact everyone in an industrial community does come into contact with it by the time early adult life is reached. By improving living and working standards and by raising the level of nutrition it means that only those who have a low inborn resistance develop the disease. The great majority of the families of this country have developed a high resistance as a result of long contact with the disease and the survival only of those most resistant to infection, a process of natural selection which weeds out the most susceptible. All the Brontë children died at an early age and as a result none of them survived to pass on the lethal trait. Natural selection is operating all the time in raising the level of resistance of the race to such dangers.

There are a number of conditions which are transmitted in a definite and clear-cut manner by inherited factors alone. Such things as the blood groups are of great practical importance in medicine and we can forecast accurately what will be the result of certain matings and even use the method to disprove disputed paternity.

These blood groups are transmitted by genes present in the cells of the parent body and the science of genetics involves a study of the way in which these genes are transmitted, whilst eugenics concerns the practical application of this information for the welfare of mankind. Unfortunately, the application of eugenics involves a wide understanding of genetic theory, which is rarely possessed by many well-meaning but uninformed persons who profess to practise eugenics.

One of the most striking conditions transmitted by an abnormal gene is the disease known as Huntington's chorea. It was originally imported into the U.S.A. from the small village of Bures in Suffolk, when in 1630 the John Winthrop fleet sailed to New England with about 700 immigrants. Amongst them were 3 illiterate men released from jail who were suffering from this condition. Nearly 1000 cases of the disease in direct descendants of these immigrants have been traced since that time in America and there are probably 1000 family groups in England and Wales with the same disease. It is one of the most distressing of all inherited diseases, and many who suffered from it were regarded as being possessed of the devil and burnt for it. Usually the disease does not develop until adult age is reached, by which time the dread defect may have already been passed on to future generations. Unfortunately, such people usually have large families, passing this terrible curse on to half their offspring. The mode of inheritance is called dominant because it expresses itself whenever the abnormal gene is present. The members of these families live in constant dread of the condition and even those not affected suffer from great mental anguish and anxiety. Needless to say, depression, suicide, and alcoholism are very frequent. As the disease develops the victims develop peculiar twitchings and grimacings, with spasmodic movements of the head and limbs. The involuntary jerkings of the limbs were once supposed to represent the sufferings of Christ on the Cross. Gradually the patients deteriorate mentally and finish up in mental hospitals.

A great deal can be done to help these families by health education. First of all there should be adequate ascertainment of all such families in the country so that suitable advice can be given. Children of affected parents, if Roman Catholics, should be advised against marriage; others, if they wish to marry, should be instructed in methods of birth control, whilst termination of pregnancy is strongly indicated if either parent is suffering from the disease. There is great ignorance in these families about the method of transmission of the trait, and a constant dread of passing this disease on to future generations. It is to be hoped that in the future some means will be devised for distinguishing in early life between those children who have received the gene and those who have escaped it. The latter could then be told that they had nothing to fear and could freely marry and have children.

One form of inheritance which is fairly well known to most people is the type of dwarfism seen in many circus clowns and known to the medical profession as achondroplasia. It was first described in 1878 by Parrot. The growth of the long bones is arrested so that the arms and legs are short; there is a large head, waddling gait, bending of the spine, and short broad feet. The condition is transmitted in the same way as Huntington's chorea; in most cases half the offspring of an affected person suffer from the condition, the other half being normal and free from the taint.

Another condition which is sometimes seen in the circus is that known as pie-balding in which the human skin becomes coloured in light and dark patches; it is very rare in the general population, but since a number of cases from one family may all finish up in the circus it may appear more common than it really is. It is most dramatic when it occurs in a negro

family; several such cases finished up in freak shows under such names as
'The Striped Graces' and 'Tiger Lilies'. One negress born in Louisiana in
1853 had 15 children of whom 8 were piebald.

Another very fascinating inherited condition is haemophilia, often called
the 'Royal disease' because it was transmitted by Queen Victoria to the
Russian and Spanish royal families. In this particular mode of inheritance
the condition is shown by males and carried by females, although a few true
cases have recently been recorded in females. It results in a tendency to
bleed from the slightest cut and many of the sufferers from this condition
have bled to death from trivial wounds, such as those acquired in some small
street accident or the extraction of teeth.

Queen Victoria of England was the first known carrier of the lethal gene.
It is difficult to trace back farther than that because the disease was only
described in 1803. It could have originated in Queen Victoria by a process
known as 'mutation', in which a normal gene is converted into an abnormal
one. It is a well-known occurrence in plants, animals, and in human beings.
Atomic radiation is an important cause of increasing the mutation rate.
As harmful genes are constantly being eliminated by natural selection so new
ones are being formed by mutation, usually maintaining an equilibrium. We
usually find that the greater the loss by natural selection the greater the
mutation rate. We can only wonder at the precise mechanism by which this
is brought about. If the abnormal gene for haemophilia arose originally in
Queen Victoria, we do not know the cause.

Ten of Victoria's male descendants have suffered from the disease and 7
of her female descendants have been proved to be carriers. The mode of
inheritance is such that half her sons would suffer from the disease and half
her daughters would be carriers. King Edward VII did not suffer from the
disease and so cannot have transmitted the lethal gene to any of his descendants. On the other hand, Leopold, Duke of Albany, her youngest son, was
a haemophiliac, and transmitted the defect through his daughter to his
grandson, Lord Trematon, who died in a motoring accident. Through two
of her daughters the disease was transmitted to the Russian and Spanish
royal families, and what a remarkable effect that must have had upon the
recent history of Europe! The disastrous influence of the 'mad monk'
Rasputin upon the Tsar Nicholas II was due to his alleged hypnotic control
of the Tsarevich Alexis, who suffered from haemophilia. The affliction of
the Crown Prince of Russia with the 'Royal disease' may well have played
a decisive part in the overthrow of the Russian Imperial régime. The two
sons of the last King of Spain, Alfonso XIII, suffered from haemophilia.
Prince Alfonso Pio died in a car accident in Florida in 1938 and the younger
son, Prince Gonzalo Manuel, died from haemorrhage as a child. (*Fig.* 41.)

Both the present Queen of England, Elizabeth II, and her husband Prince
Philip are descended from Queen Victoria. Queen Elizabeth cannot have
inherited the gene as her grandfather, Edward VII, was perfectly normal in
this respect. Prince Philip is not haemophiliac himself and the pedigree
shows that there is no chance of his having the abnormal gene, the Battenberg

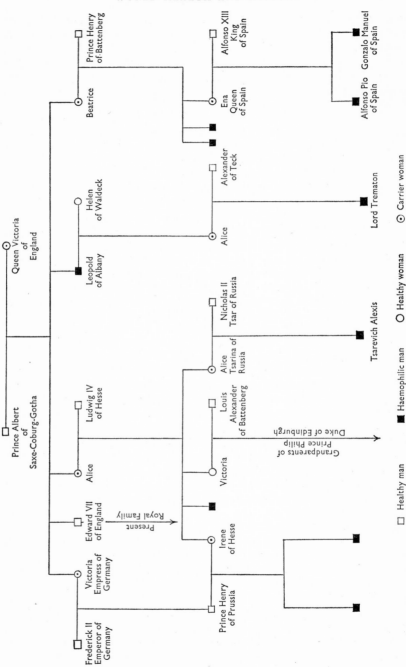

Fig. 41.—Pedigree and family tree (incomplete) of Queen Victoria showing those descendants affected by haemophilia.

☐ Healthy man ⦾ Carrier woman ○ Healthy woman ■ Haemophilic man

family, of which he is a member, being free from the trait. Again in this disease a great deal can be achieved by giving the correct advice; from a perusal of the family tree it is possible to detect on which side the lethal trait will be carried. Half the daughters of an affected man will carry the gene. It is now possible by appropriate tests to determine those who are carriers and those who are free from the taint. A woman shown to be free from the abnormal gene can be reassured as far as marriage is concerned that there is no danger of transmitting the taint to her offspring. Women who are carriers should be warned that half their sons will be affected. It should be noted, however, that nowadays prompt hospital treatment will usually prevent the haemophiliac from bleeding to death. Moreover, if an operation is necessary, suitable precautions can be taken. In this, as in all inherited disease, knowledge is power, and a great deal of apprehension can be avoided and suitable arrangements made to cope with any risk that may arise.

. The common form of colour blindness is transmitted in the same way as haemophilia, the defect being shown by men and transmitted by half their daughters. Four per cent of all men are colour blind; it is extremely rare in women.

Probably the most striking of all inherited defects was the famous case of the porcupine man. It occurred in the Lambert family who lived near Euston Hall in Suffolk. A country labourer's son was the first to suffer from the condition, though his father was normal. The defect was transmitted from father to son through five further generations, all the sons being affected and the daughters being free from the taint. The boy, then aged 14 years, was exhibited before the Royal Society in 1731. An earlier account described the condition as follows: 'The boy's skin, which was covered with rough scales chiefly about the belly and flanks, looked and rustled like the bristles or quills of an Hedge-Hog, shorn off within an inch of the skin.' These men were strong and alert and might well have founded a race of a new species of mankind, but they were destined to die out because their condition was a bar to mating. Their appearance must have been against their acquiring a wife and the actual effort involved in mating must have been quite painful to the other party. The only wonder is that so many offspring were in fact produced. One of the great-grandsons of the first case was exhibited in 1833 at a meeting of the Westminster Medical Society, and he seems to have been the last of the race.

Another form of inheritance of great interest is albinism. This is a well-known phenomenon in circus horses, in which the skin, hair, eyebrows, eyelashes, and eyes are white; the horses often also show defects of vision. Albinism occurs in human beings and is most striking when seen in Negroes. It is fairly common in Lagos, West Africa. In Europe it occurs with a frequency of 1 in 10,000. The most striking example is that of the so-called White Indians from Darien; there are said to be over 300 of them out of a population of 20,000.

The form of inheritance of albinism is most likely to show itself when there is intermarriage between closely related persons, such as first cousins. It is usually due to the marriage of two carriers of the disease who are both outwardly normal, because this particular gene is what is known as 'recessive'; it does not show itself in the carrier state. Once the defect has appeared in a pedigree, usually 1 in 4 of the brothers and sisters will suffer from the condition. Of course, this ratio may only be seen in large families.

The offspring of the persons suffering from albinism, provided they marry normal persons, are usually normal. We have therefore the anomaly of an inherited condition arising out of the blue and disappearing again, the only positive evidence that it is due to an abnormal gene being the following:—

1. There is a greater incidence of the condition in brothers and sisters than in the normal population. Thus whilst the incidence in the general population may be 1/10,000, the incidence in brother and sister will be 1 in 4.

2. There is a greater incidence of marriage between closely related persons in the parents of albinos than there is in the normal population. Thus the incidence of first-cousin marriages in the general population will be usually about 1 per cent; in the parents of persons with albinism, about 6 per cent.

The greater the degree of inbreeding between related persons the more likely it is that two persons will be carriers of the same abnormal gene, which will produce abnormality in the offspring. That is one reason why incest is taboo in most societies, although it was a normal practice for some Ancient Egyptian kings to mate with their sisters. This is the accepted practice in animal matings where abnormal offspring can be eliminated, because by this means especially good genes can be brought together to produce beneficial results, which can then be reproduced in the offspring. The founder of the 18th Dynasty of the Egyptian kings, Thotmes I, married his sister and produced offspring of outstanding ability. His daughter, Queen Hatshepsut, was a remarkable woman, her mother being descended from two successive marriages of full brothers and sisters. In this case good genes were brought to the fore, but there are few stocks which do not contain some deleterious genes and close inbreeding will bring them to light. One of the first to appear is infertility, as many stock breeders have found to their cost. This, in fact, seems also to have affected some of the highly inbred strains of the Pharaohs. The most fertile stocks are those which are mixed, producing greater vigour in the hybrids. Close inbreeding, then, as happens in some small island communities, often results in the disappearance of the race because of infertility. For the same reason it is usually considered undesirable for first cousins to marry, particularly if there is some rare lethal trait in the family which may be transmitted in this way. In former times such intermarriage was sometimes heavily penalized; thus in A.D. 390 Theodosius the Great prohibited cousin marriage under penalty of death.

It is too early as yet to be able to do anything about destroying abnormal genes, but one day it may be possible. We still need to know more about what produces them, and a great deal of research is required in the field of genetics. Most of our efforts in the past have been directed towards research into curative medicine and into control of the environment. If we are to advance, we must have much more intensive research in the fields of human genetics, which up to the present has been a neglected science.

No account of genetics would be complete unless it included a description of the work of that remarkable man, Sir Francis Galton, who founded the Eugenics Society. He defined eugenics as 'the science which deals with all influences that impair the inborn qualities of the human race; also with those that develop them to the utmost advantage'.

Sir Francis Galton died on 17 Jan., 1911, a fit and virile figure at the age of 89. He was fortunate in that at an early age he was left a large sum of money on the death of his father; he was thus able to gratify his passion for travel, making anthropological observations in many parts of Europe and Africa. He was awarded, in 1854, one of the Royal Geographical Society's annual gold medals for his explorations in Africa. His early training was in mathematics and medicine although he never qualified as a doctor. He had an outstanding intellect, publishing over 200 papers and books on a wide variety of subjects. Professor Lewis Terman, a distinguished American psychologist, has estimated that Galton, as a child, had an intelligence quotient of about 200. By the age of 5 years, he could read almost any English book and he could tell the time. Apart from his work on eugenics, he wrote on the following subjects: exploration, meteorology, geography, blood transfusion, composite photography, the sterility of heiresses, and high-pitched whistles. He developed the study of finger prints as a means of identification and was responsible for the use of the correlation coefficient in statistical analysis.

He had a remarkable bent for mechanical devices and invented, amongst others, the following highly complicated instruments: the compound drill pantograph, a pocket zeometer, an altazimuth, and a wave-engine.

It was his work in the field of human measurement, however, for which he has become most famous. His published work includes the following books: *Inquiries into Human Faculty, Hereditary Genius, A Life History Album, Natural Inheritance, Noteworthy Families, English Men of Science, Their Nature and Nurture,* and *Memories of My Life.*

One of his most controversial papers was 'Statistical Enquiries into the Efficacy of Prayer', which caused considerable controversy in Victorian England.

Galton's last effort was a book of Utopia entitled *Kantsaywhere* which he submitted to the publisher a few weeks before he died; it was refused, and Galton, as a result, told his niece to destroy the manuscript. Almost one of the last things he wrote was, 'It has cleared my thoughts to write it, so now let it go to "Won't-say-where".' Some parts of it were fortunately preserved and are reproduced in Professor Karl Pearson's third volume of *The Life, Letters and Labours of Francis Galton.*

In Galton's Utopia only those well endowed with desirable qualities were allowed to have children. Prospective parents had to sit an examination. The joint marks obtained determined the number of children that each couple could have. The following is an extract from the book.

My batch had to present itself at 12 noon. At that hour I handed in my Pass Certificate to an official, who sat in the Hall, by the entrance to a long enclosure of latticework, through which everything was easily seen from the outside. The enclosure contained a row of narrow tables ranged down its middle, on which most of the measuring instruments were placed, the heavier ones standing on the ground between them. Those instruments were duplicated that required a longer time for their use than the rest. A passage ran between each side of the tables and walls of the enclosure. Five attendants, each having one candidate in charge, were engaged all day long making a tour of the tables in succession. The candidate emerges and is dismissed at an exit door, which is separated from the entrance by a low gate, over which the official can lean while he sits.

Immediately after entering the enclosure, my attendant made me sign my name and impress my blackened fingers on a blank schedule. It contained numerous spaces with printed headings, which the attendant filled in with pencil as he went on. He took me round the enclosure testing me in turn by every instrument and recording the results. They referred to stature, both standing and sitting, span of arms, weight, breathing capacity, strength of arm, as when pulling a bow, power of grip, swiftness of blow, reaction time, discrimination (blindfold) between weights, normality of eye, acuity of vision, colour sense, acuteness of hearing, discrimination of notes, sensitivity to taste and of touch, and a few other faculties. Lastly the state of my teeth, which are particularly good, and of my mouth were inspected.

There then follows a passage about how the various measurements were translated into marks.

I was then taken to another part of the hall and submitted to an examination for aesthetics and literature. I was given both prose and poetry to read before the examiners, a copy of these extracts having been handed to me to peruse beforehand. Then a simple singing was asked for. After this, a few athletic poses were gone through as well as some marching past, and the examiners noted their opinion on my schedule. Then I was allowed an hour to write four short essays on given subjects. This was the only literary test.

I should say that they lay much stress on the aesthetic side of things at Kantsaywhere. 'Grace and Thoroughness' is a motto carved over one of the houses for girls in the College, and I have seen it repeated more than once in embroidery and the like. A loutish boy and an awkward girl hardly exist in the place. They are a merry and high-spirited people, for whose superfluous energy song is a favourite outlet. Besides, they find singing classes to be one of the best ways of bridging over the differences of social rank. Musical speech and clear but refined pronunciation are thought highly of; so is literary expression, and this examination is intended to test all these. . . .

I was then medically examined in a private room very strictly indeed, and much was asked about my early ailments and former state of health. Here again I need not go into details, for they can be easily imagined, even in a general way, even by a layman. . . .

Lastly came the consideration of my ancestry. . . . I lay under a difficulty here. The official records made at Kantsaywhere are so minutely kept, that the requirements of the examiners have grown to be exceedingly rigorous as regards the evidences of ancestral gifts and maladies. All immigrants are more or less suspected. Besides this, such evidences as would require little confirmation in England, owing to public knowledge . . . may and does require more confirmation here than can easily be collected at home. I deeply resented my own ill-luck in this matter. The examiners told me only what I was prepared to hear, but expressed at the same time much regret that they were unable to give as many marks for my Ancestral Efficiency as I possibly, or even probably deserved. In fact I only got five marks for my ancestry.

This concluded all that I had to undergo. I had spent about one hour under anthropometric tests and from half an hour to one hour under each of the other three, besides the hour in essay writing, or about four hours in all, exclusive of intervals. . . .

The maximum number of positive marks that could be gained by each candidate is four times 30 or 120. A star might also be gained in each subject. The marks were totalled, and about half of these totals usually range between 45 and 70. . . . The names and marks of those who gained 70 marks and upwards are published in the newspaper together with such brief notes as each case might call for. . . . I learnt that supplementary marks might be and often were, accorded for specially good service to the community after the examination. They had to be proposed by the Board of Examiners, and the grounds of the proposal had to be set forth in their Annual Report. . . . These supplementary marks are supposed to attest that the natural capacity of the person who receives them really exceeds that which was expressed by the number of marks he had received at the original examination.

I do not know much in detail about the examination for girls. It is carried out by women examiners, who had taken medical degrees elsewhere, and is, I was assured, as thorough as that which I had myself undergone, and was considered to be as trustworthy. . . .

I inquired minutely whether they were unable to devise some test for endurance or staying, which seemed to me one of the most important of those they had to consider. It seemed that they had not as yet succeeded in eliminating the effect of practice. Neither were they enabled to examine into character, directly as a separate subject, partly because it was not fully developed at the usual age of examination, and partly because of the extreme difficulty at that age of estimating it justly, the teachers or comrades of a girl or boy often making sad mistakes of judgment.

The book possibly expresses Galton's views on how a eugenically selected community could be organized; we know now that the applications of eugenics to improving the race can lead to very dangerous consequences, as seen, for example, in Nazi Germany. Galton's earlier writings show that he definitely deprecated overzealous and hasty action in this field.

The question of 'quality versus quantity' will be discussed in more detail at the end of this chapter.

METHODS OF STUDY

In 1883 Galton first called attention to the study of like and unlike twins as a means of distinction between the effects of heredity and environment. Like twins arise by the subsequent division of a single fertilized ovum and share the same genetic material. Unlike twins are no more similar than brothers and sisters born at different times; they merely happen to be born together. By studying unlike twins living in the same environment, it is possible to distinguish between two individual persons of different genetic make-up brought up under the same environment. By the study of like twins brought up in different environments, it is possible to study the effects of environment, uncomplicated by differences in genetic structure. In all these studies it is first necessary to prove that the twins under study have in fact arisen from one or two ova respectively. As a result of these studies, it has been shown that heredity is of considerable importance in the determination of intelligence, whereas body-weight, for example, is more dependent on environment.

There are some interesting examples of how identical twins, even though brought up apart, often have identical histories. One example is the case of identical twin sisters in New York. One married and reared a family, the other remained single. Both became blind and deaf in the same month and although in different hospitals both suffered a stroke on the same day.

In 1950 Science Service carried out a talent contest in which 16,000 schoolchildren in the U.S.A. entered. There were severe eliminating contests and the names of the winners were known only after the semi-finals. Out of the 9 girl winners, 2 were identical twins from different schools. One chose for her subject the study of birds and the other that of ant behaviour.

There is the remarkable story of the Giles brothers, who were identical twins, graduating from different colleges in the U.S.A. They both pursued very similar careers in the Army Air Force, both reaching the rank of General, although they spent most of their service life apart.

The work of Kallmann and Reisner (1943) showed, by the twin family method, that hereditary predisposition was of importance in the development of pulmonary tuberculosis. They studied 308 pairs of twins and estimated the tuberculosis morbidity-rates in other members of the family. They found that the chances of developing tuberculosis varied with the degree of blood relationship. These differences could not be explained on the result of greater exposure and were obviously related to hereditary factors.

A similar study was carried out on 691 cases of split personality (schizophrenia) by Kallmann (1946) in New York, and he estimated the incidence of the same condition in blood-relationship relatives of the twin who developed it. This disease is the commonest form of insanity in our mental hospitals and schizophrenics comprise about half of our mental hospital inmates. When one realizes that over 40 per cent of our hospital beds are for mental cases the seriousness of this problem will be realized. Kallmann found, as in tuberculosis, that the chances of developing the disease increase in proportion to the degree of blood relationship. The incidence of the disease in other members of the families is given by the following percentages: Like twins, 85·8; unlike twins, 14·7; full brothers and sisters, 14·3; parents, 9·2; half brothers and sisters, 7; and approximately 2 for step-brothers and sisters and marriage partners.

The difference in rates between like and unlike twins is in the ratio of 6–1 and an analysis of environmental factors makes it difficult to explain these differences on non-genetic grounds. The predisposition to mental disease known as split personality, therefore, appears to depend on the presence of a recessive gene, which gives the organism the ability to respond to certain stimuli with a certain type of reaction.

The following case histories quoted by Dr. I. Atkin of the Park Prewett Hospital, Hampshire, illustrate the remarkable way in which two like twins can develop the same symptoms at the same time although educated at different universities.

Twin B, born one hour later than twin A, suffered a severe scalding of her legs with shock at the age of 2½ years. Up to the age of about 10 the twins did not show significant differences, but differentiation became marked after twin B developed an eye ulcer which kept her away from school for a while, and she had to be moved to a lower form. Twin A began to forge ahead. Twin B became frustrated in the competition with A; however hard she tried, twin A always came first. Finding she could not beat her sister in arts, she took up science, entering a university in October, 1950. She had an attack of shingles in December, 1952, but some weeks earlier had become excessively religious. The acute breakdown occurred in March, 1953, at the age of 20. She began to pray for the conversion of her parents and was alternately elated and depressed. At times she would describe herself as the Virgin Mary or Queen of the Realm, talked of opening up the Kingdom of Heaven, and wanted to get married to the Lord Jesus; at other times she called herself Judas Iscariot, thought she had sold herself to the devil and ought to be crucified. After undergoing a course of treatment she made an excellent recovery. In October, 1953, she resumed her studies, and took her B.Sc. in August, 1954.

Twin A developed the first signs of split personality about a year later. In December, 1953, she became intensely self-critical, accused herself of laziness and apathy, maintained that she had led a deplorable life, described herself as despicable and a menace to everybody. On admission to hospital about a month later she claimed that she had seen God in the form of a light, was told that she would give birth to a child who would be called 'Love', and thought that she had a special mission on earth. After a course of treatment she made a good recovery. Early in 1955 she obtained an honours degree.

Twin A was the more dominant and stronger character, but it was twin B who first developed schizophrenia. Though as children they were often confused because of similarities, as time passed differences of environmental strains and stresses determined differences in their personalities, and they soon grew away from each other. Nevertheless, a strong genetic factor doomed each of them to schizophrenic breakdowns with similar psychic patterns and subsequent recoveries.

The twin-family method of the study of disease is a very useful way of comparing and contrasting the effects of heredity and environment. Other methods of study are by a pedigree or family-history method. As we have seen, these give very limited information except in the case of well-recognized conditions which are transmitted by dominant genes with a high penetrance. The other method is to compare the percentage of blood relatives who develop the condition with the percentage in the population as a whole. We can also use the frequency of first-cousin marriages as a method of comparison. In this method it is essential to have accurate incidence rates by age and sex, and a precise knowledge of the population and the distribution of disease amongst it is an essential preliminary to any work of this nature. Moreover, degrees of severity of the various conditions have to be taken into account. It is important to realize that research work into the science of genetics depends upon carefully carried out morbidity surveys in the general population.

Practical Considerations.—Many workers in the health field as well as parents and teachers should be able to give some practical advice in relation to the problems of inherited disease. It must be admitted that in the majority of cases it is not possible to do very much in the way of prevention and treatment compared with the results which can be achieved by an attack on environmental factors. This, however, should not mean that we should regard the study of genetics as unimportant. On the contrary, it is quite clear that heredity plays an important part in predisposition to ill health and disease. A clearer knowledge of genetic susceptibility very often leads to a clearer identification of the controllable factors. The study of genetics and eugenics is in its infancy, and it may be possible in the future to control these factors much more efficiently than at present. If we could devise some method which would detect the carrier of a recessive gene, our advice to such persons might be much more effective in controlling disease. The knowledge that a special hereditary susceptibility existed might lead to the earlier management of a case than would otherwise occur. This knowledge would be particularly important if routine health examinations became the general practice in this country. A campaign for prevention or early treatment would be more effective if it were applied to a small susceptible portion of the population than if it were applied indiscriminately to the population as a whole.

It is very important that the doctor should be able to explain to his patients in simple terms the way in which hereditary factors operate. We have already seen that in the case of a recessive gene it is quite hopeless to try to eliminate it from the population by preventing persons who exhibit the disease from breeding. By this means we are leaving untouched the much commoner carriers. It appears that sterilization or the prevention of breeding will have very little effect in general in removing harmful genes from the population. The most useful advice we can give in relation to genetics is in the possibility of harmful conditions occurring in the offspring of a given mating and, if we know, for example, that there is a harmful gene in a particular family, it is important that the degree of blood relationship should be considered. In matings of close relatives, the two people contain many genes in common and it is much more likely that a harmful hidden character may produce an adverse effect with such matings. In animal breeding, the stock breeder particularly selects such breedings so that harmful genes can be brought to the fore and eliminated and the animals bearing beneficial genes can be developed to provide the breeding stock. This process is, of course, quite impossible in human matings. In general, advice should be given against first-cousin marriages especially if there is any evidence of a harmful gene within the family. If a person suffers from a defect known to be due to the inheritance of an abnormal gene it is possible to give advice on the possibilities of offspring being abnormal. Similarly, if a couple have had a child exhibiting a defect which is known to be due to the inheritance of a harmful gene, it is possible to give advice on the chances of other offspring being abnormal. In dominant inheritance it is known that in the great majority of cases 50 per cent of the offspring will inherit the particular trait. In recessive inheritance, if the affected person marries a normal person, the offspring will probably be normal, and in the sex-linked recessive inheritance, in which the defect is only shown by the male, the marriage of such a person with a normal female will result in normal sons and daughters who are carriers. It must be admitted, however, that it is only in certain rare conditions that we are able to give advice which is of any value in this respect. In the majority of common conditions in which hereditary predisposition plays a part, the genetic mechanism is still not determined; nevertheless, it is possible to give parents an estimate of the chances that further children will be affected, based on statistics from collections of families where further children have been born.

Advice on genetic problems can be given at genetic clinics; so far only a few have been set up, notably at the Hospital for Sick Children, Great Ormond Street, London, and at Leeds and Bristol. Many of the conditions which are transmitted by single genes are diseases of the eye, skin, or central nervous system, and they will in each case probably have been seen and referred by the appropriate consultant in those specialities.

What of the future? Premarital investigation could yield a great deal of information and advice. Who knows but that in the future at parties young people may exchange their premarital medical dossiers prior to making a date?

QUALITY OR QUANTITY, THAT IS THE QUESTION

It now remains to consider the question of quality. There has been a great deal of talk recently on the idea that we are breeding down, that the general level of intelligence is falling due to differential fertility; the more highly intelligent the parents, the smaller the family, whilst those of lowest intelligence have the largest families. The social problem group, the submerged tenth, as it is sometimes called, is characterized by very low intelligence, high fertility, and mental instability. The mental disabilities are transmitted to the offspring and there is a high infant mortality. Nevertheless, sufficient survive to outnumber those from parents of higher intelligence. Finally, as far as intelligence is concerned, like tends to marry like; this ensures that by and large members of similar social groups marry one another. On the face of it, it would appear that there are ample theoretical grounds on which to expect a national lowering of fertility. This view is expressed by Dr. Julian Huxley in his foreword to a book called *Human Fertility*, by Robert C. Cook, published in 1951. I quote from the foreword as follows: 'The situation as regards quality is almost equally gloomy. In almost all the socially and industrially advanced countries, the level of innate intelligence, and probably of other desirable genetic qualities, is decreasing generation by generation. Furthermore, we can be certain on theoretical grounds that the relaxation of natural selection brought about through our medical knowledge and social care must be causing slow degeneration of the stock, through the accumulation of harmful mutations.' Mr. Cook elaborates this thesis in his book. Now this is a remarkable statement to come from a person like Dr. Julian Huxley. There is very little positive evidence to show that national intelligence is, in fact, falling; on the other hand, one of the most thorough investigations which has yet taken place, that of Thompson in Scotland, shows that there has been a slight rise in intelligence in the last twenty years. One explanation may be that the pupils had become used to the intelligence tests used. Turning now to the informed opinion of Dr. Penrose, who, as head of the Galton Laboratory, has studied the problems of *human* genetics for many years as distinct from animal genetics, I quote from a lecture given by him to the Eugenics Society on 25 Jan., 1949:—

I hope to make those who will study and teach human genetics in the future aware of the immense complexity of the subject. The results of experimental animal genetics must be fully appreciated, yet great caution is required in their application to human problems. The human race resembles a wild population and is not a herd of domestic or laboratory animals. It has often astonished me that advocates of race improvement are so often unaware of the difficulties in the tasks which they set themselves. Eighty years ago it seemed reasonable to Galton, on the analogy with the breeding of dogs and horses, to expect to be able to produce a superior race of men in a few generations. But knowledge of medicine and of genetics has increased enormously since that time, and with it has grown the perception of our ignorance. To lay down any general rules for improvement of the human stock in the light of modern knowledge, however, is pretentious and absurd. It is my personal opinion, after much experience in research work, that active eugenical propaganda is, on the whole, inimical to the advance of scientific knowledge. It is premature and assumes that knowledge is a static and not a growing structure. Before attempting to improve on nature and defeat her at her own game, we must understand her methods very thoroughly.

Dr. Penrose has devised a highly ingenious theoretical population model in which the defectives with increased fertility are the backbone of the population. If an efficient sterilization programme were brought in against this submerged tenth, it would diminish the fertility of the group as a whole and eventually lead to its complete extermination. Now of course this might not necessarily apply to our human society, but it may well do, and it should give us food for thought before we discriminate against certain races and classes with insufficient knowledge. Hitler, of course, introduced sterilization for those of low intelligence and also for those who are usually endowed with an intelligence above the average, the Jewish race.

The father of eugenics, Galton, wrote the following words in 1904: 'Over-zeal leading to hasty action would do harm, by holding out expectations of a near golden age, which will certainly be falsified and cause the science to be discredited. The first and main point is to secure the general intellectual acceptance of eugenics as a hopeful and most important study. Then let its principles work into the heart of the nation, who will gradually give practical effect to them in ways that we may not wholly foresee.' These words are as true today as they were nearly sixty years ago. That is why the quoted statement of Dr. Julian Huxley is to be regretted. There is no evidence that the level of innate intelligence is falling, although on certain theoretical grounds we might at first sight expect this. A detailed analysis of the problem reveals that there are theoretical grounds for assuming that there is in fact an equilibrium, part of which is contributed to by the lower tenth; to discriminate against them *might* upset that equilibrium. In the words of Penrose: 'A nation with a social problem group is not necessarily silently rotting at the core; it might even be improving.' Moreover, there also arises the moral problem of what qualities are desirable and how much of each quality we should have. The ideal in some societies may be a small nucleus of intellectuals against a large background of fertile labourers. We are far too ignorant to be dogmatic in these matters. We should therefore tread warily and proceed by evolution rather than by revolution.

The difficulties and complexities in the field of practical eugenics, where even the experts disagree, are enormous. This subject provides another example of fools rushing in where angels fear to tread.

CHAPTER XIV

DEATH CONTROL

Human population is probably the gravest problem of our time—certainly more serious in the long perspective than war or peace.—JULIAN HUXLEY

EACH country has its own particular population problem; let us begin with a study of the population of England and Wales.

During the Middle Ages the size of the population often fluctuated widely; for example, when there was large-scale famine and pestilence in the land, the population fell, but at other times when there was prosperity it rose. It has been estimated, for example, that one-sixth of the people of England were killed by plague in the year 1664–5. It is probable, however, that the population had never risen above 7,000,000 before 1760. Between 1768 and 1820, during the Industrial Revolution, there was a rapid growth of the population from about 7,000,000 to 14,000,000. During the nineteenth century this rapid growth continued and the 9,000,000 of 1801 had become 32,500,000 by 1901. The rate of increase, however, has slowed down considerably during the twentieth century. This remarkable increase was accounted for by the large excess of births over deaths. The reasons for these changes are dependent upon the changes in the social and economic life of the community. In the early nineteenth century there was a very high birth-rate and large families were the rule. Indeed, in the early days of the Industrial Revolution the large family was an asset in that children working in the factories and mines could augment the family income. However, with the passing of the Factory Acts, the growth of humanitarianism, and the higher standards of living, large families became less common. In the words of Crew (1948): 'In the first half of the nineteenth century the masses accepted poverty as a natural concomitant of their lowly station, in the second half they realized it was man and not God who was responsible for poverty.' They learned that thrift and the control of the size of the family were ways of improving this lowly station. This limitation in the size of the family was further stimulated by the growth of competitive individualism. Undoubtedly it first became apparent in the higher-income groups who wished to give their children a better start in life. At the same time there was a decline in the traditional religious beliefs and the importance of the family circle. The cult of the small family which had begun in the higher-income groups soon spread to the thriftier members of the lower-income groups.

Whilst the birth-rate was falling, the death-rate was also falling due to improvements in public health. This was particularly so with infant and child mortality, and was due to the control of the epidemic diseases. Despite the dramatic fall in both the death-rates and birth-rates, the birth-rate still remained higher than the death-rate and the population continued to increase. The expectancy of life has increased during the last hundred years and particularly in the young, but in the very old it has changed very little. Preventive and curative medicine have enabled many people who formerly would have died at an earlier age to live longer. The population is growing, chiefly by increasing the expectation of life in the younger age-groups and keeping more people alive longer. It is a process which has been associated with urbanization and industrialization.

AGE AND SEX COMPOSITION OF THE POPULATION

The increased expectation of life and the reduced birth-rate have resulted in fundamental changes in the structure of the population which are of great social and medical importance. The falling birth-rate has meant that there are relatively fewer children in the population, but the increasing expectation of life has meant increases in numbers in the older age-groups, because many children born in an era when the birth-rate was high are now surviving to old age. In other words, the average age of the population of England and Wales is increasing. At the present moment about 12 per cent of the population is aged 65 and over; in 1900 this figure was less than 5 per cent. Similar trends have occurred in the rest of Western Europe, in North America, Australia, and New Zealand. In parts of Africa and Asia only 2–3 per cent of the population is aged 65 and over.

The sex composition of the population is determined by two things, the sex ratio at birth and differences between the male and female mortality-rates in the different age-groups. There have been several theories propounded about the cause of the particular sex produced, and a number of laymen have proclaimed that they know the secrets of sex determination and are, of course, much sought after. Since the chances of boy or girl are roughly 50 : 50, any theory will be correct half the time and the failures can be put down to not carrying out instructions correctly. Science has found no evidence in favour of any known theory. The sex ratio at birth is in favour of males and in 1948 it was 1061 males to every 1000 females. It is interesting to note that the male over female ratio increased after the two world wars. The mechanism of this increase in male births following a period of excessive male mortality is difficult to explain. The male death-rates, however, are greater than the female death-rates in all age-groups. The ratio of male to female mortality in 1948 was, for example, 1·4. The sex ratio gradually falls until in the age-group 15–19 years the number of males and females in the population is about equal. With the increased mortality in males the ratio begins to be in favour of females until over the age of 85 there are approximately twice as many females as males. This increasing preponderance of females in the older population has an important bearing on the provision of medical services in the older age-groups. Women marry at an earlier age than men and there are more widows than widowers.

216

FUTURE TRENDS OF THE POPULATION

The future trends of the population will depend largely on the future trend of national fertility. It is probable that the death-rate will fall slightly, but no great improvement is to be expected. If fertility remains unaltered the total numbers will continue to grow slowly. If fertility falls we shall soon reach a peak in the population and the total numbers will begin to fall. If fertility increases, the population will continue to increase. Undoubtedly in the next thirty years there will be a steady growth in the percentage of old people in the population. This increase is almost inevitable because of the large percentage of people in the middle age-groups, and any fall in the death-rate will only aggravate the situation. The social and economic well-being of the country depends to a large extent on the age and sex structure of the population. For this reason and because of the marked changes in the composition of the population which have taken place in recent years, a Royal Commission on Population was appointed in 1944 to investigate the problem and in 1949 issued its Report. Its terms of reference were as follows: 'To examine the facts relating to the present population trends in Great Britain; to investigate the causes of these trends and to consider their probable consequences; to consider what measure, if any, should be taken in the national interest to influence the future trends in population; and to make recommendations.'

This report considered that the falling population was largely due to lowered fertility following the increasing use of birth control. The investigation showed that there was on the average a decrease in intelligence with increasing size of family, and that those of lower intelligence tended to have larger families, whereas the higher-income groups with a higher level of intelligence tended to have the small families. This differential fertility may lead in the future to a lowering of the level of intelligence, as it has been shown that intelligence is partly inherited. For a more detailed discussion of this see Chapter XIII. The Royal Commission on Population concluded that the population of working age is likely to remain constant, whereas the number of young people will decline and the number of old people will increase. The population will probably go on growing slowly until about 1977 and then decline.

The question whether an increase or a decrease is desirable is very debatable, and depends upon strategic, economic, social, medical, and psychological factors. The danger of a rapidly growing population is that the amount of land and resources per head falls as the population increases; on the other hand, it tends to increase the nation's economic power and produces a young and virile nation. A falling population affects the vitality of a nation and tends to lower national prestige, particularly as the population is an ageing one. The average number of children per family is at present 2·2, which is 6 per cent below replacement level. The average family size is not capable of rapid alterations as it is due to long-term habits which cannot be changed quickly. The Royal Commission on Population concluded that a replacement size of family was desirable at the present time. In order to bring this about it recommended that efforts should be made to encourage somewhat larger families by reducing the financial burden to young married couples and to promote family welfare. This could be brought about in the following ways: The increasing of family allowances; free grants to parents and greater income-tax rebates for children; provision of more family services, such as home helps, day nurseries, nursery schools, residential nurseries, child minders; better provision for mothers in the form of assisted family holidays, washing and laundry services, children's playgrounds, mobile house cleaning units, and the provision of household appliances on hire, such as vacuum cleaners, refrigerators, washing machines, prams, cookers, and furniture. Some of these services might well be provided by local authorities.

The Commission recommended also that increasing attention should be paid to the maternity and child welfare services and the various problems associated with them. The present housing programme does not meet the urgent need for larger families, and larger houses should be provided with more than three bedrooms to cater for the larger family.

The Commission finally recommended that there should be increasing attention paid to research into the various problems of fertility and population, and particularly into the social, economic, medical, and psychological factors concerned.

BIRTH CONTROL

People all over the world have been alarmed by too rapid rises in the population which have threatened food supplies; primitive peoples have usually met the situation by infanticide, but probably the first scientific treatment of the subject was by Malthus, who wrote his *Essay on the Principle of Population* in 1798 and recommended late marriage and moral restraint as a means of controlling the population. Francis Place published his *Illustrations and Proofs of the Principle of Population* in 1822 and advocated contraceptive measures. His book made little impression on the prim Victorians. In 1876, however, a Bristol bookseller altered the course of history. He was sentenced to two years' hard labour for offering for sale what was considered in those days to be obscene literature; in this case it was a small pamphlet entitled *The Fruits of Philosophy or the Private Companion of Young Married People*. It was really a treatise on birth control, one of the first, in fact, in this country. It could hardly be called a best seller, and was evidently little known before the court case, selling about 700 copies a year. Charles Bradlaugh and Mrs. Annie Besant, however, shocked Victorian morality by taking up the cudgels in defence of the Bristol bookseller and republished the book and informed the police. Their trial and appeal attracted enormous publicity. Overnight the book became a best seller, the sales jumping to 120,000 a year. This was the beginning of a widespread interest in birth control and from 1880 the birth-rate fell steadily. In those days it was 34 births per 1000 of the population; today it has fallen to 15. There have been two periods when it has risen, but only temporarily after each of the two world wars, due to the return of the conquering heroes.

Between the two world wars there was widespread unemployment in Britain and a feeling developed that the country was over-populated. Dr. Marie Stopes in her books probably did more than anyone to transform the sex habits of a nation. Her work is now carried on by the Family Planning Association. Just before the Second World War fear of depopulation became common in Britain and Sweden, particularly in view of the expansionist policies of Hitler and Mussolini. France, of all Western countries, is in a unique position because her fertility fell much sooner than anywhere else. In view of the upsurgence of Germany she is now pursuing an expansionist policy for her ageing population. The sale of birth control appliances is illegal and abortion is heavily punished. At the same time family allowances have been increased and child welfare services developed. Similar trends have occurred in other highly developed countries, although in North America and Australia there have been recent marked increases in birth-rates; this, together with a high rate of immigration and very low death-rates, has resulted in rates of increase higher than anywhere else in the world.

The idea that conceptions should be regulated in the interests of the mother, child, and community appears to be acceptable to six of the chief religions of the world, Buddhism, Hinduism, Mohammedanism, Confucianism, Judaism, and Christianity. The Roman Catholic Church, however, condemns the use of appliances and recommends that birth control should be by abstinence and the exercise of self control; coitus interruptus is known as the sin of Onan and is condemned by the Roman Catholic Church. Despite this it is still the most commonly used method, probably because it doesn't cost any money; it also avoids the embarrassment of shopping. It is a method, however, which is harmful psychologically. Pope John XXIII commented on the need for birth control and the use of the rhythm method; unfortunately it is not always reliable. Various efforts have been made to provide an effective method using a drug which may be taken orally, but although several drugs have been suggested it is only recently that oral contraceptives have become available which appear to be reliable.

Navajo Indian women in Mexico have for generations caused sterility by taking orally an infusion of the desert plant *Lithospermum ruderale*; attempts are being made to isolate the active principle. Drugs of the nitrofuran group will inhibit male fertility, but unfortunately in doses which are effective they produce nausea and vomiting. In any case, a drug which has to be taken morning and night is hardly likely to be taken entirely reliably over long periods of time. Sterilization can be performed safely and quickly by a very simple operation in the male, although to many males such a procedure would be repugnant. It can also be performed fairly easily in females.

Turning to the Eastern countries, the position is similar to what it was one hundred years ago in this country. There is a high birth-rate with low standards of living for many, and the death-rate is beginning to fall, at a greater rate, however, than it did in the West, because those countries have all the knowledge for the prevention of disease which it took the West two hundred years to acquire. Public health has come in a big way to India and

China, removing many causes of death which formerly kept the population in control. In Ceylon, for example, malaria has been wiped out by the use of DDT and in seven years the death-rate has fallen from 22 to 12 per 1000; this fall took seventy years in England and Wales. There is widespread control of death, but as yet, little control of birth. Each day the population of the world is increasing by 88,000 and each year by 34,000,000. In 1955 the world population was, at a conservative estimate, more than 2,600,000,000; within fifty years, if it increases at the same rate, the population will be doubled. Imagine the problem of feeding, clothing, and housing another 2,600,000,000 people in the next fifty years. That is probably the most important problem facing the world today and it is likely to have a greater effect upon health than any other factor. Malthus in the eighteenth century first propounded the theory that population begets population and increases in geometrical progression, but the food resources can only increase in arithmetical progression, so that eventually the population of the world will outstrip the food resources.

It looks as though public health can now make this possible, and we have already seen evidence of this in India where in recent years there have been serious famines, and we have witnessed the appalling spectacle of people lying down to die from starvation in the streets of Calcutta, whilst in other parts of the world there has been a superabundance of food.

The Food and Agricultural Organization (F.A.O.) of the United Nations is very much concerned with this problem of feeding the masses. Probably three-quarters of the people of the world are already on diets inadequate for optimum health, and an increase of one-quarter in the world's food resources would only raise the average diet of the present population to an adequate diet. In the next fifty years, then, we must more than double the food resources of the world. In 1954 estimates by the F.A.O. indicated that whereas the population of the world is increasing by 1·5 per cent per annum, the food resources are only increasing by 1 per cent, but in the East, food resources are only increasing by 0·04 per cent per annum. In 1956 Mr. Dag Hammarskjoeld reported a much improved situation; the food resources were increasing by 2½ per cent; only in Latin America were the food resources lagging behind the population growth. Increases in the future will depend mainly on increasing effort and on the availability of modern equipment and techniques. Experts in various branches are needed badly, in addition to irrigation schemes for water, tractors, fertilizers, insecticides, and seed in large quantities. One of the greatest drawbacks to agricultural productivity in the past has been the lethargy, lack of energy, and apathy of the inhabitants of many of the backward countries, due largely to the effects of disease, such as malaria, yaws, syphilis, and so on. Yaws is a case in point, for it causes severe ulcers on the palms of the hands and the soles of the feet so that the sufferer cannot till the soil, whilst the person with malaria knows quite well that a period of hard work will result in an unpleasant bout of fever. The alleviation of many of these conditions has created a great demand for land and the old lethargy is disappearing. As a result the price of land is rising.

In some parts of Afghanistan the value has increased twentyfold and the income of many families is rising at the same time. Although public health has produced the problems, it is possibly contributing towards their solution.

We in England should not delude ourselves into thinking that the problem is one which we can ignore; quite apart from the humanitarian aspect, it must affect our food supplies. We have to import more than 50 per cent of our food from other countries, and there is little chance of our altering that figure by traditional methods of food production, yet we have to compete in the food markets of the world with the ever-increasing demands of those countries like India and China where the population is increasing rapidly; and let us not forget that, as in prehistoric days, food is still the most important thing for health and happiness.

The production of many of the raw materials of industry, of which cotton is a typical example, is in direct competition with the use of land for food; for as standards of living increase everywhere there are also other increasing demands on the use of land.

One thing is certain: unless birth-rates are quickly reduced, there will be a growth of world population on a vaster scale than anything which has ever been seen before. Of course, Nature usually finds the answer; widespread starvation could very soon occur on a wider scale than ever before, and it may be that the atomic bomb would certainly be more effective in destroying people than past wars have been. The total European losses in World War II were put at about 15,000,000. This was made good in less than six months.

The importance of the control of population has long been recognized by primitive island communities. The isolated island of Tikopia in the Pacific Ocean is an example; because of its isolation it is of fundamental importance to adjust the population to the limited food available. The policy is laid down by the chieftain and heads of families who decree whether young men can marry, conception is prevented by coitus interruptus, and the father of a newly born child smothers it at birth if food supplies are short. Sometimes despite these measures there have been too many mouths to feed. On two occasions a section of the population has been forcibly driven from the island, i.e., forced migration. It would appear that Tikopia has solved its population difficulties successfully. In some of the Pacific islands, however, there are problems of under-population, caused largely by the common practice of abortion which renders females sterile, so that in later life when they want babies they are unable to have them.

Barbados and Mauritius are examples of islands which have not solved their difficulties; they are densely populated and overcrowded. In 1954 the Government of Barbados made the following statement: 'The first objective of the health programme should be the development of means whereby the birth rate is reduced as rapidly as modern science and services have reduced the death rate.'

In recent years financial help has been available for a number of under-developed countries, often with tragic results. Puerto Rico is a case in point. For the last forty years the U.S.A. has poured money into the island for health services to try to increase the standard of living, with the result that the population has doubled. But there has been little increase in the standard of living and the agricultural resources of the island are now insufficient for its needs. Its people have only been saved from starvation by the importation of food.

Egypt and Java have similar difficulties, the latter being the most densely populated island in the world with over 1000 people to the square mile. India and Japan are two Eastern countries which are endeavouring to do something about the problem. Japan has now made abortion and sterilization legal, and this has already had a marked effect on the population problem. Dr. Yoshio Koya, Director of the Institute of Public Health, Tokyo, stated in 1953 that there were then well over 1,000,000 abortions a year. Infanticide has been practised for over a hundred years, but today birth control is the official policy recommended. India is in a special position; her standards of living are much lower than those of Britain even two hundred years ago, but she has at her command all the accumulated knowledge of those two hundred years and the population of 400,000,000 is now increasing by 5,000,000–8,000,000 per annum. The Indian Government has realized this and in its second five-year plan has made proposals for definite action in limiting the growth of population. It has allocated 50,000,000 rupees for family planning schemes.

China is the most interesting of all; her 1953 census revealed a population of 602,000,000, a quarter of the world's total. The Census Commissioner, Mr. Pai Chien-hua, said in 1955 that the growth of agricultural production far exceeds the growth of population and he looks forward to the time when the population will be 800,000,000. The task for China is enormous, requiring the support of 15,000,000 extra people each year. By 1957 even this view had changed. On 7 March, Madame Li Teh-Chuan, the Minister of Health, announced in Peking that abortion and sterilization were to be made legal in China. She said that strenuous efforts had been made to popularize birth control methods but this work was far from enough. It will be interesting to see how China fares compared with India.

The U.S.S.R., at the World Population Conference in 1954, said that she had no population problems because of the application of the theories of Karl Marx. She was pursuing an expansionist policy. In January, 1955, Mr. Khrushchev said: 'The more people we have the stronger will our country become; if we added 100,000,000 to our 200,000,000 inhabitants it would still be too few.' Contrast this with a recent remark made by Mr. Nehru: 'We should be a far more advanced nation if our population were about half what it is.'

Eire is the solitary example of a country whose population has declined from a high emigration rate which has continued since the disastrous famine of 1845, which was itself due to overpopulation.

It would appear that there were two opposing views. The Communist one was that expansion of populations is a good thing, at any rate in countries which are still underdeveloped, and that the proper organization of the economic resources of a country will see that sufficient food is produced. This view appears to have been held by Russia (though recent reports indicate that she is also beginning to change her views to come into line with the rest of the world) and until recently by China, who have populations of 800,000,000 between them. On the other hand, India and Japan hold the view of Malthus that the populations of their countries are too large for the available food resources. They are taking active steps to reduce the birth-rate. It is obvious that what is good for one country is not necessarily good for another. In contrast to the young, quick-growing population of Asia, the Western countries have populations which are growing slowly but which are ageing rapidly. In order to counteract this trend France is pursuing a policy aimed at drastically increasing the birth-rate.

Apart from the question of a population policy we should not forget that family planning is based on the healthy notion that child-spacing is an indispensable part of individual preventive medicine and is necessary for a healthy and harmonious family life. This fact has been acknowledged by the Roman Catholic Church. In 1956 the International Catholic Institute for Social Research in Geneva announced a prize of $5000 for the best essay which would answer the population problem within the requirements of Catholic principles. All over the world there is a climate of opinion favourable to the idea of family planning, but there are still great stumbling-blocks to a widespread acceptance of the idea. The greatest of these are lack of understanding of the problem by the majority of people and apathy. Teachers and obstetricians are generally still not aware of the urgency of the problem. There is still a taboo on discussion of sex matters even in medical circles. One of the greatest advances in the teaching field has occurred in North America where, in 1956, 50 professors of obstetrics distributed to their medical students over 7000 copies of Dickinson's *Techniques of Conception Control*.

One thing is abundantly clear; the development of the food resources of the world is the most important requirement for future health, welfare, and happiness. Perhaps sooner than we realize we shall begin to witness the evil effects of too rapid overpopulation, brought about by cramming into a few years all the accumulated knowledge of two hundred years. The world has applied death control without taking into consideration the enormous poser of human fertility; this has resulted in what we might call 'an explosion of people'. This force, in my opinion, is likely to be more dangerous even than the atom bomb, because it is, as far as our experience goes, to a considerable extent uncontrollable, and therein lies the danger!

Attempts to bring birth control measures to primitive communities have in the past never been wholly successful because due consideration has not been given to the cultural, social, and religious attitudes of the people themselves.

A most important field study into motivation for family planning is being carried out in a village near Ludhiana in the Punjab, India. This is being conducted by Dr. John Wyon and is a project-cum-action survey sponsored by the Government of India and the Department of Epidemiology of Harvard University, under the supervision of Dr. John Gordon. This study is providing most useful data on the fundamental attitudes and feelings of village people to family planning.

The origin of these fundamental difficulties can be pinpointed by a quotation from Sir William Osler: 'Natural man has but two primal passions—to get his sustenance and to beget his kind.'

SICK SOCIETY

Between the two world wars British medicine was more concerned with the problems of the younger age-groups than with those of the elderly. Since the end of the Second World War a remarkable change has taken place. The infant death-rate has fallen to extremely low levels, lower than many people twenty years ago would ever have thought possible. The late Lord Horder has referred to these changes in the following words: 'The problem of the care of the elderly person becomes not only more and more topical, it is of increasing urgency. Whether in sickness or in health, the problem is formidable.' This sense of urgency has been expressed even more forcibly by Bernard Baruch, who, when asked to comment on the most significant events which had occurred in the first half of the present century, replied that he considered the increase of the life span to have had more profound medical, economic, and social implications than such discoveries as atomic energy and air transport. We have seen in our lifetime a virtual elimination of many of the physical hazards of existence, and we have better housing, improved nutrition, and healthy working conditions, but in their place we have become also conscious of the ever-increasing importance of mental ill health and to realize that here is a great field for prevention. The majority of the complaints with which the general practitioner has to deal have a psychological basis; they include such things as indigestion, headaches, muscle pains, irritability, and mental tension, quite apart from the so-called psychosomatic disorders, such as gastritis, peptic ulcer, high blood-pressure, asthma, disordered action of the heart or effort syndrome, anxiety states, and hysteria. We can speak today of our sick society, of the increase in juvenile delinquency, of sex crimes and perversions, of alcoholism, suicide, and broken families. All these are a product of the way of life in the Western world, problems which are on the increase. Margaret Mead (1954a,b) has studied the way of life of several primitive tribes and has shown that mental ill health as we know it in the West is almost unknown in Samoa and New Guinea. During the last century Western man has become more and more deprived of those basic emotional satisfactions which are necessary for normal mental development. Let us consider for a moment what these are. First of all, adequate mothering is necessary; the infant not only has certain physical needs such as food and warmth, but also requires love, affection, and security. We are only just beginning to realize, in fact, that lack of this maternal love and affection can have far-reaching results, producing physical, intellectual, emotional, and social defects. The infant or child who does not himself receive real love and affection is incapable

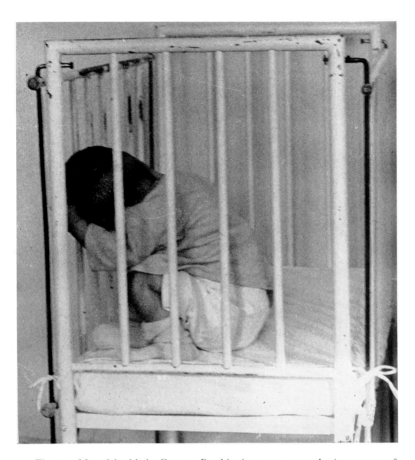

Fig. 42.—Mental health in Greece. Psychiatrists agree upon the importance of mother love and care for a young baby. Such love and care, they insist, soon create affectionate ties between mother and child—ties which are essential to its normal physical and mental development. But where a child for one reason or another is deprived of this mother love and care, especially where, abandoned or orphaned, he is placed in an institution and has no one person to care for him in a personal and loving way, a child is considered to be suffering from 'maternal deprivation'. The effects of this are most noticeable and most disastrous where children of under 12 months are concerned. The effect on children of 6–12 months is one of depression similar to that observed among adult patients in mental hospitals. The child retires from those around him, his activities are retarded. He will stay, completely immobile, for hours at a time, sitting up or lying down in an attitude of complete listlessness. Insomnia is frequent and invariably there is a lack of appetite. Loss of weight is inevitable, together with high susceptibility to any and every infection.

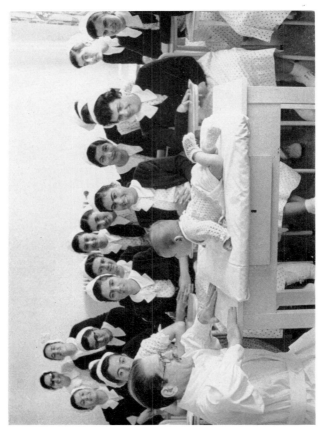

Fig. 43.—There can be no substitute for real mother love, but a solution to the tragedy of the unloved child—orphaned or abandoned—is to provide a mother-substitute and a way of living as near as possible to normal family life. Such is the aim of the Metera ('mother' in Greek) Babies Centre in Athens. This home for abandoned children was opened recently with international help. It has two aims: to provide temporary mother-substitute love and care with the help of specially trained 'mother nurses', and to locate permanent foster homes. The Director of the Metera Children's Home, Dr. Doxiadis, explains to some student nurses what it means to be a 'mother nurse'. He is assisted by an 18-month-old inmate of the home.

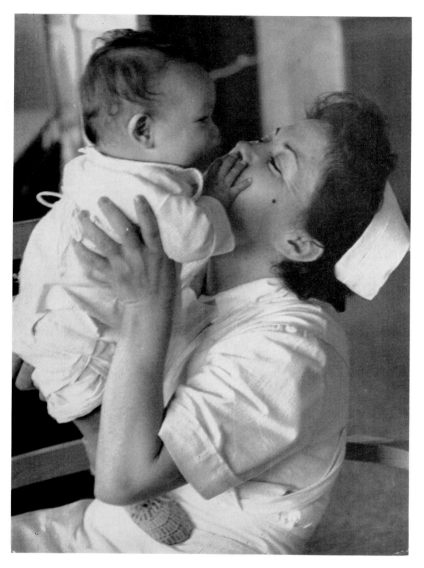

Fig. 44.—Each 'mother-nurse' cares for a maximum of four children. She not only takes care of their material needs, but also gives them a tenderness and love they need so badly.

of giving love or of feeling affection and grows up callous and indifferent to the feelings of others. This produces the delinquent, the problem family, and eventually the criminal.

A study of the deprivation of mother love and its effects has been made recently by Bowlby (1951) on behalf of the World Health Organization, because of the large number of homeless children resulting from the war. All wars produce homelessness and large numbers of children deprived of mother love and affection; probably none has been so serious in its effects as World War II. The physical damage was terrible enough but there is every possibility that the mental ill health produced will far outweigh this in importance, nor shall we see the end-results until the present generation of children has reached adult age.

Unfortunately, we know of no really effective treatment. As in other diseases, control is dependent upon striking at the root of the trouble.

In the first few months of life the child needs close body contact with its mother; the baby should be held firmly, fondled, rocked, and talked to. Adequate sucking at the breast is terribly important apart from the physical value of breast milk. This primitive instinct is the first action of a newly born animal—the need to continue the close physical relationship with the mother. In some primitive tribes, breast-feeding continues for as long as two years. In Western communities, breast-feeding has become less frequent and often only lasts a few months. The importance of all this has been illustrated in the following animal experiment. One-half of a litter of puppies was brought up from birth on the bottle and the rest of the litter, the control group, was allowed to suckle normally. Those reared from the bottle showed very definite differences in character, such as restlessness and viciousness.

Later on, the warmth of motherly love stimulates and enriches the emotional life of the child, when it begins to walk and talk and when regular habit formation begins. There is a marked difference in the extent to which the growing infant receives this attention in the different social classes.

In Aberdeen, for example, 60 per cent of the wives of professional and business men (Registrar-General's Class I and II) are breast-feeding at three months compared with 20 per cent in the wives of semi-skilled and unskilled workers (Registrar-General's Class IV and V). The standards of maternal care and attention which are so important for proper habit formation also vary with social class; for example, 72 per cent of infants belonging to well-to-do mothers are 'potting' regularly at the end of the first month and only 28 per cent in the poorer-class mothers. All this is reflected in a higher infant and foetal death-rate in the poorer classes, not only because of poorer standards of parental care, but also because of overcrowding, bad housing, increased risk of faulty nutrition, and so on. The mothers also have poorer physique, lower intelligence, less education, lower incomes, and more frequent pregnancies. The infant mortality-rates and stillbirth-rates are particularly high in coal-miners compared with clerks, for example, despite the fact that miners now get much larger wages; another reason for the abolition of the task of coal-mining! (*See* Morris, 1955.)

Those of us who have seen the care and attention which some African natives bestow on their offspring cannot help but compare the lack of affection seen in some white mothers, not only those living in the slums, but quite often in the houses of the wealthy, where the nannie is brought in to try and replace the love and affection of the natural mother.

Bowlby studied children brought up in institutions and those adults who developed mental illness and produced abundant evidence of this thesis. In other words, mother love is just as necessary as suitable food for normal growth and development. (*Fig. 42.*) If the child is deprived of the latter he will develop physical defects; if deprived of the former, he will develop defects in mental health; these will show themselves by abnormal behaviour, such as emotional instability, cruelty to animals or children, persistent truancy from school, and later by such things as stealing or lying, which may bring him to the juvenile court as a delinquent. Unfortunately, the delinquent makes a bad parent and tends to reproduce the conditions in the next generation; thus a vicious circle is set up, ever-increasing in its circumference. The truth of the phrase 'there is no place like home' is more important today than ever. Bad homes are nearly always better than good institutions; that is a sentiment which may shock many of our well-meaning councillors who can view with pride the clean clothes and good physical condition of the long line of children from the cottage homes. They do not always realize that the adverse physical environment from which they have been 'rescued' is nothing like so dangerous as the emotional vacuum into which they have been forced.

Under what conditions does maternal deprivation arise ? First of all, unwanted pregnancies, not only in unmarried mothers, but in those who have been made into honest women by marriage. Again there are social class distinctions; in Aberdeen, 15 per cent of first pregnancies were conceived pre-nuptially in the 'well-to-do', but it was as high as 37 per cent in the poorer classes. This means that there must be a considerable number of unwanted babies; how many it is difficult to say. At any rate, some mothers have a subconscious hatred of their firstborn which has stopped a life of gaiety and freedom and they are quite likely to take it out of the child, particularly if they are unstable and lacking in emotional maturity and the capacity for love and affection. Such occasions are likely to be more common in wartime, with quick romantic courtships and the anticlimax of prolonged separations.

Hospital life also tends to produce the same ill effects as life in institutions. In African, Indian, and Lapp societies mothers go to hospital with their babies and sleep by their cots. Until recently children's hospitals in the Western world only allowed occasional visiting.

How then are we to utilize this all-important knowledge ? One of the greatest needs at the present moment is the thorough inculcation of these ideas into all potential mothers and all those connected with the care of children. It is important to realize that there can be adequate substitutes for the real mother and that satisfactory adoption is the best solution; a good foster parent may also be a reasonable solution, but committing a child to life in an institution is a serious social crime. Dickens knew the dangers of life in institutions and was well aware of its evil effects. (*Figs.* 43, 44.)

The present problem for mental health is similar to that which faced public health a hundred years ago. The cause of physical ill health was known but prejudice and the attitude of *laissez-faire* prevailed; it needed a Benjamin Disraeli to break down the conservatism of people, which, in the words of *The Times*, 'would rather take the risk of cholera and the rest . . . than be bullied into health'.

Today we know an important way of tackling mental ill health, but there are strong forces of prejudice at work; members of committees find more satisfaction in seeing a docile crocodile of well-cared-for children wending their way back to the cottage homes than in those grubby children of Mrs. A. playing football in Paradise Row.

The education of those responsible for child care is not, of course, the only need in our mental health programme. The education for adolescence, marriage, and motherhood is just as important. The Eskimo child learns about sex at a very early age and in other primitive tribes it is a common feature of the way of life for young children to witness the sexual act. The initiation into manhood and womanhood is an important part of the preparation for adult life in primitive communities.

Most Western children do not learn the facts of life until puberty approaches. In Victorian days the servant girl played an important part in the sexual initiation of many children. Today, however, the earliest lessons may be learnt from the parents or more often at school from the older students. Sex is something to be talked about in whispers and in dark corners; smutty stories and dirty pictures provide an interesting background. Usually the information acquired is incorrect; some girls even today believe that contact with the male sex is dangerous and avoid men. Small wonder then that many girls grow up with a fear of sex and many boys marry with a supreme ignorance of what the sexual act means to the woman. Many marriages are irretrievably ruined on the first night of the honeymoon by ignorance and fear. Many wives are sexually frustrated and dubbed as 'cold'. It is disturbing to find that one-third of all women are inadequate in this respect. The fault, however, usually lies in the husband; indeed, Balzac in his *Physiologie du mariage* compared the average husband to an orang-utan trying to play the violin.

These relics of Victorian days are, alas, too often still prevalent amongst our genteel middle classes. Dickinson and Beam (1949) quote a typical case of a married woman whose mother told her: 'No good woman ever has pleasure; passion is for the vile . . . I'd be ashamed if I enjoyed it.' No doubt this extreme attitude is a good deal rarer in young people today than formerly, but any doctor knows what a common thing it has been in his middle-aged and elderly patients. Knowledge of the techniques of sexual intercourse required in marriage in Western cultures is not acquired automatically. It must be learnt either by experience or by informed education. Presumably the latter method is to be preferred. Unfortunately, in the majority of our successful marriages the former is the usual method.

Figures for premarital intercourse have risen over the last decades and Terman predicts that virginity at marriage will be close to vanishing point for boys born after 1930 and for girls born after 1940; he considers that premarital intercourse with the future spouse is now almost universal. It should be noted that he is referring to American society!

At any rate, we should at least try and see that parents-to-be should receive their education in some other way. Already in some schools the facts of life are taught in biology classes, but I doubt whether any school-teacher has yet had the nerve to teach the arts and techniques of coitus. In any case probably few have sufficient knowledge to give the information. Undoubtedly the best person to give such advice is a happily married wife with a large family of her own. Most people would prefer, I expect, to get their information from the sort of books that Dr. Marie Stopes has written and perhaps one day she will be acknowledged as one of the greatest benefactors of mankind.

Perhaps of even greater importance is the art of bringing up children. The health visitor has been the chief exponent of health education in this field, but only in those recently qualified has the training included the new ideas mentioned here. All mothers-to-be and health visitors should study the books by Gesell (1948) and by Illingworth (1957) on this subject.

Our hospital authorities should see to it that arrangements are made for mothers to accompany their children into hospital. The prejudices of hospital sisters who view these ideas with alarm must be brushed aside, and, of course, nurses should be trained in the correct handling of children.

At school, in industry, and in the armed forces mental hygiene is just as important as physical health, perhaps even more so, and whereas the latter is well cared for in all but a few special instances, there is very little in the way of positive effort to prevent mental ill health. Physical factors are obvious and can be readily appreciated, and have been and are being controlled; on the other hand, psychological factors are less easily understood and are becoming increasingly important as a cause of sickness absence and accidents in industry. Before the Industrial Revolution men were largely craftsmen employed in villages, working for themselves and seeing the fruits of their own labour. They had a pride in their work and could develop a sense of achievement. William Morris considered that the introduction of machinery into industry had taken away the sense of gratification and sense of achievement which was largely responsible for happiness in work. Today, the majority of people are employed in large-scale industries in which they perform a routine job, and in which they hardly ever see the final results of their labours. There is no feeling of gratification or sense of achievement, and as a result there is often a general feeling of frustration and lack of pride in work. The worker has lost the sense of independence engendered by the possession of his own tools and by the ability to himself produce the finished article. At the beginning of the Industrial Revolution, with the growth of the small workshop, there was still an immediate personal relationship, in which the owner-employer often spoke to his employees by name. With the large-scale organization in industry this happy state of affairs is often lost, but it can be replaced by something else—by loyalty and a sense of participation in a great enterprise.

Let us look for a moment at the reasons why people work; in other words, their incentives. First of all, they must work as a means of earning a livelihood; that has always been an important reason. Secondly, because of the feeling that they should work, that work is an essential part of the life of a human being, and the feeling of guilt if the individual is not performing a useful function in society. Thirdly, and this is a more fundamental and perhaps not such an obvious reason, people work as a means of self-expression and all work should, therefore, wherever possible be made intrinsically interesting. Fourthly, people work because it is socially attractive. Many people work because it is a means of meeting people and a means of social intercourse. This is especially so where the home life of the individual is solitary and lonely. In the war it was a strong incentive, particularly in young women, because of the companionship and company which they got from their association with others and it is a very strong incentive today in keeping older people at work. Unfortunately, during the last one hundred years, the economic motive has been the driving force behind work. If we are to get the best out of workers in industry we must try and develop the other incentives, incentives which are social rather than economic.

But in all events our industrialists cannot know too much about man management and human relationships. I think most of us are beginning to realize that manpower is the most expensive and precious commodity we have; it certainly needs looking after! The problems of mental ill health have largely been created by conditions of life in our cities. Can the new social age provide the answers which will enable us to prevent, rather than cure? I think the answer must be yes, if we will pursue a policy of universal health education with strength and determination and remember Metchnikoff's words that 'ignorance must be counted as the most immoral of acts'.

CHAPTER XV

WORLD HEALTH AND THE FUTURE

The secret of world health is to be found ultimately in the homes of the people

IN the beginnings of time when man first walked the land, personal health depended upon the ability of the individual and the law of the survival of the fittest. The basic need for existence was food, which could only be obtained by hard work, initiative, and valour. Time has not altered that fundamental concept, although paradoxically the emphasis has changed; whilst there are still many people in the world who are sick because of insufficient food, increasing numbers are ill because they are getting too much. Since early times many civilizations have fallen into ruins, destroyed initially by plague, typhus, malaria, and the rest.

The civilizations of the Western world have grown in power because they have learnt how to control these, the captains of the men of death. The history of that growth reveals time and time again that lessons learnt by bitter experience can easily be forgotten and disaster result. The prime lesson, to which many give voice but few follow, is that prevention is better than cure as far as community health is concerned. Whereas in this field the individual person can do much to help, his efforts are of little avail unless the community does a great deal. The State then has a responsibility in community health, and all its power and wealth depend upon a healthy people. The scientist has played a great part in these conquests, but his contributions would be useless unless there were some means of applying this knowledge to the common good. In the first place, laws were needed to enforce action against the evils of inertia and apathy. When trouble threatened, people were only too eager to do all in their power to remedy the immediate disaster, but as soon as the evil was past they lapsed back into lethargy and the attitude of *laissez-faire*.

To the common herd, sufficient unto the day was the evil thereof, and palliative medicine their creed, but men of vision realized that the rooting out of the cause was the only answer for future health. Fortunately in the twentieth century there have been and are men of this calibre in our law makers and administrators.

By the turn of the century the only important sanitary nuisance which was left unabated in Britain was air pollution, and, as we have seen, this sanitary evil is still as prevalent as ever it was. The problems of public health were tackled with vigour and determination by men of action, albeit also of tact. Similar problems now beset the underdeveloped countries, which need more than anything adequate finance to foster their schemes and a literate public to accept them. Prejudice and inertia are difficult to overcome when poverty, illiteracy, and ignorance are rife.

One of the greatest difficulties of stopping illness at its source is knowing how to weave the discoveries of medicine into the pattern of daily life. In order to do this it is necessary in the first place to have an intimate knowledge of the people in the community. Many public health programmes have failed for the very reason that the expert did not understand the ideas and modes of behaviour of the community for which he was responsible. The first step for successful health education is often re-education in attitudes, and in order to do this the health educator must himself be prepared to learn. We should remember the words of Dr. Samuel Darling: 'If you wish to control mosquitoes, you must learn to think like a mosquito.'

For these reasons, the World Health Organization has appointed social anthropologists to investigate ways and means of adapting public health programmes to the specialized activities of different communities. The State can do a great deal but no plan can ever be wholly successful unless the individual plays his part.

Future public health programmes will depend more and more upon routine health examinations and health education.

ROUTINE HEALTH EXAMINATIONS

The first routine health examination should be carried out during pregnancy in order to detect a whole host of conditions which affect not only the health of the mother but also the child to be born later. Infections during the first three months of pregnancy are particularly important, because even a quite trivial disease like German measles can cause serious defects in the developing infant such as deafness, blindness, heart disease, and mental defect. We have very little knowledge, however, of the long-term effects of such disorders. Early deviations from health can be detected by routine weighing, examination of the blood and urine, taking the blood-pressure, and by examination of the abdomen, which includes radiography. In infancy a similar routine is carried out at the well-baby clinic or infant welfare centre. In the school health service the work begun by the child welfare service is continued and routine health examinations are carried out, supported by all the special facilities required to cope with children who are blind, deaf, crippled, mentally defective, epileptic, diabetic, defective in speech, malnourished, and emotionally maladjusted.

On entering industry, it is the duty of the Appointed Factory Doctor to examine all juveniles once a year up to the age of 18 years and to advise on the proper placing of each child in a job suitable to his capacities. He must also examine at regular intervals men who are engaged in specially dangerous jobs, such as handling lead, chromium, or radioactive substances. Since World War II there have been extensions in the spread of health services to industry; the nationalized industries have all developed medical services to provide not only emergency treatment of injuries but also the routine examination of men and their fitness for certain jobs, and real attempts are made to fit disabled men into jobs best suited to their capacity. It is particularly important in road, rail, and air transport and in coal-mines, and in such jobs as crane driving, where a defect of vision or an undetected condition like diabetes could have a serious effect upon the health and safety of others. Many of the large private industries have followed the example of the nationalized industries—for example, the large motor manufacturers, the steel works, Lever Brothers, I.C.I., and Boots. Many smaller firms have followed suit, appointing local practitioners to act as advisers in a part-time capacity. Some firms have gone further and realize that the employment of the elderly will be an ever-increasing problem in industry, and have made special arrangements for the routine health check-up of their older workers. An interesting development for small firms is the scheme run on the Slough Trading Estate, where over 140 firms, employing some 17,000 workers, have combined together to provide a comprehensive industrial medical service for their workers. The Disabled Persons Employment Act of 1944 did the same sort of thing for persons permanently disabled, realizing that they were at a disadvantage when competing with fit workers. An orthopaedic surgeon, Sir Reginald Watson-Jones, described it as the most important social reform of our time.

In America and Britain there are several schemes afoot for the early detection of degenerative disease in older persons by routine health examinations and by health education. The following is an extract from a recent Annual Report of the Chief Medical Officer of the Ministry of Health for England and Wales:—

> The Minister is advised that earlier diagnosis and prompt treatment of most cancers improve the chances of cure and survival, and the object of any such scheme would be to explore the question whether a wider knowledge among the public of the early signs or symptoms of certain cancers, especially those in accessible sites, would lead to a gradual increase in the number of patients presenting themselves to their family doctors as soon as possible after noticing such signs.
>
> Accordingly he invites local health authorities to consider what action in their area can practically be taken under the powers provided in the Public Health and National Health Service Acts.

The armed forces are using to an ever-increasing extent various methods of examination which will fit the individual into the right job. The civilian health services are lagging behind in this matter because most politicians seem to be unaware of this changing emphasis. But for them, Britain could have had a medical service today which might have been called with truth a 'health service'. Unfortunately, it has become more and more an 'ill health service', with the whole emphasis placed on the hospital and all that surrounds it, drugs, super specialists, and increasing costs. Some voices were raised meekly in protest when the Bill was under discussion. Mr. A. W. J. Greenwood said in a maiden speech in Parliament:—

> I wish the Bill had been a more positive health Bill than it is at the present time. It seems to concentrate not on the promotion of health, and not even on the prevention of disease, but upon the cure of disease when it has developed. It is an unfortunate

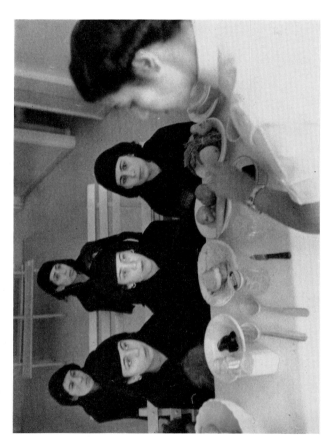

Fig. 45.—Health education for mothers. Bad feeding in the early years may rob a child of its rightful heritage of health and strength. An important part of the work of Maternal and Child Health Centres established in many countries with the assistance of W.H.O. and U.N.I.C.E.F. is to teach mothers how to plan a correct diet for their children and for themselves during pregnancy and weaning. This picture was taken at the Maternal and Child Health Centre at Damascus, Syria, where Moslem mothers attend a demonstration on how to make the best use of inexpensive foods.

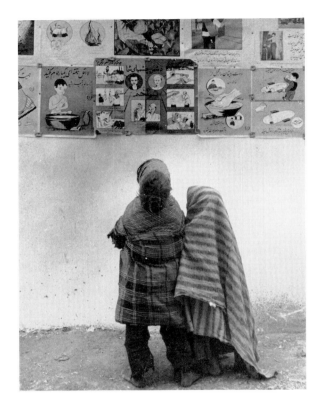

Fig. 46.—Iran. Health education in the control of insect-borne diseases. Two children study health education posters issued by the Iranian Ministry of Health, which have been put up on the village's one white-washed wall.

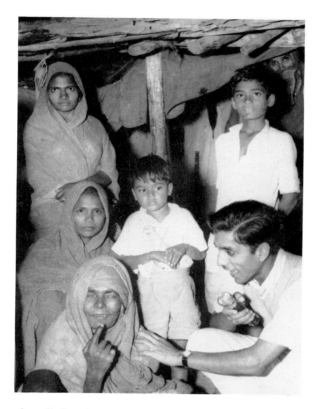

Fig. 47.—A medical student examines a blind woman as part of Nagpur Medical College rural teaching practice.

fact that very few people in this country, or perhaps in any other country, realise that they are ill until fairly late in the course of their disorder. . . . I am sure that in due course we shall be forced to the conclusion that periodic health overhauls are essential to the health and wellbeing of the people of this country.

HEALTH EDUCATION

This will be in the future our most important weapon in the prevention of disease and the maintenance of health. As we have already seen, many of the diseases of the world can be tackled and prevented by attention to personal habits; as public health solves the problem of the adverse environment so does personal health become more and more important. Now that the State has done so much, the efforts of the individual can bear fruit abundantly.

Health education starts in infancy when the mother teaches her offspring clean habits and it continues through childhood, with the school gradually taking over this function. Unfortunately, the standard of intelligence and of knowledge varies enormously in the different countries of the world, but in most countries there are skilled workers available to help. In the U.S.A. and working with W.H.O. there are trained health educators, but so far little has been done in Europe to train professional advisers in health education. (*Figs.* 45, 46.) The health visitor, or public health nurse, as she is called in the U.S.A., is a nurse specially trained to teach and to give instruction in health matters in the home. Her original purpose was to advise on the health of infants in an attempt to combat the enormous infant mortality. That campaign has achieved remarkable success; the infant mortality-rates have fallen from 150 per 1000 at the beginning of the century to the new low level of 25 per 1000 in 1955. Her chief difficulties today are dealing with the problems of the elderly. Unfortunately there are nothing like sufficient of these valuable people to go round. As in all branches of nursing, there is a grave shortage even in Britain.

Education for parenthood and for marriage is enormously important and should be part and parcel of education for citizenship and all that it entails. These subjects are just as important as reading, writing, and arithmetic.

In Great Britain there is an important organization concerned with health education; this is the Central Council for Health Education. In the international field there was created in 1951 the International Union for Health Education of the Public, whilst much of the work of W.H.O., F.A.O., and U.N.E.S.C.O. is concerned with this subject. In January, 1958, the *International Journal of Health Education* was launched. It fills a very real need and will help to develop the principles of this doctrine throughout the world.

Health education should be continued in universities, technical colleges, and in industry itself. In fact, one of the main functions of the Student Health Service is to give personal advice on health, whilst in many apprenticeship schemes, instruction in health forms an important part of the curriculum.

Much has been said of counselling the older worker on how best he can utilize his abilities, but this advice must take into account the state of his physical and mental health. Preventive geriatrics should begin in middle age or even earlier.

Perhaps the job in which health education matters most of all is that of being a soldier. In the Army there is a directorate of Army Health which is really concerned with health, unlike our Ministry of Health which seems to concern itself mostly with disease. All that has been said about prevention applies with added force in the services. It is gratifying to know that in the British Army the greatest attention is paid to prevention; as a result, this policy paid handsome dividends in the last war, resulting in an army which was healthier than ever before, not only physically but mentally. Here are the words of the Secretary of State at the end of the Second World War: 'The Health of the Army has exceeded all reasonable expectations. . . . The deaths from disease of all kinds were negligible throughout this campaign. These remarkable results have been achieved by the development of improved methods of maintaining health and preventing disease, by the careful training of the Army in the application of the principles of hygiene, and by the discipline and understanding of the British soldier.' Could there possibly be a more eloquent vindication of the value of health education than this ?

If the health of our industrial workers today was anything like as good as that of our army in wartime, there would be an enormous saving in lost time and accidents.

Clearly what is needed is a comprehensive industrial health service organized for all occupations in the same way that the Army organizes its health services for the occupation of being a soldier. Note, by the way, that this is a separate and distinct organization from the Army Medical Service which is concerned with hospitals, consultants, drugs, nursing services, etc. In fact, Sir Ralph Glyn, in discussing before the Houses of Parliament the National Health Service Bill, regretted the fact that there was no mention of industrial health in the Bill. Unfortunately, many young doctors only get their first experience of preventive medicine if they enter one of the armed services as a unit medical officer. This experience will stand them in good stead when returning to civilian practice.

It is true that the Dale Committee was set up in 1941 to consider and advise on the provision of an occupational health service. Its report, issued in 1951, recommended a comprehensive provision of occupational health services, including non-industrial occupations, by the gradual extension of existing medical services. At a time when forthright and sweeping changes were needed it was so lukewarm and non-committal in its proposals that it was hardly worth the paper it was written on.

Clearly health education is not a prerogative of the doctors; it is a subject for the health visitor, nurse, school teacher, army officer, shop steward, works foreman, manager, first-aid worker, and, most important of all, for parents and politicians.

Unfortunately, too many people regard health education as a simple matter of telling people what to do and what not to do. To be successful, however, a much more imaginative approach is required to replace the archaic didactic attitude which is so common today. It is no easy task; in the first place the health educator must know what people are feeling, thinking, and believing about health matters and he must have an intimate knowledge of their attitudes. Health education is a process of learning and a person's main reason for learning is to further his own interests; it must be concerned, therefore, with the goals, interests, and purposes of the people. A useful method with village people is the Socratic approach in which there is group discussion and active co-operation with the persons to be taught. It is important also to avoid generalizations and to be specific. In other words, the methods of teaching must attract and hold the interest of the people and a number of methods are always more successful than a single one. Thus one should use posters, films, radio talks, group discussions, and lectures illustrated by film strips or the epidiascope. Health education which deals with an individual's personal problems is usually more successful than the mass approach. The doctor or nurse both have ample opportunities to practise this in the clinic or hospital, but how rarely is it done? The main criticisms of the clinic by patients are: (1) Lack of tact on the part of the doctor; (2) loss of time by the patient because of long hours of waiting; (3) failure on the part of the doctor to treat adequately or to give proper instructions.

In fact, I have seen doctors in antenatal clinics and tuberculosis dispensaries who never speak to the patient at all, but merely examine and write out a prescription. When a person is sick, one has an ideal chance of practising comprehensive medicine; in fact all medicine should be comprehensive, combining treatment and prevention, so that at the same time as the doctor is treating the sick, he should seize the opportunity to educate a receptive patient in the ways of health.

Doctors and nurses invariably reply to this criticism by saying that they have too many patients and not sufficient time. In India there are several field research projects being carried out to try and find out the best ways of educating illiterate village people. The Ford Foundation, for example, is sponsoring three research and action projects in rural health centres, aimed at finding out how to get people to use latrines; in another project the aim is to find out how best to get people to adopt birth control measures. The general practitioner visiting patients in their homes has the most rewarding chances of anyone to practise health education. Over one hundred years ago, in 1859 to be precise, Florence Nightingale drew attention to this point of view in the following words: 'Hospitals are at best a necessary evil . . . the secret of national health is to be found in the homes of the people.'

In the early part of the present century there was considerable apprehension of interference by local authorities on medical matters and a great dread of bureaucratic control. The freedom of the profession was at stake! The individualistic outlook of many doctors was antagonistic to anything which aimed at the prevention of disease. As a result there developed a gap between the medical officers of health who stood for treatment of the patient. What a pity that the Dark Ages supervened upon the ideas of Hippocratic medicine!

235

If that tradition had developed without interruption, general practice might have developed more in sympathy with the idea of prevention rather than of cure. In the last fifty years there has been an ever-increasing utilization of the services of the general practitioner and the consultant in the field of preventive medicine. They are employed in antenatal, child welfare, and school health services, and this is all to the good. In industry also the majority of appointed factory doctors and works medical officers must come from the ranks of general practitioners, and specialists are being employed in ever-increasing numbers by industry and the various Ministries of, for example, Health, Labour, National Insurance, and Education.

The revolution began in 1911 and came to its climax in 1948. Thirty-seven years is a long time, but the organization of medicine and all the administration associated with it are now so complicated that it is quite impossible to expect any medical student to 'pick it up', so to speak, in the course of his clinical teaching. The student of medicine must first of all be a good clinician, and by that I mean experienced in the art of diagnosis, but unless his teachers realize that something more is required in the application of this knowledge to modern conditions then much of his usefulness will be lost. The importance of the prevention of disease and the promotion of health is taught in our provincial medical schools as a subject worthy of study not only in its own right, but also as an important practical help to the future doctor. Unfortunately, this is not the position in some London schools.

Scope in the research field is, of course, enormous and many of the field surveys which are now needed in the study of social medicine require a large staff. These studies collect their information from every branch of society, from hospitals, general practitioners, clinics, industry, medical officers of health, the Registrar-General, and even householders. Since the war we have learned as a result a great deal about the cause and prevention of the following conditions: coronary heart disease, leukaemia, tuberculosis, chronic bronchitis, dust disease of the lungs, poliomyelitis, cancer of the lung, stomach, and uterus, stillbirths, infant mortality, blindness in premature babies, congenital malformations, and a whole host of occupational diseases.

We have gained also a great deal of information about genetic factors as a cause of disease and about the ageing process. Similar methods are used in testing the efficacy of such immunizing agents as BCG, poliomyelitis, influenza, and whooping-cough vaccines. These results could not have been obtained in any other way except by the large-scale survey method. Brilliant research of this kind has been organized by the Department of Epidemiology and Medical Statistics at the London School of Hygiene and Tropical Medicine, the Pneumoconiosis Research Unit in South Wales, the Social Medicine Research Unit of the Medical Research Council, and by many university departments.* The purpose of these studies has been admirably

---

* The first University Department of Social Medicine was set up at Oxford under Professor John Ryle, already well known as a consultant and writer on medical topics. This department has carried out research which is of the greatest importance on such subjects as tuberculosis, child health, leukaemia, and genetics.

described by Dr. J. Morris, head of the M.R.C. Unit for Research in Social Medicine:—

Medicine as a whole needs more epidemiology, for without it cardinal areas have to be excluded from the consideration of human health and sickness. Epidemiology, moreover, is rich with suggestions for clinical and laboratory study, and it offers many possibilities for testing hypotheses emerging from these. One of the most urgent *social* needs of the day is to identify rules of healthy living that might do for us what Snow and others did for the Victorians, and help to reduce the burden of illness in middle and old age which is so characteristic a feature of our society. There is no indication whatever that the experimental sciences alone will be able to produce the necessary guidance. Collaboration between clinician, laboratory scientist, and epidemiologist might be more successful. The possibilities are at present unlimited, if often neglected.

From the teaching and research point of view social medicine must rank in importance with such subjects as clinical medicine, physics, chemistry, and zoology. Nobody ever questions that such departments should have whole-time Professors at their head and yet there is only one single Professor of social or preventive medicine in the twelve London teaching hospitals. Compare this with the provinces, where there is at least one Chair in every medical school except Oxford. Moreover, the majority are whole-time professors. At conferences held in India in 1955 on medical education it was recommended that every medical college should have a separate department of preventive and social medicine, with a full-time staff. In the U.S.A., too, there are over eighty departments of preventive medicine or public health, many of them having more than one Professor. In New York alone there are at least eight, whilst in the East, new departments of preventive medicine and public health are naturally enough increasing. (*Fig. 47.*) The W.H.O. Expert Committee on Professional and Technical Education has also had something to say on teaching and research in preventive and social medicine. It considered that the following conditions were essential for the proper organization of this teaching:—

1. Status as an independent department, with professorial rank for the head of the department (holder of the chair).
2. Support by the administration of the university and the school, including the provision of an adequate budget.
3. Support and co-operation from the other members of the medical faculty.
4. Research facilities in some field related to activities in preventive and social medicine.
5. Responsible participation in a clinical programme, interpreting the word 'clinical' as covering any activity with human beings.

To make the teaching of preventive medicine vital and interesting it must be based on work with people; preventive medicine cannot be taught in a vacuum. The world as a whole is turning more to constructive and preventive medicine. The hospital consultant is the last person to understand the importance of this subject; the more specialized he becomes, the less he can see the whole. Sir James Mackenzie wrote in 1919: 'There is not an individual on a teaching staff, qualified from experience, to see all the branches of medicine in their proper perspective.' That statement is a good deal truer today. They organize things a little better in Norway where every specialist must have spent at least a year in general practice.

The days of our general physicians, as a result of the new order, are passing. Sir William Osler, Professor John Ryle, and Lord Horder were three of the greatest of all these. They had wide interests in preventive medicine and could see medicine as a whole in relation to other human activities. The super-specialist sees little of the natural history of disease or the importance of studying man in relation to his environment. Let us remember the words of Trousseau, a great French physician, who said, 'To know the natural progress of disease is to know more than the half of medicine.'

The social aspects of disease must always be taken into account by the clinician in arriving at a correct application of the diagnosis, not only in terms of what is wrong with the patient but also to explain why this person became ill in this way on this particular occasion, which, of course, has also an important bearing on prescribing the management of the case. Unfortunately, many clinicians who are adept at interpreting the social aspects of individual disease in diagnosis and treatment are not fully alive to the wider implications involved in the prevention of disease and the promotion of community health.

There are four questions which should be asked when a patient is ill:—
1. What is the matter with him? (Diagnosis.)
2. Can he be relieved of his sickness? (Treatment.)
3. Why did he become ill in the way he did? (Aetiology.)
4. How can other people avoid getting the same sort of illness? (Public health.)

The patient himself is only really interested in the second question, and it is not much use telling him that he has got disseminated sclerosis or a glioma of the brain if we can't do anything about it. The doctor himself is usually most interested in the first, the diagnosis, and in the second, the treatment, and usually that is as far as the case goes. Every sick person is a challenge to the community, of something which has occurred which should not be, but preventive medicine is not an exclusive right of the medical profession, as is clinical medicine; it is a subject of vital interest to all. The doctor, because of his special training and experience, however, should be in a better position than anyone to advise about cause and prevention; in this respect there is sometimes a clash between the interests of the individual and the interests of the community. Should the doctor reveal that the food handler is a typhoid carrier or that the school-teacher is suffering from open tuberculosis? That is a question for the community to decide. The doctor has a duty, not only to his patient, but also to the community to which he belongs—to safeguard the health of that community.

There are many countries in the world which are experiencing the same troubles that Britain went through one hundred years ago, but they will compress in the space of a few decades change and progress which took her

238

a hundred years; mistakes and difficulties will be inevitable, but they will be minimized if those countries will take note and digest some of the lessons revealed by a study of history. Let them learn from our mistakes! We have seen that the achievement of world health is no simple matter but a most complicated affair which, if it is to be a reality, requires not only knowledge but the application of financial and technical assistance on a large scale. One of the greatest hopes for the future health of the world is the World Health Organization.

THE WORLD HEALTH ORGANIZATION

Health is a state of complete physical, mental, and social well-being and not merely the absence of disease or infirmity..—FROM THE W.H.O. CONSTITUTION

The W.H.O. came into being in September, 1948, in order to solve health problems on a global basis. At the moment there are eighty-nine nations in the Organization, and Russia has returned as an active participant. The head-quarters are at Geneva (*Fig.* 48), with regional offices in Washington for the Americas, at Alexandria for the Eastern Mediterranean, at Copenhagen for Europe, at New Delhi for South-East Asia, at Brazzaville for Africa, and at Manila for the Western Pacific.

The Constitution of W.H.O. emphasizes the need for international co-operation and stresses two important conditions for the achievement of World Health:—

1. The health of all peoples is fundamental to the attainment of peace and security and is dependent upon the fullest co-operation of individual states.

2. Unequal development in different countries in the promotion of health and control of disease, especially communicable disease, is a common danger.

The functions of the Organization are as follows:—

1. To direct and co-ordinate international health work.

2. To establish and maintain effective collaboration with the United Nations.

3. To assist Governments in establishing, maintaining, and strengthening health services.

4. To furnish appropriate technical assistance and in emergency to provide necessary aid at the request of Governments.

5. To establish and maintain such services as may be required, including epidemiological and technical services.

6. To stimulate and advance the work of eradication of epidemic, endemic, and other diseases.

7. To promote inquiry into the prevention of accidents.

8. To promote the improvement of the following: Nutrition, housing, sanitation, recreation, working conditions, and other aspects of environmental hygiene.

9. To propose conferences, agreements, and regulations with regard to international health.

10. To promote maternal and child welfare.

11. To foster activities in the field of mental health.

12. To promote improved standards of teaching and training in the health, medical, and related professions; this it does by giving fellowships (nearly 1500 a year) and arranging courses.

13. To study and report on administrative and social techniques affecting public health and medical care from preventive and curative points of view, including hospital services and social security.

14. To provide information, advice, and assistance in the field of health.

15. To establish and revise as necessary international nomenclatures of diseases, of causes of death, and of public health practices.

16. To standardize diagnostic procedures as necessary.

17. To develop, establish, and promote international standards with respect to food and for biological, pharmaceutical, and similar products.

It publishes weekly, monthly, and annually information and statistics on infectious disease as a means of controlling the spread of epidemic disease. In addition there are daily broadcasts from Geneva to all parts of the world on the so-called pestilential diseases (plague, typhus, cholera, yellow fever, and small-pox). The idea behind this is the total eradication of certain diseases. The most striking achievements are the eradication of the yellow fever mosquito from South American cities, of malaria from Brazil, Egypt, Sardinia, and Cyprus, and the international control of small-pox; it also has given emergency aid in Morocco, Chile, and the Congo, for example. In addition, statistics are published on the incidence and mortality of other diseases. It publishes several journals, including the *Bulletin* and *Chronicle* of the W.H.O., in addition to a great many monographs on a wide variety of subjects from mental ill health to the cost of the health services. It also runs an extensive library.

Technical aid has been given on a large scale to many countries, and it holds frequent conferences and seminars on subjects of public health importance; it also has an extensive research programme. One of its fundamental principles is that without mental health there can be no physical health.

It is obvious that the battle for world health cannot go on without money. It has been estimated that four of the worst diseases could be eradicated for less than it would cost the world to finance a war for one week, and yet the budget of W.H.O. is little more than that spent by many large cities on their health services. The scheduled budget of 1963 is nearly $30,000,000. At this moment the world is spending thousands of millions of pounds on armaments; if only we could spend that money on health, what an enormous return we could get in terms of human happiness! W.H.O. is still short of sufficient funds to carry out its tasks, and has to turn to various methods in order to raise money. In 1962, for example, it launched a postage stamp campaign to obtain publicity and funds for the malaria eradication programme (*Fig.* 49). The F.A.O. (Food and Agriculture Organization), U.N.I.C.E.F. (United Nations International Children's Emergency Fund), and I.L.O. (International Labour Organization) all help in improving world health by giving assistance in their respective spheres.

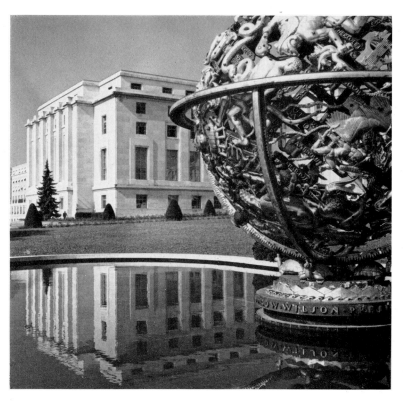

Fig. 48.—Headquarters of the World Health Organization. Palais des Nations and pond
with armillary sphere. A new building is being erected in Geneva.

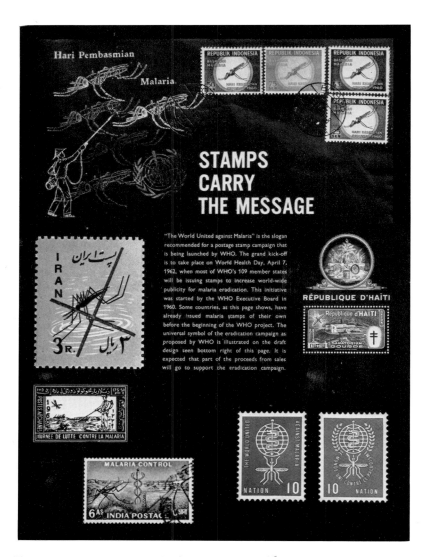

Fig. 49.—A postage stamp campaign is one of the methods used to raise funds for W.H.O.

THE BILL OF SICKNESS

There is an overwhelming relationship between poverty and sickness: sickness is a cause of poverty and poverty is a cause of sickness. Lord Beveridge's schemes aimed at breaking this vicious circle by attacking poverty. As a result in Britain today poverty is no longer an important cause of sickness; probably it is truer to say that old age is the most important general factor causing ill health. It is not so in many less fortunate countries. In China, Egypt, and India only 50 per cent of children born reach the age when they themselves can contribute to the national economy; moreover, many of them are permanently damaged in the process.

The economic loss to such countries is enormous, but even in the U.S.A. it has been estimated that the cost of illness and disability is equivalent to $38,000,000,000 a year, or £13,000,000,000.

The economic cost of preventing disease is trivial in comparison; the saving in hospital beds for diphtheria and tuberculosis in recent years has been enormous. In New York, for example, in 1920, the hospital bill for diphtheria alone was over $1,000,000 dollars; in 1939 it was $44,000.

The experience of the Metropolitan Life Insurance Company illustrates this point. Between 1911 and 1925 they spent $20,000,000 on health education, stressing early diagnosis and providing nursing services for their policy holders. The death-rate during this period fell by 30 per cent, a decrease double that of the population as a whole. The saving in terms of finance was $43,000,000.

The loss in production in tropical countries is fantastic; in the Middle East, for example, something like 90 per cent of the population are affected with worm infestation contracted from wading in infected water. It probably costs Egypt £20,000,000 a year. The most important requirements are pure water supplies and eradication of insect vectors, particularly the mosquito. The cost of such measures is a fraction of the money saved in increased production.

The Surgeon-General of the United States Public Health Service, Dr. L. A. Scheele, estimated in 1951 that 50,000,000 people had already been protected from malaria and the expenditure of 2s. a year per inhabitant would produce a startling decrease in the incidence of the disease.

The control of disease due to personal contact is more expensive, particularly where hospitals and trained personnel have to be provided, but since the advent of the antibiotics a relatively cheap form of treatment has come into use which for the first time has enabled important groups of disease to be brought under control by curative methods.

The cost of health services varies a great deal depending upon the extent of the services provided. In the United Kingdom, the cost of preventive and treatment services is about 5 per cent of the national income. In 1949–50, the National Health Service net cost was £371·6 million with an average of £8 12s. per person per year by comparison. The total cost of the preventive services was only £67,500,000 in the same period. By 1953–4 the cost had risen to £430·3 million, but the cost per head was almost exactly the same, namely £8 15s., the increased cost being due mainly to the increase in the population. In America medical services are so costly that most people take out some form of voluntary medical care insurance. This costs about £13 per year per person whilst the preventive services cost about 30s. per year. At St. Bartholomew's Hospital the cost per patient per week is almost £30; it is about £16 in the provinces. It is clearly much cheaper to spend £5 a week on help in the home than to have to admit an old man to hospital simply because there is no one to look after him. These figures illustrate the high cost of hospital treatment today. Unfortunately, the poverty of many countries precludes them from providing comprehensive medical care programmes, and they are more likely to get value for money in terms of health by spending it on prevention rather than on treatment.

The cost of medical services, however, is not the only or indeed the chief item in the bill of sickness; the loss of national income in terms of wages and productivity is enormous; not only that, there is a terrific bill for National Insurance. Another important factor is the ageing of the population which means a bigger bill for sickness and pensions. Thus in England and Wales the expenditure in 1955 for all National Insurance purposes was £660,000,000. It is estimated that in 1979 it will be £1,000,000,000. The extra £340,000,000 will be due to the large number of persons drawing old-age pensions and is based on the assumption that the rate of pensions will not go up. Truly an ageing population imposes an enormous economic burden on the community.

There is a great shortage of trained personnel in all branches of public health. The greatest needs are for doctors, sanitary inspectors, health visitors, and nurses. The *World Directory of Medical Schools*, published by W.H.O. in 1959, gives the latest figures available for physicians. In the U.K. there was 1 physician to every 1149 persons and in the U.S.S.R. 1 to every 784, whereas in Indonesia there was 1 physician for every 70,768 persons. Details relating to other health personnel are to be found in the *Second Report on the World Health Situation, 1957–1960*, published by W.H.O. in 1963. It would appear that health is very much a question of economics.

The twentieth century faces on a global scale the overwhelming burden of large numbers of people handicapped by poverty and sickness. The World Health Organization considers that 'the enjoyment of the highest attainable standard of health is one of the fundamental rights of every human being'. But from time immemorial man has been plagued by disease which left him little opportunity for developing those highest standards of well-being which we deem to be so important.

Health will depend not only on efforts in the medical field but also in agriculture, industry, and economics, so that higher crop yields and bigger incomes will often do more than hospitals and doctors. The bill of sickness is great, but however we settle it, let us remember that health *could* be purchased at a reasonable price if people would *act* as if they *believed* prevention to be better than cure.

Dr. Oliver Wendell Holmes read a paper in 1842 before the Boston Society for Medical Improvements on 'The Contagiousness of Puerperal Fever'. At that lecture he said: 'The time has come when the existence of a private pestilence in the sphere of a single physician should be looked upon not as a misfortune but a crime.'

Perhaps one day we shall reach such a state of affairs that the only diseases which occur are those due to some fault in the individual person; when we can stop all illnesses at their source, then there will be no need for surgeons. But even if those days do come to pass we shall still need teachers to tell us how. In the future the doctor will become more and more a teacher, a teacher of how to keep fit, and any illness that does occur will be due to neglect. This will be the public health of the future. Unfortunately, human nature being what it is, we cannot ever expect to be perfect in these matters, and, sad to relate, the public and the doctors themselves are usually far more interested in the few cases which are cured by the skill and daring of a great surgeon than the thousands of deaths which did not occur because they were prevented. The healing knife appeals to the sense of drama which is in all of us, but the millions of healthy people who now walk our streets are taken for granted. Epidemics which do not occur are of little news value.

There is plenty to do in the underdeveloped countries in the old traditional public health fields, but as the epidemic diseases are conquered so too will the rest of the world face similar problems to those which face the ageing peoples of the Western world today.

Enormous advances have been made in our scientific and technological knowledge, but still the greatest bars to progress are ignorance, selfishness, and suspicion. Advances in world health need to be based on an understanding of the four truths propounded by Gautama Buddha 2500 years ago:—

1. There is disease and suffering in the world.
2. There is a cause.
3. There is a means of removing the cause.
4. There is the path by which this can be accomplished.

The world today has almost too many scientific facts and too much information, but too little knowledge of how to apply it. Our efforts in the future, by which disease and suffering can be eliminated, must be based on a new form of international co-operation and the idea of world citizenship. Dr. Frank Boudreau, formerly of the Milbank Memorial Fund, has expressed this hope for the future in the following words:—

The World Health Organization is peculiarly fitted to become the spearhead of a world revolution which will have as its aim not the destruction of present civilization, but the organization of a peaceful world. . . . W.H.O., above all other agencies, is fitted to show the way, for its jurisdiction is one of the few areas where men of all races and creeds can work together.

*   *   *   *   *   *

On a huge hill,
Cragged, and steep, Truth stands, and he that will
Reach her, about must, and about must go.
JOHN DONNE (c. 1595), Satyre iii. l. 79.

REFERENCES AND FURTHER READING

AMERICAN PUBLIC HEALTH ASSOCIATION (1960), *Control of Communicable Diseases in Man*, 9th ed. New York.
BARRY, F. W. (1889), *Report on an Epidemic of Smallpox at Sheffield during 1887–1888*. London.
BEVERIDGE REPORT (1942), *Social Insurance and Allied Services*. London: H.M.S.O.
BOOTH, CHARLES (1891–1903), *Life and Labour of the People in London*. London.
BOWLBY, JOHN (1951), *Maternal Care and Mental Health, Wld Hlth Org. Monogr. Ser.*, No. 2.
BOYD-ORR, JOHN (1937), *Food, Health and Income*. London.
BROCKINGTON, F. (1958), *World Health*. Harmondsworth.
BRYANT, A. (1950), *The Age of Elegance*. London.
CHADWICK, EDWIN (1842), *The Sanitary Condition of the Labouring Population*. London.
COOK, ROBERT C. (1951), *Human Fertility*. London.
CREW, F. A. E. (1948), *Measurements of the Public Health*. Edinburgh.
CRUICKSHANK, E. W. H. (1946), *Food and Nutrition*. Edinburgh.
DANIEL, CLARENCE (1946), *An Illustrated Account of Eyam Plague*. Tideswell, Sheffield.
DAVEY, T. H., and LIGHTBODY, W. P. H. (1961), *The Control of Disease in the Tropics*, 2nd ed. London.
DICKENS, CHARLES (1854), *Hard Times*. London.
—— (1867), *The Uncommercial Traveller*. London.
DICKINSON, R. L., and BEAM, L. (1949), *A Thousand Marriages; a Medical Study of Sex Adjustment*. Baltimore.
DISRAELI, BENJAMIN (1845), *Sybil, or the Two Nations*. London.
DIXON, C. W. (1962), *Smallpox*. London.
DOLL, R., and HILL, A. B. (1956), 'Lung Cancer and other Causes of Death in Relation to Smoking', *Brit. med. J.*, **2**, 1071.
DRUMMOND, Sir JACK, and WILBRAHAM, A. (1939), *The Englishman's Food: A History of Five Centuries of English Diet*. London.
DUBOS, R. J., and DUBOS, J. P. (1953), *The White Plague*. London.
ELLIS, HAVELOCK (1946), *Sex in Relation to Society*. London.
ENGELS, F. (1892), *Condition of the Working Classes in 1884*. London.
FARR, WILLIAM (1852), *Report of the Cholera Mortality in England 1848–9*. London.
FRANK, JOHANN PETER (1779–1818), *System einer Vollständigen Medicinischen Polizey*. Berlin.
FRAZER, W. M. (1950), *A History of English Public Health, 1834–1937*. London.
GALEN, see in GREEN, R. M. (1951), *A Translation of Galen's Hygiene (De Sanitate Tuenda)*. London.
——, see in MAJOR, RALPH (1954), *A History of Medicine*, vol. 1. Oxford.
GESELL, A. (1948), *Studies in Child Development*. London.
GILLETT, E., and HUGHES, J. D. (1955), 'Public Health in Lincolnshire in the 19th Century', *Publ. Hlth*, **69**, 34, 55.
GORDON, JOHN E. (1948), 'Louse-borne Typhus Fever in the European Theatre of Operations. U.S. Army, 1945', in *The Rickettsial Diseases of Man*. Washington.
—— WYON, JOHN B., and INGALLS, THEODORE H. (1954), 'Public Health as a Demographic Influence', *Amer. J. med. Sci.*, **227**, 326.
GROTH-PETERSEN, E., KNUDSEN, JØRGEN, and WILBEK, ERIC (1959), 'Epidemiological Basis of Tuberculosis Eradication in an Advanced Country', *Bull. Wld Hlth Org.*, **21**, 5.

HAMILTON, A. (1943), *Exploring the Dangerous Trades*. Boston.

HAMMOND, B. C., and HORN, D. (1958), 'Smoking and Death Rates', *J. Amer. med. Ass.*, **166**, 1294.

HECKER, J. F. C. (1844), *The Epidemics of the Middle Ages*. London.

HIPPOCRATES, see in CHADWICK, JOHN, and MANN, W. N. (1950), *The Medical Works of Hippocrates*. Oxford.

HOBSON, W. (1961), *The Theory and Practice of Public Health*. London.

HOLLAND, G. CALVERT (1843), *The Vital Statistics of Sheffield*. London.

HOOD, THOMAS (1843), *Punch*, **5**, 260.

HUNTER, DONALD (1962), *The Diseases of Occupations*, 3rd ed. London.

HYGE, T. V. (1947), *Acta tuberc. scand.*, **21**, 1.

ILLINGWORTH, R. S. (1957), *The Normal Child*, 2nd ed. London.

JENNER, EDWARD (1798), *An Inquiry into the Causes and Effects of the Variolae Vaccinae*, 1st ed. London (reprint Milan, 1923).

KALLMANN, F. J. (1946), 'An Analysis of 691 Schizophrenic Twin Index Families', *Amer. J. Psychiat.*, **103**, 309.

— — and REISNER, D. (1943), 'Twin Studies on the Significance of Genetic Factors in Tuberculosis', *Amer. Rev. Tuberc.*, **47**, 549.

KINGSLEY, C. (1863), *The Water Babies*. London.

LEGGE, Sir THOMAS (1934), *Industrial Maladies*. London.

LEIGH, Rev. W. (1833), *Cholera at Bilston in 1832*. Wolverhampton.

LINDELL, B. O., and DOBSON, R. LOWRY (1961), *Ionizing Radiation and Health*. Geneva. (World Health Organization Public Health Papers, No. 6.)

LOGAN, W. P. D. (1956), 'Mortality from Fog in London', *Brit. med. J.*, **1**, 722.

LUCIA, SALVATORE P. (1963), *Wine as Food and Medicine*, 2nd ed. New York.

M'GONIGLE, G. C. M., and KIRBY, J. J. (1936), *Poverty and Public Health*. London.

MACKINTOSH, J. (1953), *Trends of Opinion about the Public Health 1901–5*. London.

MALTHUS, T. R. (1798), *An Essay on the Principles of Population*. London.

MEAD, MARGARET (1954a), *Growing Up in New Guinea*. Harmondsworth.

— — (1954b), *Coming of Age in Samoa*. Harmondsworth.

MEDICAL RESEARCH COUNCIL (1956, 1960), *The Hazards to Man of Nuclear and Allied Radiations*. London: H.M.S.O.

MORRIS, J. N. (1955), 'Uses of Epidemiology', *Brit. med. J.*, **2**, 395.

PAMPANA, EMILIO (1963), *A Textbook of Malaria Eradication*. London.

PARACELSUS (1567), *Von der Bergsucht*. Dillingen.

PAUL, BENJAMIN D. (1955), *Health, Culture and Community* (ed.). New York.

PEARL, R. (1928), 'Alcohol and Life Duration', *Internat. Clinics*, 38th ser., **3**, 28.

— — (1938), 'Tobacco Smoking and Longevity', *Science*, **87**, 216.

PEARSON, KARL (1914), *The Life, Letters and Labours of Francis Galton*. Cambridge.

PENROSE, L. S. (1949), 'The Galton Laboratory: Its Work and Aims', *Eugen. Rev.*, **41**, 17.

PICKLES, W. H. (1939), *Epidemiology in Country Practice*. Bristol.

PLACE, FRANCES (1822), *Illustrations and Proofs of the Principles of Population*. London.

POLLITZER, R. (1954), *Plague, Wld Hlth Org. Monogr. Ser.*, No. 22.

— — (1960), *Cholera, Ibid.*, No. 43.

PORRITT COMMITTEE REPORT (1962), *A Review of the Medical Services in Great Britain*. London.

RAMAZZINI, B. (1713), *De Morbis Artificium Diatriba*. Geneva. (Trans. W. C. Wright, 1940, Chicago.)

ROBERTS, J. A. FRAZER (1959), *An Introduction to Medical Genetics*, 2nd ed. London.

ROSS, R. (1911), *The Prevention of Malaria*, 2nd ed. London.

ROUECHE, BERTON (1955), *Eleven Blue Men*. New York.

ROWNTREE, B. S. (1901), *Poverty; a Study of Town Life*. London.

ROYAL COMMISSION ON POPULATION (1949), *Report*. London: H.M.S.O.

RUSSELL, Sir JOHN (1954), *World Population and World Food Supplies*. London.

RUSSELL, P. F. (1955), *Man's Mastery of Malaria*. London.

RYLE, JOHN A. (1948), *Changing Disciplines*, 2nd ed. London.
SHAPTER, THOMAS (1849), *The History of the Cholera in Exeter 1832*. London.
SIGERIST, HENRY E. (1933), *The Great Doctors; a Biographical History of Medicine* (English translation). New York.
SIMON, Sir JOHN (1890), *English Sanitary Institutions*. London.
SMILLIE, WILSON G. (1952), *Preventive Medicine and Public Health*, 2nd ed. New York.
SNOW, JOHN (1855), *On the Mode of Communication of Cholera*. London. (Reprinted 1936, Cambridge, Mass.)
STOCKS, PERCY, and CAMPBELL, JOHN M. (1955), 'Lung Cancer Death Rates among Non-smokers and Pipe and Cigarette Smokers', *Brit. med. J.*, **2**, 923.
STOKES, JOHN (1921), *History of the Cholera Epidemic of 1832 in Sheffield*. Sheffield.
STRODE, G. K. (1951), *Yellow Fever*. New York.
THACKRAH, CHARLES TURNER (1831), *The Effects of the Principal Arts, Trades and Professions, and of Civic States and Habits of Living, on Health and Longevity, with Suggestions for the Removal of many of the Agents which Produce Disease and Shorten the Duration of Life*. London.
THOMPSON, G. H. (1947), 'The Trend of National Intelligence', *Occasional Papers on Eugenics*, vol. 3. London.
TOWNSEND, J. G. (1950), 'Investigation of the Smog Incident in Donora, Pa., and Vicinity', *Amer. J. Publ. Hlth*, **40**, 183.
TOWNSEND, PETER (1957), *The Family Life of Old People*. London.
TREVELYAN, G. M. (1942), *English Social History*. New York: Longmans Green.
TROLLOPE, F. (1840), *The Life and Adventures of Michael Armstrong, the Factory Boy*. London.
UNITED NATIONS (1951), *Bulletin of Narcotics*, vol. 3. New York.
VERNON, H. M. (1939), *Health in Relation to Occupation*. London.
WILLIAMS, WALDEN (1956), *Vest Pocket Calorie Counter*. New York: Garden City Books.
WEBB, B. (1948), *Our Partnership*. London.
WINSLOW, C. E. A. (1951), *The Cost of Sickness and the Price of Health*, Wld Hlth Org. Monogr. Ser., No. 7.
WORLD HEALTH ORGANIZATION (1957), *Effects of Radiation on Human Heredity*. Geneva.
— — — (1958), *The First Ten Years of the World Health Organization*. Geneva.
— — — (1959), *World Directory of Medical Schools*. Geneva.
— — — (1963), *Second Report on the World Health Situation*. Geneva.
WU LIEN-TEH (1959), *Plague Fighter*. Cambridge.
YOUNG, ARTHUR (1771), *Eastern Tour*, vol. 4. London.
ZINSSER, HANS (1935), *Rats, Lice and History*. London.

INDEX

The more important sections are in heavy type

INDEX

249